Circulatory Physiology
—the essentials
THIRD EDITION

James J. Smith, M.D., Ph.D.

Professor of Physiology and Medicine
The Medical College of Wisconsin
Milwaukee, Wisconsin
Director, Human Performance Laboratory
Zablocki Veterans Administration Medical Center
Milwaukee, Wisconsin

John P. Kampine, M.D., Ph.D.

Professor of Anesthesiology and Physiology
Chairman, Department of Anesthesiology
The Medical College of Wisconsin
Milwaukee, Wisconsin
Director of Anesthesiology
Milwaukee County Medical Center
Wauwatosa, Wisconsin

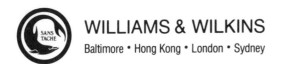

WILLIAMS & WILKINS
Baltimore • Hong Kong • London • Sydney

Editor: Timothy S. Satterfield
Associate Editor: Victoria M. Vaughn
Copy Editor: Anne Schwartz
Designer: Bob Och
Illustration Planner: Ray Lowman
Production Coordinator: Barbara J. Felton

Copyright © 1990
Williams & Wilkins
428 East Preston Street
Baltimore, Maryland 21202, USA

Accurate indications, adverse reactions, and dosage schedules for drugs are provided in this book, but it is possible that they may change. The reader is urged to review the package information data of the manufacturers of the medications mentioned.

Printed in the United States of America

First Edition, 1980
Reprinted 1980, 1981, 1983
Second Edition, 1984
Reprinted 1985, 1986, 1987, 1988, 1989

P024514

Library of Congress Cataloging-in-Publication Data

Smith, James J. (James John), 1914–
    Circulatory physiology: the essentials / James J. Smith, John P. Kampine. — 3rd ed.
    p.   cm.
    Includes bibliographical references.
    ISBN 0-683-07775-9
    1. Cardiovascular system. 2. Blood—Circulation. 3. Cardiovascular system—Diseases. I. Kampine, John P., 1934–   . II. Title.
    [DNLM: 1. Blood Circulation. WG 103 S651c]
    QP102.S64   1990
    612.1—dc20
    DNLM/DLC
    for Library of Congress   89-70708
                                                                                         CIP

90 91 92 93 94
1   2   3   4   5   6   7   8   9   10

Dedicated to our parents

James W. and
Catherine Smith

and

Dr. Clifford and
Florence Kampine

They showed us the way.

Preface to the Third Edition

It is the logical purpose of any textbook of medical physiology to describe and interpret the functions of the normal circulation—how it works and why it works. This we have tried to do in our text.

But in preparing the *"Essentials,"* we have always had a second objective, which to us was of equal importance, that is, to extend the scope of the book to an analysis of circulatory dysfunction and disease. Consequently, about half of the text is concerned with cardiovascular pathophysiology. Students in health sciences often measure the value of a course on the basis of how it may ultimately help them to understand disease better. It is our belief that an introduction to pathophysiology early in the curriculum might add a further dimension to their medical education and perhaps encourage them to look at disease through the eyes of basic science. Residents and young clinicians have told us they found this approach useful, and some have used it as a review for American Board examinations.

To achieve the second purpose, clinical applications have been stressed throughout; in addition, the final chapters include capsule descriptions of some of the most prevalent and crippling of the circulatory diseases, namely, ischemic heart disease, congestive heart failure, hypertension, and circulatory shock. We are fully aware that ours is by no means a complete treatise on cardiovascular pathophysiology, which is an immense subject. But we believe it is a beginning, from which the student or physician may profit.

Dr. Harold Brooks, Chief of Cardiology at our medical school, has recently pointed out that the practice of medicine in the next few decades will be far different from that of the past and present. There will be far more attention given to preventive medicine than to crisis management, more concern with outpatient than inpatient care, a shift from invasive to noninvasive diagnostic methodology, and strong emphasis on basic science research, including cellular and molecular biology. This means that physicians and other health scientists need to be firmly grounded in the basic science and pathophysiology of their fields. This will be of benefit not only to themselves but also to their patients, who today are much better educated and continually seek information as to how they can best order their lives so as to protect themselves against circulatory disease. Such explanations require a sound and updated knowledge of the pathogenesis of cardiovascular disease.

Aside from pathophysiology, we have—as in previous editions—incorporated sections on the physiology of exercise; physical training; the circulatory effects of nonexercise stresses such as postural change, cold, hemorrhage, and fainting; the general nature and purpose of exercise stress tests; and the cardiovascular effects of aging. We believe an introduction to such areas will acquaint the student with how environmental stresses may affect the circulation and how patterns of daily living can play an important role in the incidence of circulatory disease.

In fashioning these sections on circulatory stress and disease, we have added anatomical, biochemical, pharmacological, pathological, and clinical aspects where we felt it appropriate for the analysis of the pathophysiology. We have done this because the manifestations of disease are manifold and often involve different systems and different disciplines. We have also added brief descriptions of the treatment of some of the circulatory disorders; these descriptions are definitely not intended to be guides to therapy but have been included since treatment is often an attempt to reverse the pathophysiology, and aside from its intrinsic objective, the method of treatment may provide the student valuable insight into what is possible or practical in dealing with the conflict between the patient and the disease.

In order to use this broader pathophysiological approach, we relied on assistance from other scientists and clinicians in allied fields who have carefully reviewed sections of the book, made corrections, and offered helpful suggestions. In past editions as well as in the present one, we gratefully acknowledge our debt to these individuals.

The unprecedented pace of cardiovascular research continues at an ever-increasing rate. We have made a considerable effort to assimilate the most important of these advances into this edition. There are extensive revisions and some expansion of the sections on electrical and ionic events of cardiac contraction, contractile properties of the myocardium, physiology of the microcirculation, regulation of peripheral blood flow and venous return to the heart, physiology of exercise and exercise training, circulatory response to postural change, the physiology of aging, and the physiology of shock. In accord with these changes some old figures have been discarded, and new figures and tables have been added. However, our basic objectives and approach are unchanged. Since the teaching of physiology is an ever-changing art and there is no universally acceptable method of presentation, we would welcome comments not only regarding specific items and topics but also on the general approach used in the book.

James J. Smith   **John P. Kampine**

Preface to the First Edition

This book—which is intended for medical students—has evolved from our lectures in cardiovascular physiology to the medical and graduate classes. However, we have also been influenced in the method of presentation by our teaching sessions with nurses and allied health students as well as with residents and physician groups. It seems that all of us share the perennial problem of the increasing volume of material and the pressing need to cull out the relevant in the time allotted. As a consequence we have tried to confine ourselves to the essentials.

We have two primary aims in the preparation of this book; the first was to present the basics of circulatory physiology mainly for those who are (or will be) charged with the diagnosis and care of cardiovascular patients. As a result, many interesting topics dealing with fundamental mechanisms have usually been omitted or treated only briefly. In further accord with this objective, clinical applications have been emphasized throughout the text and two chapters on the pathophysiology of certain cardiovascular disorders have been included. Physicians and others involved with coronary care units and circulatory stress testing may find this approach useful.

A second objective has been to develop some of the more difficult concepts in an orderly, stepwise and hopefully intelligible manner. Diagrams have been liberally used and physical, chemical and biological principles and analogies incorporated when they seemed useful.

In developing topics rather briefly and bypassing some of the complex issues, the danger is that the student may feel that the subject is straightforward and that most problems are resolved, which of course is far from the truth. Not only on questions of diagnosis and treatment but on a number of basic concepts, there is still intensive investigation and considerable controversy.

But it is sometimes helpful to have a small-scale map of the battlefield, which is why we undertook to write this book. And, in any event, for the student, the classroom and the laboratory may be better places to air the unsolved problems. We also hope that the references we have included, many of them reviews by leading authorities, will help to focus attention on current research in this field.

We wish to acknowledge, with very real gratitude, our many colleagues and our own students who have made helpful comments and valuable suggestions. However, in the final analysis, the selection of content and method of presentation must be our own responsibility; such selection is a highly individual process and no doubt others would have made different choices. We would, therefore, very much welcome comments, not only regarding specific errors or omissions but also general impressions and suggestions.

James J. Smith   **John P. Kampine**

Acknowledgments

In this edition, as in the previous ones, we were fortunate to obtain the advice of outstanding scientists and clinicians in a number of allied fields. We sought help from those who were not only excellent investigators but also were experienced teachers in medical and other health sciences. We believe the latter to be important because the selection, from the wealth of material, of that which is most relevant for the student is obviously of critical importance.

It is a pleasure to acknowledge the assistance of the following from other disciplines and other institutions: Dr. Tom P. Aufderheide, Dept. of Surgery (Emergency and Trauma), Milwaukee County Medical Center; Dr. Virinderjit S. Bamrah, Chief of Cardiology, and Dr. C. Vincent Hughes, Medical Director, Cardiopulmonary Rehabilitation Center, Zablocki VA Medical Center; Dr. James P. Filkins, Professor and Chairman, Dept. of Physiology, Loyola University, Stritch School of Medicine, Chicago, IL; Dr. Mahendar S. Kochar, Director, Hypertension Section and Assistant Chief of Staff for Education, Zablocki VA Medical Center; Dr. Joel A. Michael, Professor of Physiology, Rush Medical College, Chicago, IL; Dr. Lois M. Sheldohl, Director, Exercise Physiology Lab, Zablocki VA Medical Center; Dr. Philip W. Smith, Associate Professor of Medicine (Infectious Diseases), University of Nebraska School of Medicine, Omaha, NE: Dr. James D. Storey, Chief, Clinical Chemistry (Pathology), Zablocki VA Medical Center, and Dr. V. Thomas Wiedmeier, Professor of Physiology, Medical College of Georgia. From the Physiology Department of the Medical College of Wisconsin, the following faculty members provided very valuable advice and assistance: Dr. Jean F. Liard, Dr. Julian H. Lombard, Dr. Jeffrey L. Osborn, Dr. Richard J. Roman, and Dr. William J. Stekiel. We, however, accept final responsibility for the content and method of presentation.

We would also like to extend special thanks to our secretaries, who skillfully and patiently typed the manuscript, especially Mary Frescura, Penny Parker, and Karen Searle; to the Medical Media Service of the Zablocki VA Medical Center for preparation of the figures; and to the publisher, Williams & Wilkins, for continued encouragement and assistance.

Contents

CHAPTER 7. VENOUS RETURN
AND CARDIAC OUTPUT

CHAPTER 10.   REGULATION OF ARTERIAL BLOOD
                         PRESSURE

CHAPTER 11.   CIRCULATION TO SPECIAL REGIONS

CHAPTER 12. PHYSIOLOGY OF EXERCISE
AND THE EFFECT OF AGING

chapter 1

Blood and the Circulation: General Features

General Characteristics

In man, as well as in higher animals, the circulation plays a special role. It is the transport system for the delivery of oxygen and the removal of carbon dioxide, and this carrier function makes it indispensable for the survival of every cell and organ of the body. The circulation also delivers nutrients from the gastrointestinal tract to all the body parts, carries waste products of cellular metabolism to the kidney and other excretory organs, transports electrolytes and important chemical regulators called hormones, and serves to maintain body temperature. In addition, it is instrumental in converting certain inactive materials into active compounds and transports cells and immune substances that are concerned with the defense mechanisms of the body.

Since the storage capacity of tissues for oxygen is small, the body requires an adequate minute-by-minute supply. Under ordinary circumstances the survival times of the "vital organs" (*i.e.*, the brain and heart) without oxygen are only a few minutes, so that even a brief failure of the circulatory or respiratory system may have a serious or fatal outcome.

1

Another significant characteristic of the circulatory system is its vulnerability to disease. The incidence of cardiovascular disorders is particularly high in the so-called "developed" nations of the western world. While rheumatic and coronary heart disease as well as cerebrovascular accidents (stroke) have become prevalent, the most common of all circulatory disorders is hypertension; it is estimated that in the United States 35 million have the disease and require therapy, and an additional 25 million have borderline hypertension that warrants surveillance.

Although there has in recent years been a modest decline in mortality from cardiovascular disease, there are currently still about 2 million deaths per year from cardiovascular disease—more than cancer (20%), trauma (6%), and all other causes combined. The majority of these deaths are associated with atherosclerosis of the coronary, cerebral, or renal arteries. Although the specific cause of atherosclerotic disease in unknown, major "risk factors" such as high blood pressure, cigarette smoking, and increased blood cholesterol are known to predispose to its development. A world-wide research and educational effort has been mounted in recent years in an attempt to deal with the immense problem of cardiovascular disease.

Functional Divisions of the Circulation

There are two main components of the circulation, the smaller pulmonary division consisting of the pulmonary artery, capillaries, and pulmonary veins, and the much larger systemic division consisting of the aorta, arterial branches, capillaries, veins, and vena cavae: The systemic vessels supply and drain all the organs and tissues of the body. These two divisions are serially connected hydraulic circuits and form a closed system; each consists of a pump, a distributing system, an exchange system, and a collecting system (Fig. 1.1). Whereas the two divisions function in a generally similar manner, they have some important differences; the pulmonary division has a much lesser volume, its vessels are shorter and thinner walled, and it operates under lower pressure and with less resistance to flow.

The heart, which propels the blood through both divisions, has four chambers, a right and left atrium and a right and left ventricle. The atria are, in essence, auxiliary pumps which assist the flow of blood into the ventricles and help fill these chambers properly so they will be better primed for the subsequent power stroke. The ventricles are the main pump elements. The right ventricle propels blood through the pulmonary artery to the lungs (pulmonary circulation) and the left ventricle through the aorta and systemic arteries to the remainder of the body (systemic circulation). Each ventricular chamber has inlet and outlet valves which act reciprocally, that is, one closes before the other opens, thus preventing backflow (Fig. 1.2).

During ventricular contraction (*i.e.*, systole) the internal ventricular pres-

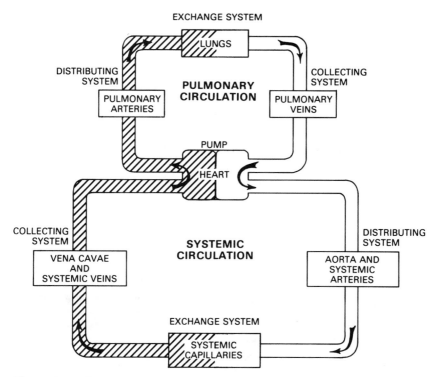

Figure 1.1. Functional divisions of the circulation. The *pulmonary circulation* delivers blood to the lungs for the elimination of carbon dioxide and the acquisition of oxygen. The *systemic circulation* transports oxygen (as well as nutrients and other substances) to all tissues of the body.

sures rise rapidly to a peak; the ventricles then relax, the internal pressures fall quickly to near zero followed immediately by the ventricular filling phase (*i.e.*, diastole). In the ventricles and large arteries, the pressures continually fluctuate between the higher levels which prevail during contraction (systole) and the lower levels during relaxation (diastole). Clinically, however, systolic pressures in the ventricles and large arteries are usually designated as the highest (during systole) and diastolic pressures as the lowest (during diastole), expressed in millimeters of mercury. Thus in the left ventricle, which is a high-pressure pump, typical pressures would be 120/0, while in the right ventricle, which is a low-pressure pump, the corresponding pressures would be about 25/0. Normally the two ventricles are in almost identical phase and rhythm because they are compressed simultaneously by the muscular myocardium which envelops both chambers. The myocardium of the left ventricle is usually 8 to 10 mm thick, that of the right ventricle about 2 to 3 mm. Since the overlying muscle mass is an important factor in determining the internal

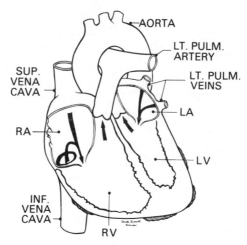

Figure 1.2. Right and left side of the heart (semidiagrammatic). When the right and left atria (*RA* and *LA*) contract, they propel blood into the respective ventricles. When the latter contract, the right ventricle (*RV*) forces blood toward the lungs and the left (*LV*) toward the periphery. All the valves—the right and left atrioventricular (AV) valves and the pulmonary and aortic valves—are unidirectional. With the onset of systole, both ventricles contract simultaneously, the AV valves close, the aortic and pulmonary valves open and blood is ejected. Note the greater wall thickness of the left ventricle.

pressure developed in a hollow organ, it is logical that the ratio of the peak internal pressures of the two ventricles would be similar to the ratio of their muscle thicknesses.

Distributing System. The arteries are branched, hollow cylindrical tubes. In the systemic division, the aorta (the largest artery) and its arterial branches are long, rather thick-walled, high-pressure conduits that transport blood over the systemic circuit to the small arteries and arterioles. Their internal pressure diminishes from about 120 mm Hg (systolic) and 80 mm Hg (diastolic) at the beginning of the aorta to a constant mean pressure of about 25 mm Hg at the arteriolar end of the capillaries. The pulmonary artery pressure, normally about 25/10 mm Hg, decreases to a mean pressure of about 10 mm Hg at the entrance to the lung capillaries. Aside from blood distribution, the arterial systems have two additional, important functions; the first portions serve a pressure-storing or ''Windkessel'' function and the terminal arteries, a resistance or ''stopcock'' function. These are described later in this chapter.

Exchange System. Capillaries are numerous, tiny, highly branched, microscopic tubes. Their very large surface area facilitates the transfer of oxygen, carbon dioxide, water, nutrients, and electrolytes through their walls. The internal pressures in the capillaries range from values of approximately 25 mm Hg on the arterial side to about 10 mm Hg at their confluence on the venous side. The combined volume of the capillaries is small but their surface and cross-sectional areas are immense.

Collecting System. The collecting system, which extends from the smallest venules to the largest terminal veins in the chest (vena cavae), drains blood back to the atria. Veins are large capacity, very thin-walled cylindrical vessels; veins below the heart have one-way valves which prevent reflux and thereby assist in the transport of blood back to the heart. Their internal pressure is low, ranging from about 10 mm Hg near the capillaries to about 0 mm Hg at their entrance to the heart. In the erect subject, the vascular pressures in the lower extremities are increased due to the effect of gravity as will be discussed in Chapter 6.

Blood

Formed Elements

Blood is essentially a two-phase fluid consisting of formed cellular elements suspended in a liquid medium, the plasma. The formed elements are red cells (erythrocytes), white cells (leukocytes), and platelets. If a blood sample from a normal adult is centrifuged in a graduated test tube of uniform bore, the relative volume of the packed red blood cells, termed "hematocrit," will be about 40 to 45% of the total, as shown by the height of the packed cell column (Fig. 1.3). Thus, the red cells occupy about 40 to 45% of the total volume of blood in the body. The white cells, being less dense, will settle on top of the red cells in a thin so-called "buffy" layer. The remaining 55 to 60% is plasma, sometimes called the "plasmacrit."

The erythrocytes are biconcave discs about 2.4 μm in thickness and 8 μm in diameter which are produced in the bone marrow through a process known as erythropoiesis. Their biconcave shape increases the total surface area available for diffusion. The red cells owe their characteristic color to the presence of the pigment hemoglobin, which has a remarkable capacity to combine with and transport oxygen. In the normal adult there are about 4.5 to 6.0 million red blood cells per cubic millimeter of peripheral blood. A greater than normal red cell volume in the blood is called polycythemia. A deficiency of red blood cells is known as anemia, which has pathophysiological consequences because of the accompanying hemoglobin deficiency (Fig. 1.3).

In the normal individual, there are 5,000 to 10,000 white blood cells per cubic millimeter in normal peripheral blood; an excess is usually termed leukocytosis and a deficiency, leukopenia. The white cells are mainly concerned with combating bacterial infections, with immune processes, and with bodily defense. Platelets are vital elements for blood coagulation. There are about 150,000 to 300,000 platelets per cubic millimeter in normal peripheral

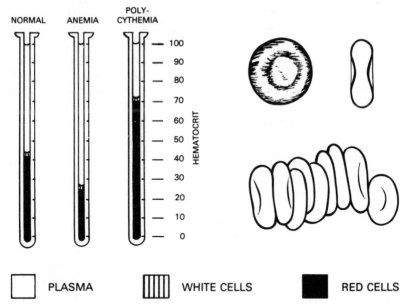

Figure 1.3. Hematocrit and red blood cells (RBCs). *Left,* The percentage of packed RBCs in the centrifuged blood samples, termed the hematocrit, is increased in polycythemia and decreased in anemia. The corresponding changes in hemoglobin content alter the oxygen-carrying capacity of the blood. *Right,* Surface and cut views of red cells. RBCs sometimes gather into stacks called rouleaux which tend to offer increased resistance to flow.

blood, but because of their small size (2–3 μm) they occupy only an insignificant fraction of the blood volume.

Plasma and Constituents

The plasma or fluid fraction of the blood normally occupies about 55% of the blood volume and carries a variety of substances including plasma proteins (which are the major portion of the plasma solids), nonprotein nitrogen, electrolytes, hormones, enzymes, and blood gases. The normal concentrations of some of the more important constituents of plasma are given in Table 1.1.

Blood Volume

The total blood volume is the sum of the volume of the cells and plasma, both of which are usually determined by dilution methods. This involves (in the case of plasma) the injection of an amount (A) of a test substance such as ^{125}I-labeled human serum albumin (HSA). After about a 10-minute mixing period, a sample of blood is withdrawn, the red cells removed by centrifu-

Table 1.1.
Normal Concentration of Plasma Constituents

Per dl (deciliter) Plasma	
Total protein	6.0 to 8.5 g
Albumin	3.0 to 5.5 g
Fibrinogen	0.2 to 0.4 g
Glucose (fasting)	65 to 110 mg
Total lipids	400 to 1000 mg
Cholesterol	150 to 300 mg
Triglycerides	50 to 150 mg
Nonprotein nitrogen (NPN)	20 to 45 mg
Blood urea nitrogen (BUN)	10 to 20 mg
Uric acid	3 to 7 mg
Creatinine	0.4 to 1.4 mg
Electrolytes (serum) mEq/liter	
Na^+	136 to 145
K^+	3.5 to 5.0
Ca^{2+}	4.3 to 5.1
Cl^-	98 to 106

gation, and the plasma concentration (C) of the test substance determined. The total plasma volume (V) is then determined as: $V(\text{ml}) = A(\text{mg})/C(\text{mg/ml})$.

The red blood cell volume can similarly be estimated with red cells labeled with radioactive chromium (^{51}Cr) using the same principle. The plasma volume, at any particular moment, represents a temporary balance between the intake of fluid and its output via kidneys, gastrointestinal tract, etc. While it may temporarily fluctuate over a period of time, in a relatively steady state, an individual's total blood volume usually remains remarkably constant. Since values in the normal adult generally range from 70 to 75 ml/kg of body weight, a 70-kg adult might therefore have a total blood volume of about 5000 ml with about 55% or 2,750 ml of the total as plasma volume and about 45% or 2,250 ml as total red cell mass.

The dilution principle assumes that none of the indicator material is lost and that perfect mixing occurs. This is not entirely true since some of the plasma protein (with indicator attached) is slowly eliminated during the test period and some ^{51}Cr is sequestered in the spleen and other reticuloendothelial organs. For more accurate determinations of cell and plasma volumes, the blood concentrations of the indicator material are followed over a 30- or 60-minute period, plotted against time on log graph paper, and the original concentration estimated by extrapolating backward to zero time.

Volume and Pressure

Volume and Pressure Distribution

The most important physical characteristics of the circulation are volume, pressure, and flow. Volume and volume-pressure relations comprise the *statics* of the system and define the basic qualities that distinguish important functional properties of arteries and veins. Pressure and flow relate to the moving stream of blood and so characterize the *dynamics* of the circulation.

Total blood volume is, in most primates, a reasonably linear function of body weight and in the healthy human adult averages 75 ml/kg (*i.e.*, about 2.5 to 3.0 L/M^2 of body surface area). Individual variations depend mainly on age, climate, and degree of physical activity. Continued orthostatic stimulation is necessary for the maintenance of adequate total blood volume, since forced bed rest, prolonged water immersion, and exposure to the weightlessness of space will all lead to decreased blood volume and orthostatic hypotension. In recumbent man, about 25 to 30% of total blood volume (*i.e.*, about 22 to 26 ml/kg) consists of "thoracic" or "central" blood volume. Upon assumption of the upright posture, about 500 to 700 ml of blood, (*i.e.*, about 6 to 8 ml/kg and 26 to 30% of the central blood volume) is rapidly displaced from the thorax to the lower portion of the body and lower extremities. The physiological effects of this postural dislocation of blood are discussed further in Chapter 13.

It has been estimated that in a normal 70 kg adult with a total blood volume of about 5000 ml and thoracic (or central) blood volume of about 1250 ml, about 350 ml would be contained in the vena cavae and right heart and thus serve in a sense as the right heart reserve. This means that in cases of stress, when more cardiac output may be needed, this volume can be drawn upon to increase right ventricular filling and filling pressure. About 900 ml are contained in the pulmonary artery, lungs, pulmonary veins, and left heart and similarly serve as immediate reserve for the left ventricle. Thoracic blood volume thus constitutes an immediate source of filling pressure and volume for the two ventricles. This ready reserve is highly important, since ventricular filling is a critical determinant of stroke volume and cardiac output (see Chapter 5, Intrinsic Regulation of Heart).

Volume-Pressure Relations in Blood Vessels

From the standpoint of the distribution of blood volume among the functional systems of the circulation, about two-thirds of the total blood volume is normally in the venous system and about one-sixth is on the arterial side (Fig. 1.4). However, the pressure distribution is quite different, being in an almost inverse relation to the volume distribution (Fig. 1.5). This disposition of pressure and volume is due in large part to the structure and relative elasticity of the arteries and veins, that is, to their pressure-volume relations. While it is true that the entire arterial tree serves as a distributing conduit, all arteries are not alike. From an anatomical and functional standpoint they may be divided into two main groups that differ structurally and functionally from each other, and both of which, in turn, differ notably from veins.

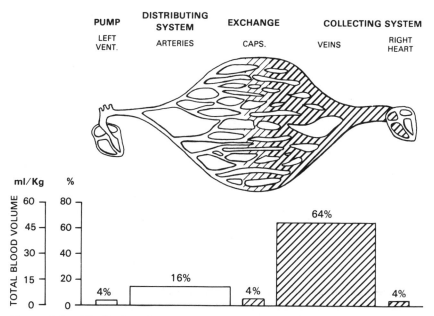

Figure 1.4.   Distribution of blood volume in the systemic circulation. Not shown is the 8% fraction in the pulmonary vessels.

1. Aorta and Large Arteries.   All blood vessels have an endothelial lining and contain varying proportions of smooth muscle, elastin, and collagen; however, the aorta and the large arteries have unusually large amounts of elastin in their walls and thus are capable of considerable expansion and recoil. This quality enables them to store pressure energy as their walls are stretched during ventricular systolic ejection; with subsequent rebound of the vessel wall, this pressure energy can then be released as kinetic energy of flow in the succeeding diastole. This helps to propel the blood toward the tissues during the diastolic phase of the cardiac cycle and promotes a more even flow to the capillaries. The large arteries are therefore the "pressure storers" of the circulation. As previously mentioned, the internal pressure in the large arteries is normally about 120/80 mm Hg.

2. Small Arteries and Arterioles.   These vessels have fewer elastic fibers and more circular smooth muscle fibers. They have, therefore, contractile capabilities which, when activated, serve to constrict their lumen, dam back the flow, increase the pressure centrally (toward the heart), and decrease the pressure peripherally (toward the capillaries). These vessels thus serve as the "stopcocks" of the circulation and are usually called the "resistance" vessels. Their pressures generally range from 60 to 90 mm Hg in the small arteries to 40 to 60 mm Hg in the arterioles.

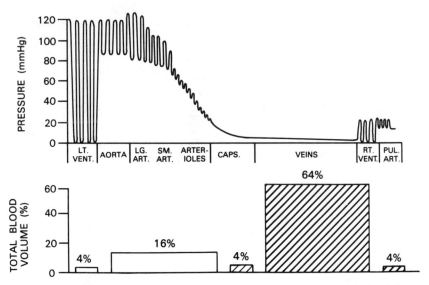

Figure 1.5.   Pressure and volume distribution in the systemic circulation. Illustrating the inverse relationship between internal pressure and volume in different portions of the circulatory system.

3. Veins.   The veins are very thin-walled vessels with only small amounts of elastin and limited smooth muscle in their walls. Their pressures are low, ranging from about 10 mm Hg at the venular ends of the capillaries to about 0 mm Hg at the entrance of the vena cavae to the heart. As indicated in Figure 1.5, the venous system normally contains about four times more blood than the arterial system; yet, if more fluid or blood is infused into the vascular system, 90% of the new fluid will be taken up by the veins because of their great distensibility. Because of this property, the veins are known as the "volume storers" of the circulation.

Distensibility and Compliance of Blood Vessels

In order to compare more precisely the volume and pressure characteristics of blood vessels, their "distensibility," that is, the increase in volume necessary to induce a unit pressure change, may be determined. If a large artery or vein is removed, tied at both ends, and blood or fluid injected slowly into the lumen, the internal pressure will increase progressively as volume is added. If the percentage of volume change is plotted against the internal (transmural) pressure, pressure-volume or distensibility curves similar to those in Figure 1.6 will result.

The slope of the curve at any point (ratio of percentage of volume increase to pressure increase), which is a measure of the distensibility, varies with the

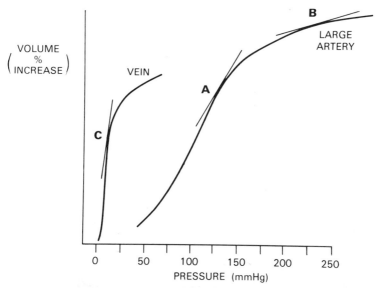

Figure 1.6. Distensibility (percentage of volume increase per unit pressure change) in a normal large artery and vein. Note the decreased slope of the arterial curve at higher pressure (*B*). Also note the steep slope and much higher distensibility of the veins (*C*) at their physiological pressures (0–10 mm Hg) compared to the slope and distensibility of arteries (*A*) at their usual pressures (75–150 mm Hg).

degree of filling. The normal young aorta has good distensibility and recoil at normal physiological pressures of about 75 to 150 mm Hg (Fig. 1.6*A*), which gives it the important property of a "pressure storer." However, at higher pressures such as 200 mm Hg, when it is "overfilled," (Fig. 1.6*B*), its wall becomes more rigid and has lesser distensibility, a smaller slope, and less recoil.

In the latter case, the expandable qualities of elastin in the arterial wall are limited by the less expandable collagen and smooth muscle which, when stretched, reaches its limits and resists further distension. Distensibility is influenced, therefore, not only by the thickness and composition of the vessel wall but also by the degree of filling of the vessel.

As illustrated in Figure 1.6*C*, veins at their physiological pressures (0–10 mm Hg) have a high distensibility, ranging from 6 to 8 times that of arteries. However, vessels do not begin to show distensibility until they are filled. Since the veins have, in addition, about 3 to 4 times more volume than the arteries, the capacity of the venous system for storage of blood is about 25 to 30 times that of the arterial system and accounts for the primary function of veins as "volume storers" of the circulation.

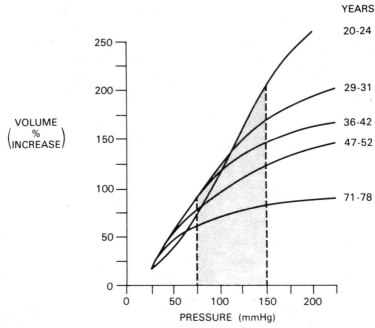

Figure 1.7. Decrease in aortic distensibility with advancing age. Note particularly the changes in distensibility within the physiological pressure range of 75 to 150 mm Hg and the greater differences at the higher pressures. (Reprinted with permission from P. Hallock and J.C. Benson, *J Clin Invest* 16: 597, 1937.)

"Compliance" and "capacitance," terms that are similar but not identical with distensibility, may be defined as the volume change per unit pressure change when fluid is added. These terms are commonly used to describe the expandability of vessels or of organ systems such as lungs. However, compliance and capacitance have the disadvantage of defining the pressure-volume relationship without reference to the size of the vessel; obviously a given increment of volume will induce a much larger pressure rise in a small vessel than in a large one, so that the smaller vessel may have an apparently lower compliance. For this reason "distensibility,"or the *percent* volume change per unit pressure, permits a more logical comparison of vessels of different sizes and types.

Distensibility may be altered by age, disease, autonomic stimulation, and various drugs. In the elderly, the arterial walls become infiltrated with less-distensible fibrous tissue, which increases their stiffness (Fig. 1.7). This can affect pressure and flow relations in the entire arterial tree. This lesser distensibility at increased age is offset to some extent by the increased volume of the aorta in older individuals, since this increased volume enables the aorta to accommodate the ejected left ventricular blood with less increase in pressure. However, the increased rigidity of the aorta coupled with the greater vascular resistance of the arteries constitutes a significantly greater impedance to left ventricular ejection in the older subject, which is undoubtedly a considerable factor in increasing cardiac work and limiting left ventricular function in the elderly (see Chapter 12, Aging).

Oxygen Transport

Although the assimilation and transport of oxygen is a definitive part of respiratory physiology, its importance to the normal and abnormal circulation warrants a brief review.

The chief constituent of the erythrocyte is hemoglobin (Hb), the primary oxygen carrier, which is normally present in a concentration of 14 to 15 g/dl of whole blood. Hb combines reversibly with oxygen to form oxyhemoglobin (HbO_2), the primary oxygen carrier. When exposed to certain drugs and other oxidizing agents, Hb is converted to a darker colored methemoglobin, which is present in only very small amounts in normal blood. Because Hb has a higher affinity for carbon monoxide, it can displace the O_2 to form carboxyhemoglobin; thus, exposure to excessive amounts of carbon monoxide can significantly reduce the oxygen-carrying capacity of the blood.

If blood is exposed to a sufficiently high oxygen pressure so that all the Hb is combined with oxygen to form HbO_2, it is "fully saturated"; under these circumstances, 1 g of Hb can combine with 1.39 ml of oxygen so that blood with a Hb concentration of 15 g/dl will then have an "oxygen capacity" of 20.8 ml/dl of blood or 20.8 vol %. The amount of oxygen with which each unit of Hb will actually combine is dependent primarily on the partial pressure of oxygen (Po_2) to which the Hb is exposed. This relationship is defined by the oxygen dissociation curve (Fig. 1.8).

In the alveoli of the lungs, where the Po_2 is normally at a high level, the blood will be about 97% saturated, i.e., 97% of Hb is combined with O_2 (A in Fig. 1.8). In this case arterial blood with a Hb concentration of 15 g/dl will have an oxygen content of 20.2 ml/dl. After the blood has given up some of its oxygen in the tissues and reached the large veins (mixed venous blood), its Po_2 value will have decreased to about 40 mm Hg. As indicated in Figure 1.8, V, at this Po_2 the blood will be only about 75% saturated with oxygen, and the blood oxygen content will be about 16 ml/dl; therefore, this blood will have released to the tissues about 4 ml of gaseous oxygen for each 100 ml of blood flow through the capillaries.

While oxygen content is determined primarily by the Po_2, it is also influenced to a lesser extent by four other factors: pH, Pco_2, blood temperature, and the concentration of 2,3-diphosphoglycerate (2,3-DPG). An increased red cell concentration of the organic phosphate, 2,3-DPG, may occur in chronic hypoxia or chronic lung disease.

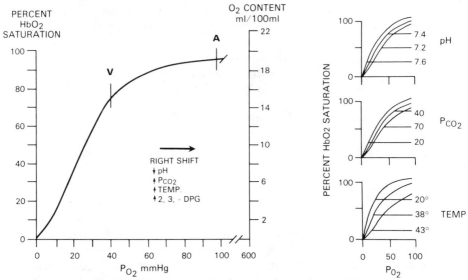

Figure 1.8. *Left*, Oxygen dissociation curve showing the relationship between the partial pressure of oxygen (Po_2) and the percentage of oxyhemoglobin (HbO_2) saturation of the blood. In the alveoli of the lungs (*A*) the Po_2 is about 100 mm Hg, which results in 97% HbO_2 saturation. In the mixed venous blood returning from the tissues, the Po_2 has fallen to about 40 mm Hg and the HbO_2 saturation is approximately 75% (*V*). *Right*, Small shifts of the curve to the right, which occur in the tissues because of the lower pH, higher Pco_2, and higher temperature, tend to lessen the affinity of Hb for oxygen and assist in release of oxygen to the tissues. (Adapted from J.B. West, *Respiratory Physiology*, Baltimore: Williams & Wilkins, 1979, p. 75.)

A decrease in pH or an increase in any of the other three factors will produce a "shift to the right" in the oxyhemoglobin dissociation curve (Fig. 1.8. The result is that at the same Po_2, less O_2 will be bound to the Hb and consequently more released to the tissues, which results in a lesser affinity of Hb for O_2. Conversely, an increase in pH or a decrease in Pco_2, blood temperature, or 2,3-DPG will have the opposite effect (*i.e.*, the dissociation curve will shift to the left, so there is greater affinity of hemoglobin for oxygen).

The shape of the oxygen dissociation curve has other implications; at the upper "plateau" portion of the curve where it is flatter, large changes in Po_2 will have relatively little effect on HbO_2 saturation and content. As a result, moderate decreases in Po_2 encountered at high altitude or other low oxygen environments result in smaller reductions in HbO_2 saturation and content than would ordinarily be the case, so that the hypoxia will be partially "buffered." On the other hand, in the capillaries, where the Po_2 falls sharply, as represented by the steep portion of the curve, the tissues have the advantage of being able to pick up a large supply of oxygen with only a small decrease in PO_2.

Suggested Readings

Babior BM and Stossel TP. *Hematology, A Pathophysiological Approach.* New York: Churchill Livingston, 1984.

Bader H. Anatomy and physiology of vascular wall. In: *Handbook of Physiology*, Section 2: *Circulation*, edited by WF Hamilton and P Dow. Washington, D.C.: American Physiological Society, 1963, vol. II, pp 865–889.

Burton AC. *Physiology and Biophysics of the Circulation.* Chicago: Year Book Medical Publishers, 1972, pp 66–67, 119–120.

Marshall RJ and Shepherd JT. Interpretation of changes in "central" blood volume and slope volume during exercise in man. *J Clin Invest* 40:385, 1961.

Sjostrand T. Volume and distribution of blood and their significance in regulating the circulation. *Physiol Rev* 33:202, 1953.

Spivak JI (ed.). *Fundamentals of Clinical Hematology.* Hagerstown, Md: Harper & Row, 1980.

Yu PN. *Pulmonary Blood Volume in Health and Disease.* Philadelphia: Lea & Febiger, 1969.

West JB. *Respiratory Physiology—The Essentials*, 2nd ed. Baltimore: Williams & Wilkins, 1979, pp 70–74.

chapter 2

Hemodynamics

Poiseuille's Law

In 1846, Poiseuille, a French physician, described the factors governing non-pulsatile flow of a homogeneous fluid through rigids tubes. He stated that if all other factors are held constant, the rate of flow, Q, through a cylindrical tube of length, L, and radius, r, was directly proportional to the driving pressure, ΔP (the difference in pressure between two ends of the tube). In addition, Q was inversely proportional to the length of the tube, L, inversely proportional to the viscosity of the flowing liquid, η, and directly proportional to the fourth power of the radius of the tube, r.

He added two necessary proportionality constants (π and 8) to elaborate "Poiseuille's law": $Q = \Delta P r^4 \pi / \eta L 8$. (Fig. 2.1).

Although blood is a nonhomogeneous fluid, which in the body flows through branching, distensible tubes in a pulsatile manner, Poiseuille's law nonetheless gives good approximations and has proven very useful in understanding the "in vivo" circulation. Furthermore most of the factors in his equation are analogous to those in an ordinary hydraulic system and lend themselves to simplifications that may profitably be applied to basic and clinical cardiovascular problems.

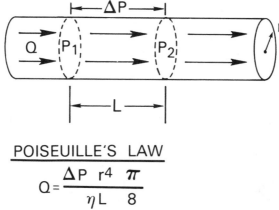

POISEUILLE'S LAW

$$Q = \frac{\Delta P \; r^4 \; \pi}{\eta L \; 8}$$

Figure 2.1. Poiseuille's law. In an artificial system, flow through a cylindrical tube or any segment of a tube is directly proportional to ΔP, the driving pressure along the tube, and the fourth power of the radius, r. Flow is inversely proportional to L, the length of the segment and to η, the viscosity of the liquid. The proportionality constant is $\pi/8$.

Resistance to Flow

If ΔP in Poiseuille's equation is considered to be the driving pressure, the remaining factors, $r^4/\eta L$, may be considered impediments to flow. If these residual factors are collected together, inverted $\left[\dfrac{\eta L}{r^4}\right]$ and designated R, as resistance to flow, the formula can then be simplified to: Q (flow) $= \Delta P$(driving pressure)/R (resistance to flow), and by transposing: R (resistance to flow) $= \Delta P$(driving pressure)/Q(flow).

In this very basic and useful hemodynamic generalization, R is defined as that resistance provided by a vessel or circulatory bed, which permits a given pressure differential to produce a unit flow. It will be recalled that this equation is an analogue of Ohm's law, which states that with direct current, the electrical resistance, R (in ohms) is the ratio of electromotive force (in volts) and the current (in amperes).

By generalizing from an isolated cylindrical tube to the intact circulation in an organ or in the entire circulatory system, the vascular resistance to flow may similarly be estimated as the ratio of the pressure gradient across the organ or system to the blood flow through it. When this method of calculation is used, resistance is sometimes expressed in PRU units (pressure-resistance units) which are defined as mm Hg/ml of flow/min. An adult human, for example, with a mean aortic pressure of 100 mm Hg and a mean right atrial pressure of 0 mm Hg, would have a pressure gradient across the systemic circulation of 100 mm Hg (ΔP). If the cardiac output were 5 L/min, the total peripheral resistance (TPR) of the system would be : TPR = 100 mm Hg/ 5000 ml/min, or 0.02 mm Hg/ml/min, or 0.02 PRU units.

Although the concept of vascular resistance is commonly employed in basic cardiovascular studies, its clinical application has been somewhat limited because measurements of flow, particularly in individual organs and tissues, are still technically rather difficult.

In comparing vascular resistances of different organs and organisms, it should be noted that blood flow (the denominator) is strongly influenced by the size and vascularity of the organ while arterial pressure (the numerator) is not. Thus an infant with a body weight and cardiac output only $\frac{1}{20}$ that of an adult will have a calculated total vascular resistance much greater than the adult, even though the relative dimensions of vessels and tissues as well as flow per unit mass may be generally similar. For this reason, when comparing organisms, vascular resistance is usually expressed on a weight basis (*e.g.*, per 100 g of tissue).

Components of Vascular Resistance

In the previous discussion of Poiseuille's law, the question of what actually constitutes resistance was temporarily bypassed. In transposing Poiseuille's law, the vascular resistance became $R = \eta L/r^4$.

It is seen that η, the viscosity, is the fluid resistance factor and L/r^4, the blood vessel resistance factor. While it seems reasonable that the viscosity and length of the system would be important in determining resistance to flow, the disproportionate role of the radius—which makes it the predominant factor in the equation—is rather surprising. The fourth power effect is due to the fact that flow in a cylinder is proportional, not to the radius of the tube, but to its cross-sectional area, which is an r^2 factor ($A = \pi r^2$); in addition, flow is a function of the velocity of the moving column, which in turn is proportional to the square of the distance from the axis to the vessel wall. The combination of these two r^2 terms and the consequent magnification of the radius factor has important implications for the control of flow in the intact organism.

Within the same vascular bed over a short period of time, neither the length of the circuit nor blood viscosity would ordinarily change appreciably; the most important adjustment of vascular resistance, therefore, is accomplished by alteration of vessel diameter. A decrease in lumen diameter is brought about by contraction of the smooth muscle of the vessel wall (vasoconstriction), which increases resistance to flow; relaxation of the tone of the muscle (vasodilation) increases the lumen size and, therefore, decreases resistance. Thus, alteration of vascular resistance to an organ is almost entirely a function of the adjustment of the caliber of blood vessels. By virtue of this radius

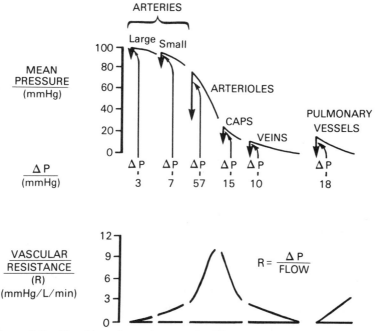

Figure 2.2.   *Top,* Vascular resistances in different segments of the circulation. The pressure fall (Δ*P*) is shown in different parts of the circulation and is least in the aorta and the greatest at the arteriolar level. *Center,* If the Δ*P* values are divided by the cardiac output (5 liters/min) which will be constant through all the segments, the vascular resistance of the different segments (*bottom*) can be estimated. As expected, it is least in the aorta and highest in the arterioles.

effect, large changes in resistance to flow can be brought about quickly with small changes in vessel diameter.

In addition to the calculation of total peripheral resistance (TPR) described above, how can we estimate the resistance (*R*) of a part of the circuit (*i.e.,* determine the distribution of the resistance)? If we assume a constant flow (*Q*) through all the collective cross sections of the entire circulation (Fig. 2.2), and if $R = \Delta P/Q$, the greatest resistance will lie in that segment in which the pressure fall is the greatest (*i.e.,* the arterioles) and the resistance is least where the pressure fall is least (*i.e.,* the aorta) (Fig. 2.2).

Series and Parallel Resistances

In a manner analogous to electrical circuits, vascular resistances may be in series or in parallel. If in series, the resistances are additive, but when in parallel they are additive as reciprocals, so that $1/R_T = 1/R_1 + 1/R_2 + 1/R_3$

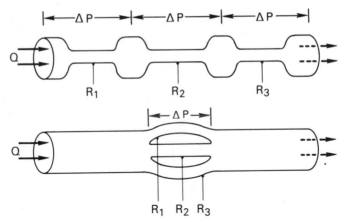

Figure 2.3.   Vascular resistances in series and in parallel. *Top*, If across each series resistance, the driving pressure, (ΔP), is 3 mm and the flow (Q) 1 ml/min, then each resistance (R) would be $\Delta P/Q$ or 3 mm Hg/ml/min and R_T (total resistance) = 9 mm Hg/ml/min. *Bottom*, In parallel resistances, if across each resistance the driving pressure (ΔP) were 3 mm Hg and the flow (Q) 1 ml/min, then the total resistance is calculated as $1/R_1 + 1/R_2 + 1/R_3$ or 1 mm Hg/ml/min. Note that when the three resistances are in parallel, the total resistance is only $\frac{1}{9}$ of that which would prevail if the three resistances were in series (*i.e.*, the ratio of $R_p/R_s = \frac{1}{9}$) so that it takes a ΔP of only 1 mm Hg (instead of 9 mm Hg) to produce a flow of 1 ml/min.

(etc.). This means that in a parallel circuit, R_T is less than any of the individual R terms.

Viewed as a total system, the large majority of the vascular resistances of the organs and tissues of the body are in parallel. For the circulatory system this provides a significant advantage, not only because greater flow can be achieved with small changes of pressure but also because parallel vascular circuits permit greater flexibility in the control of flow to individual beds (Fig. 2.3). Thus, through manipulation of resistances, flow through one circuit can be increased or decreased without necessarily affecting the proximal arterial pressure or flow through other parallel circuits. For example, in Figure 2.3 (parallel resistances), if R_1 is increased, flow through that circuit is decreased without affecting the driving pressure ΔP or the resultant flow across circuits 2 and 3. By contrast increase in R_1 in the series conduit (Fig. 2.3) will reduce flow to all the downstream circuits. Because of the awkwardness of adding reciprocals, the conductances of parallel circuits ($C = 1/R$) are sometimes used in place of resistances for hemodynamic calculations.

In the above, it was emphasized that a decreasing vessel radius greatly increases vascular resistance; however, it should be recalled that this applies only to a single tube system. In the intact organism, we know that while vessel radii decrease, the number and cross-sectional area of the vessels increase considerably as we move from aorta to capillary and furthermore, as mentioned above, their parallel arrangement decreases their resistance. Theoretical quantitative analyses of these two diverse factors indicate that despite the great increase in the number and cross-sectional area of vessels, there is a net increase in vascular resistance from the aorta down the arterial tree. This is further evidence of the disproportionate resistance effect of the smaller radii on flow. It should also be pointed out that these factors do not negate the empirical usefulness of regional or total resistance calculations done on the same organism (e.g., in pressure-flow studies described below) in which the formula $R = \Delta P/Q$ is used.

Figure 2.4 is a diagrammatic sketch of the main circulatory resistances of the body. Although the great majority of vascular circuits are in parallel, in certain organs such as the kidney and liver, the blood traverses two capillary beds in tandem, so that their resistances are in series. The result of this is that the second capillary bed has a lower pressure and lesser ability to increase its flow when such increases are needed.

Vascular Impedance

The resistance to flow (R), which was defined above as the ratio of the mean values of $\Delta P/Q$, resides mainly in the arterioles and applies only to a steady-flow system. But what about vascular resistance to pulsatile flow, for example in the aorta, where it is most marked? The opposition to this type of flow offered by the aorta and arterial bed is termed "impedance," which may, therefore, be defined simply as pulsatile resistance or the resistance to phasic flow.

The major determinants of aortic impedance are (a) the viscoelastic properties of the aorta and large arterial vessels, (b) the inertia and viscosity of the blood, (c) the reflection of the flow and pressure waves back through the arterial tree from the periphery, and (d) the peripheral vascular resistance. Thus, aortic impedance depends partly on the frequency of the arterial pressure and flow curves and their relationship. Because these are complex waves, the quantitative analysis of aortic impedance depends on precisely timed biophysical measurements of pressure and flow at multiple points in the flow tract.

Such analyses have shown that pulsatile resistance (impedance) is much higher than resistance would be at equivalent steady-flow levels. But in spite of the fact that oscillatory flow is mechanically much less efficient than steady laminar flow, numerous investigators have reported that the mammalian organism apparently functions best when blood flow is pulsatile.

Recent investigators have indicated that in normal aging and in certain circulatory diseases such as hypertension, the decreased compliance of the aorta and large arteries combined with increased peripheral resistance elevates aortic impedance to the point where left ventricular ejection is severely hand-

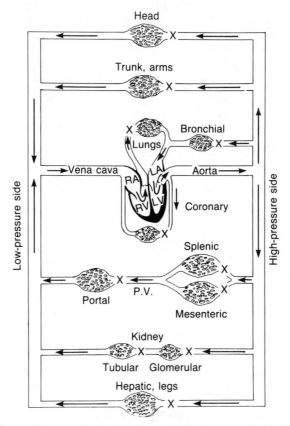

Figure 2.4. Diagrammatic sketch of vascular resistances in the body showing parallel and series circuits. The X's indicate the location of control points where arterioles control the flow (Reprinted with permission from Year Book Medical Publisher from *Physiology and Biophysics of the Circulation*, 2nd ed. Chicago, 1972.)

icapped. Some investigators have proposed that these impedance defects may be the critical factors in the declining ventricular performance in such conditions. Because of the technical difficulty of measuring vascular impedance, relatively few studies of this type have been made thus far in clinical situations. However, the increasing efforts now being expended in this direction will undoubtedly assist in determining more precisely the possible role of vascular impedance in circulatory disease.

Viscosity

As indicated in Poiseuille's equation, the resistance to flow due to the friction of molecules in the moving stream is known as the viscosity. In a homogeneous

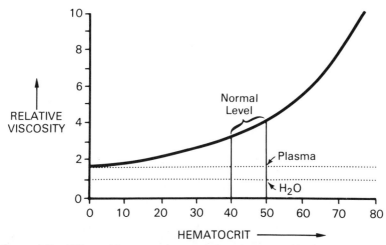

Figure 2.5. Effect of hematocrit on relative viscosity of blood. Note that as hematocrit increases, the relative viscosity increases disproportionately.

liquid such as water, in an artificial system, viscosity is a constant. However, in the case of a two-phase medium such as blood flowing in an *in vivo* circulatory system, viscosity is not constant but depends on several factors: (*a*) the concentration of the suspended medium (the cells), (*b*) the velocity of flow, and (*c*) the radius of the vessel.

If measured with reference to water, as is commonly done, the relative viscosity of plasma is about 1.3. The relative viscosity of whole blood depends mainly on the cell concentration or hematocrit as shown in Figure 2.5. At normal hematocrits of 42 to 45, the relative viscosity of blood is about 3.6 compared to water. However, because the relationship is exponential, an increase of 10 in the hematocrit from the level of 40 will increase the viscosity about 25% and an increase of 20 to the level of 60 will increase viscosity about 60%.

In low hematocrit states such as anemia, viscosity and therefore vascular resistance both fall, resulting in increased cardiac output. In high hematocrit conditions such as polycythemia and leukemia, in which hematocrit levels may reach 60 to 70%, a profound increase in systemic and pulmonary vascular resistance occurs with a resultant elevation of blood pressure.

Vessel bore and flow rate are two additional factors affecting blood viscosity in a two-phase medium. In tubes less than 200 μm in diameter—which would include arterioles, capillaries, and venules—the relative viscosity of the blood decreases and offers less resistance to flow. This phenomenon, for which there is no satisfactory explanation, is sometimes called the Fahraeus-Lindqvist effect.

A further peculiarity of two-phase fluids such as blood is that at low flow rates the apparent viscosity increases (anomalous viscosity). This phenomenon has been attributed to the disposition of red cells in the flowing stream; at higher velocities the cells accumulate in the axial part of the stream, but at low velocities they assume a more even distribution and hence offer greater flow resistance. Another factor that is probably involved in anomalous viscosity is the tendency of erythrocytes to aggregate into stacks of "rouleaux" at lower flow velocities (Fig. 1.3). This effect has been found by some investigators to be exaggerated in low flow states such as burns or shock, causing pronounced cell clumping or "sludge" in the microcirculation with severe hindrance to flow and a resultant ischemia of the tissue.

It should also be mentioned that in the capillary bed the blood hematocrit is usually about 10% less than in the large vessels for reasons that are not well understood at present.

It is evident, therefore, that in different parts of the circulation, there will be significant variations in vessel diameter, flow velocity, and hematocrit and that the net effect on viscosity is not always predictable. Present evidence suggests, however, that the hematocrit effect on viscosity is the most important and predominant one.

Under special circumstances, temperature may affect blood viscosity in a significant manner. There is about a 2% rise in viscosity per 1°C fall in temperature. During prolonged exposure to cold and high wind the extremities will become chilled, and the reduced flow effect of vasoconstriction will be enhanced by the increased vascular resistance resulting from the heightened viscosity. In addition, the shift of the HbO_2 dissociation curve to the left and consequent lesser release of O_2 to the tissues at the same Po_2 (Fig. 1.8) will intensify the ischemia and increase the possibility of frostbite and serious damage to the part.

Flow Velocity and Turbulence

The linear velocity of blood flow varies widely in the circulatory system—from a mean value of about 30 to 35 cm/sec in the aorta to about 0.2 to 0.3 mm/sec in the capillaries as illustrated in Figure 2.6. If we assume that equal volumes will be transported through the collective segments of the circulation in equal times, the mean flow velocity ($\bar{V}$) will vary inversely with the cross-sectional area; i.e., $\bar{V}$ (mm/sec) = flow (ml/sec)/cross-sectional area (πr^2 in mm²).

By transposing the factors in the above equation, the circulation time (CT) between two points (A and B) in a closed circulation can be calculated as the quotient of the volume contained between A and B and the mean rate of flow between the two points, i.e., CT in sec = volume (A to B) in ml/mean flow (A to B) in ml/sec. In states of circulatory failure, an increased CT for the systemic circulation is usually an index of decreased total flow, i.e, of low cardiac output and inadequate circulation.

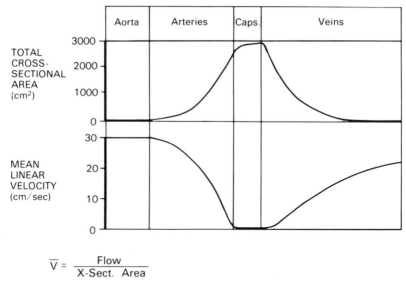

$$\overline{V} = \frac{Flow}{X\text{-Sect. Area}}$$

Figure 2.6.   Relation of cross-sectional area and mean velocity of flow in the systemic circulation.

Poiseuille's law assumes that the different layers of molecules move parallel to each other in longitudinal streamlines somewhat resembling concentric sleeves. The molecules adjacent to the vessel wall are stationary; each succeeding layer has increasing velocity, with the maximum at the axis. Under these circumstances of "streamline" flow, the frictional resistance is independent of the pressure-flow relations and thus in the case of a homogeneous fluid is linear as has been previously described.

However, under certain circumstances, particularly at high velocities, the flow is no longer streamline but becomes turbulent with swirls and eddies (Fig. 2.7). In this case flow is approximately proportional to the square root of the pressure gradient rather than the pressure itself; the turbulent stream now offers a considerable increase in resistance.

Reynolds has defined the factors affecting this phenomenon and stated that turbulence is likely to occur in a moving stream when the Reynolds ratio (R_e) exceeds a value of about 1000 for blood or 2000 for homogeneous fluids: $R_e = \alpha \times v \times D/\eta$, in which σ is the density of the fluid (g/cm^3), v is the average velocity (cm/sec), D is the diameter of the vessel (cm) and η is the fluid viscosity (g/sec/cm^2). Since blood density is relatively constant, the factors tending to increase the Reynolds number and cause it to exceed the R_e are an increased velocity of flow (such as in larger blood vessels), a decrease in viscosity such as in anemia, and a decrease in the radius of the vessel such

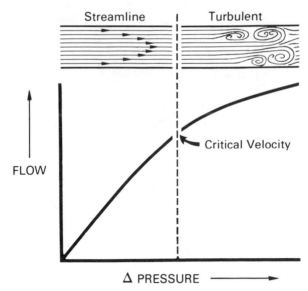

Figure 2.7. Relationship between velocity of flow and turbulence. (Reprinted with permission from T.C. Ruch and H.D. Patton, *Physiology and Biophysics*, Philadelphia: W.B. Saunders, 1974.)

as a stenosis (fixation) of a heart valve or coarctation (fibrotic constriction) of a blood vessel such as the aorta.

From the clinical standpoint, an important factor is that streamline flow is silent but turbulence produces noise that can often be heard with the unaided ear or with a stethoscope. Sounds used in the conventional determination of arterial blood pressure are audible because of the turbulence induced in the flow stream. In circulatory disease, defects in valves and constrictions of orifices will produce additional abnormal sounds that are used in clinical diagnosis (Chapter 3).

Rheology (the study of flow characteristics and deformation) and its application to human disease are important areas of current research. It is known, for example, that atherosclerotic lesions are often localized in the region of orifices, bends, and branch points of arteries. Rheological studies now indicate that in these regions the high-pressure, high-velocity stream in large arteries may subject the wall to continuous pressure stresses. These local injuries increase the permeability of the endothelium to plasma lipoproteins, thus greatly accelerating the atherosclerotic process at these sites.

Tension in the Blood Vessel Wall—Laplace's Theorem

Consideration has previously been given to the internal volume and pressure of a blood vessel but not to the vessel wall itself, which obviously is a key

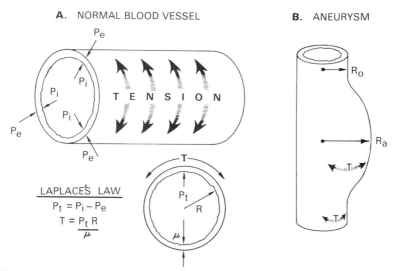

A. NORMAL BLOOD VESSEL

B. ANEURYSM

LAPLACE'S LAW

$$P_t = P_i - P_e$$
$$T = \dfrac{P_t R}{\mu}$$

Figure 2.8. Pressure-volume-tension relations in blood vessels (Laplace's law). *Left* (A), P_t the transmural pressure (dynes/cm²), is equal to the P_i (internal pressure) minus the P_e (external pressure). R is the radius (cm) and μ, the wall thickness (cm). T is the tension in the vessel wall (dynes/cm of longitudinal length). *Right* (B), Aortic aneurysm is the atherosclerotic weakening of the vessel with resultant bulging. The increased radius R_a at the aneurysm site increases tension at that point and puts further stress on the aortic wall.

factor. In a hollow cylindrical tube, the circumferential tension, T, in the wall along the linear axis of a vessel is usually measured in dynes/cm and is calculated as the product of the transmural pressure, P_t (inside pressure minus outside pressure) and the radius, R (Fig. 2.8). This relationship (first defined by Laplace) was later expanded by Frank to include the factor of wall thickness, μ, as follows: $T = P_t R/\mu$. This relationship suggests that in normal vessels in which the radius and wall thickness are in approximate proportion, the wall tension will vary with the transmural pressure and the two will tend to stay in reasonable balance. A capillary, for example, with a small radius and low pressure will require only a thin wall to sustain its lesser tension, but a large artery with a greater pressure and radius will have a higher tension and need for a thicker wall.

   Wall tension may be important in certain pathological conditions such as severe arteriosclerotic disease in which an aortic wall may weaken, gradually bulge, and become thinner at that point. With increasing radius and the progressive thinning, the tension at that site will further increase and the aorta may balloon and develop an "aneurysm," which might require surgical repair to prevent a rupture.

   In congestive heart disease the progressively increasing size of the failing heart may also produce inordinate tension in the wall of the heart. Because myocardial oxygen requirements are partly a function of myocardial tension, a reduction in heart size through medication will often promote increased cardiac efficiency by reducing wall tension and, therefore, reducing oxygen requirements per unit of mechanical work of the heart (see Chapter 14, Congestive Heart Failure).

Pressure-Flow Curves

The vascular resistance of an organ, tissue, or entire organism is determined mainly by the caliber of the blood vessels, particularly the arterioles. The caliber of the arterioles is determined by the "tonus" or contraction state of the vascular smooth muscle. The tone of the vascular muscle is, in turn, the result of a balance between the inherent tone due to the muscle itself, the sympathetic efferent vasoconstrictor impulses to the vessel, and the effects of humoral agents such as catecholamines, angiotensien, and local metabolites (Chapter 9).

In certain experimental and clinical situations, it is advantageous to measure peripheral vascular resistance. In the treatment of hypertension, for example, it is useful to know whether the high arterial pressure is due to excess vascular resistance or increased cardiac output. In peripheral vascular disease it would be helpful to periodically quantitate the degree of vascular resistance of the region in order to follow the course of the disease or the effectiveness of various types of therapy. In the development of new vasoactive drugs, it is important to assess the ability of the drugs to produce or reverse a state of vasoconstriction. Therefore, attempts are often made to determine the pressure-flow relations of an organ, tissue, or entire circulatory system.

If a homogeneous fluid is perfused through a rigid tube and the radius and length of the cylinder and the fluid viscosity are kept constant, the flow as predicted by Poiseuille's law will vary directly with the pressure gradient ΔP and a straight-line relationship will result (Fig. 2.9). However, if the tube is distensible, the radius of the vessel will increase as the perfusion and the transmural pressure increase; the resultant flow will then increase according to the fourth power of the radius.

With *in vivo* systems, resistance to flow will be influenced not only by the distensibility of the vessels but also, as previously discussed, by the effects of vessel caliber and flow velocity. Flow resistance is also influenced by the type of tissue involved. In lung or skin tissue, for example, if perfusion rates are altered gradually rather than abruptly so that the vessels are permitted to adapt, a pressure-flow curve similar to that shown in Figure 2.10a will result.

In the normal resting tissue (Fig. 2.10a) the curve is exponential and convex to the pressure axis; thus, the flow through the tissue rises disproportionately with increasing perfusion pressure (ΔP), due to the increased distention of

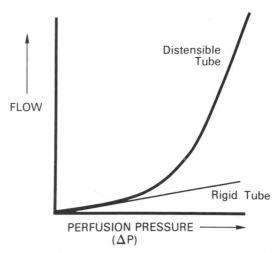

Figure 2.9. Pressure-flow curves in an artificial system using rigid and distensible tubes. Note that with increased perfusion pressure, there is a large increase in flow in the distensible tube.

the vessels as described above. This is a "passive" type of pressure-flow curve. In other tissues which show "autoregulation" the pressure-flow curve will have a different configuration (Chapter 9).

A pressure-flow perfusion system similar to this is frequently used to test the pharmacological effects of drugs on vascular smooth muscle. Injection of a constrictor agent such as norepinephrine will reduce the caliber of vessels and shift the curve to the right (Fig 2.10c), *i.e.*, there will be less flow per unit pressure and the resistance of the bed will be increased. Similarly if a vasodilating drug such as histamine is injected (Fig. 2.10d) there will be a reduction in the pressure-flow ratio and less resistance to flow.

It will be noted that these pressure-flow curves do not go through the origin, that is, flow goes to zero while there is still positive pressure in the perfusion system. The reason that this phenomenon occurs in certain tissues is not known. One theory is that as the vascular smooth muscle contracts, its inherent constrictive force and the resultant tension of the wall become greater than the distending force of the internal pressure; as the lumen becomes smaller, the tension becomes disproportionately greater than the distending pressure and the tension "wins," closing the vessel before the pressure has dropped to zero. The internal pressure that still exists when the vessel closes is known as the "critical closing pressure." Regardless of the explanation, the phenomenon is a potential hazard in low flow states such as shock in which tissues already ischemic are further threatened with sudden complete cessation of flow to certain capillary beds.

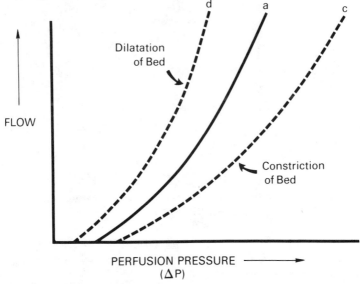

PERFUSION PRESSURE ———▶
(ΔP)

Figure 2.10.   Pressure-flow curve of cutaneous vascular bed. As perfusion pressure is increased, the flow to the vascular bed increases disproportionately, (*i.e.*, the peripheral resistance decreases). If a vasoconstrictor drug is injected, the pressure-flow curve changes from *a* to *c* indicating a general increase in vascular resistance. After a vasodilator drug, the pressure-flow curve will resemble that shown at *d*.

Suggested Readings

Badeer HS. Elementary hemodynamic principles based on modified Bernoulli's equation. *Physiologist* 28:41–46, 1985.

Burton AC. *Physiology and Biophysics of the Circulation*. Chicago: Year Book Medical Publishers, 1972.

Cokelet GR. Rheology and hemodynamics. *Annu Rev Physiol* 42:311–324, 1980.

Folkow B and Neil E. *Circulation*. London: Oxford University Press, 1971, pp 4–56.

Green HD, Rapela CA and Conrad MC. Resistance and capacitance phenomena in terminal vascular beds. In: *Handbook of Physiology*, Section 2: *Circulation*, edited by WF Hamilton and P Dow. Washington, D.C.: American Physiological Society, 1963, Vol. II, pp 935–960.

Milnor WR. *Hemodynamics*. Baltimore: Williams & Wilkins, 1982.

O'Rourke MF. Vascular impedance in studies of arterial and cardiac function. *Physiol Rev* 62:570–623, 1982.

Patel DJ and Vaishnav RN. *Basic Hemodynamics and Its Role in Disease Processes*. Baltimore: University Park Press, 1980.

Popel AS, Liu A, Dawant B, *et al*. Distribution of vascular resistance in terminal arteriolar networks. *Am J Physiol* 254:1149–1156, 1988.

Saari JT and Stinnett HO. Diameter vs number in diameter of vessel resistance. *Physiologist* 24(6):51–56, 1981.

Strandness DE and Sumner DS. *Hemodynamics for Surgeons*. New York: Grune & Stratton, 1975.

chapter 3

The Heart: Structure and Function

Functional Anatomy

The atria, whose walls consist mainly of two thin, overlying muscular sheaths arranged at right angles to each other, serve as blood reservoirs as well as pumps. The two thicker-walled ventricles pump blood from the low-pressure venous systems into the higher-pressure arterial systems.

In the pulmonary circuit, the right ventricle receives venous blood at about zero pressure and propels it into the pulmonary artery to a peak systolic pressure of about 25 mm Hg. The blood is oxygenated in the pulmonary capillaries and returned to the left heart. The left ventricle takes oxygenated blood, again at about zero pressure, and pumps it at a peak pressure of about 120 mm Hg into the aorta and systemic circuit and then to all the tissues of the body. The pulmonary circuit, because of its lower pressure and its shorter,

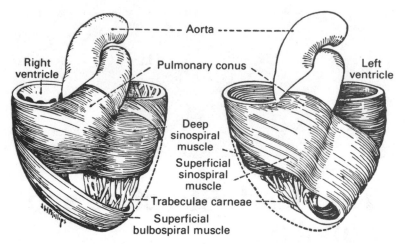

Figure 3.1.   Components of the myocardium. The outer muscle layers pull the apex of the heart toward the base; the inner circumferential fibers constrict the lumen, particularly of the left ventricle. (Reprinted with permission from R.F. Rushmer, *Cardiovascular Dynamics*, Philadelphia: W.B. Saunders, 1976.)

wider-bore vessels with thinner walls, is characterized as a low-pressure, low-resistance system.

The ventricles generate pressure energy by ejecting blood against arterial resistance, and kinetic energy by imparting velocity to the blood. Pressure work—which usually comprises more than 95% of the mechanical energy expended by the heart—can be estimated as the product of the stroke volume and the mean arterial pressure against which the ventricle works. Since the two ventricles eject similar volumes at identical heart rates, the left ventricle, because of its higher ejection pressure, performs about five to seven times as much pressure work as the right.

The myocardial muscle of each ventricle consists of three interdigitating layers (Fig. 3.1). The two outer muscle layers are oriented obliquely from the base of the heart (superior portion), which is the area of attachment to the aorta and other great vessels, to the apex, which is the tapered free portion. Upon contraction, the oblique fibers shorten the ventricular wall and pull the apex anteriorly and toward the base. The circumferential fibers constrict the ventricular diameter.

Right Ventricle

X-ray studies of the heart chambers have shown that the right ventricle has a concave outer wall and during contraction moves toward the interventricular septum with a bellowslike action, while the atrioventricular (AV) groove, or external depression, separating the right atrium and right ventricle, shortens

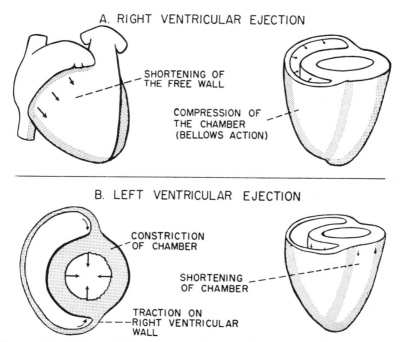

Figure 3.2. Right and left ventricles. Contraction characteristics and modes of emptying. (Reprinted with permission from R.F. Rushmer, *Cardiovascular Dynamics*, Philadelphia: W.B. Saunders, 1976).

toward the apex (Fig. 3.2). This anatomical configuration permits the thin and flexible wall of the right ventricle to eject a large volume of blood with a minimal amount of shortening against a low outflow pressure. However, if the pulmonary valve becomes thickened and stenotic, the resistance against which the right ventricle contracts will be much increased and flow into the pulmonary artery impeded. The right ventricular muscle then hypertrophies and may gradually approach the left ventricle in wall thickness.

Left Ventricle

As indicated above, left ventricular contraction involves both a decrease in diameter and a shortening of the axis between the base and apex of the heart; the net result is a movement of the apex toward the mitral valve. Simultaneously, the interaction of the various cardiac muscle groups produces a lifting effect on the apex, moving it toward the anterior chest wall and producing a palpable impulse at the left midclavicular line at about the interspace between the fifth and sixth ribs. The left ventricle with its more cylindrical outline (Fig. 3.2) has a mechanical advantage over the right ventricle in generating

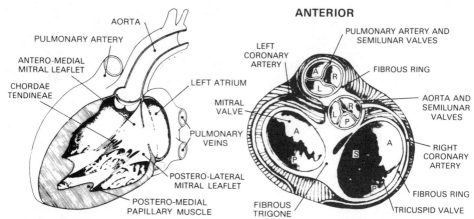

Figure 3.3.   Heart valves. *Left,* Schematic drawing of the left lateral view of mitral valve complex showing mitral annulus, the two mitral leaflets, chordae tendineae and papillary muscles. *Right,* A section through the base of the heart at the level of the fibrous ring supporting the cardiac valves. The right coronary artery arises from the anterior aortic sinus and the left coronary from the left posterior aortic sinus. (Adapted from J.W. Hurst, *The Heart, Arteries and Veins,* 5th ed., New York: McGraw-Hill, 1982, and J.T. Shepherd and P.M. Van Houtte, *The Human Cardiovascular System,* New York: Raven Press, 1979.)

stroke volume and power, because the volume it ejects through a decrease in the diameter of a cylinder is a function of the square of the radius, rather than a linear function (Laplace's law, Chapter 2). The thick-walled and heavier left ventricle is also thought to provide a type of splint against which the outer wall of the right ventricle is pulled, thus ejecting the right ventricular blood by means of a squeezing, bellowslike action.

After careful anatomical studies, Streeter has proposed that the ventricular muscle fibers are arranged in figure-eight paths similar to an unevenly folded lariat with the smaller loop around the apex and the larger loop around the base of the heart. He suggests that tightening of the lariat simulates ventricular emptying and that it is this unique arrangement that permits the remarkably rapid and energy-efficient ventricular ejection.

Heart Valves

Efficient pumping action of the heart requires a minimum of reflux as the blood is transported. This is achieved through two sets of unidirectional, reciprocating valves. One pair, the aortic and pulmonic (also called semilunar) valves are located at the exits of the right and left ventricles and open and close passively (Fig. 3.3, *right*). When open, the three-cusped aortic valve does not flatten against the aortic wall. This is important since it permits blood to flow unimpeded into the left and right main coronary arteries, whose openings are located in the aortic wall directly behind the open valve leaflets.

The two AV valves consist of the "tricuspid" on the right and the "mitral" on the left, which open toward the ventricles, permitting blood to enter from the atria. Both valves are thin walled and attached at the lower or free sides of their leaflets to papillary muscles on the ventricular walls by means of thin, stringy chordae tendineae (Fig. 3.3, *left*). The papillary muscles contract when the ventricles contract and so prevent the valves from bulging too far into the atrial chamber during ventricular contraction. A small amount of blood may occasionally regurgitate through a normal AV valve during ventricular contraction but with little effect on cardiac function. However, if one of the chordae tendineae becomes ruptured, the valve leaflet to which it is attached may bulge significantly. This produces an incompetent valve with regurgitation of a sizeable fraction of the blood backward into the atrium during ventricular systole, which results in a marked loss of pumping efficiency. This complication, which may follow a "myocardial infarction" or "heart attack," may result in rapid death.

The AV valves have larger cross-sectional areas than the semilunar valves and are subjected to less mechanical force during valve opening and closure.

Methods of Studying Cardiac Function

The pressure changes described in the following section were determined in the human subject with high-fidelity pressure transducers. The transducers were attached to long, thin tubes (catheters) threaded into the heart chambers and the large vessels through a peripheral vein or artery (cardiac catheterization). If a radioopaque contrast material is injected, the outlines of the chambers can be visualized. With high-speed fluoroscopy, rapid single or biplane photography, ultrasound, and other techniques (Chapter 7), the rate of movement of the cardiac wall, the stroke volume, and the emptying characteristics can be studied. These methods are used routinely in many cardiac catheterization laboratories. Methods of recording pressure and flow are further discussed in Chapter 6 and of cardiac output in Chapter 7.

For more precise study of heart sounds and murmurs, a small microphone is placed on the chest wall. The sound vibrations are amplified and recorded on an oscilloscope or polygraph; this *phonocardiogram* records the sounds as oscillations and, through use of filters and other special devices, permits an accurate analysis of sound frequency and intensity from which their clinical significance can be determined.

An additional technique of great clinical value is the recording of the electrical changes generated by the heart, *i.e.*, the electrocardiogram (ECG). The development of multiple leads for precise electrical recording at different points on the body has aided considerably in the diagnosis of certain cardiac irregularities (arrhythmias) and in the localization of myocardial damage. Electrical characteristics of the heart are described in Chapter 4.

The Cardiac Cycle

The cardiac cycle represents a combination of mechanical, electrical, and valvular events whose interrelationship is complex but essential to the understanding of how the heart functions and how disease processes affect it. At rest, the normal adult heart beats at a rate of about 70 to 75 beats per minute. Blood flows from the atria to the ventricles and from the ventricles to the large arteries at a velocity that is determined by the pressure differences between the chambers. Normally the valves offer no resistance and open or close as a function of the relative pressures exerted by the flowing stream and the energy imparted by the contractions of the atrial and ventricular musculature.

At a rate of 75 beats per minute, the complete cycle for filling and emptying of the chamber would occupy 0.8 sec or 800 msec (Fig. 3.4). The cardiac cycle is divided into systole and diastole. Left ventricular systole (*i.e.*, the contractile period of the left heart) extends from the early rise of ventricular pressure and the closure of the AV valve (Fig. 3.4A) to the closure of the aortic valve and the beginning of diastole (Fig. 3.4C). During most of the period from *B* to *C*, the ventricular pressure is higher than the aortic, the aortic valve is open, and the ventricle ejects blood into the arterial system. At *C* the aortic valve closes.

Diastole, which is the period of ventricular relaxation and filling, begins with the closing of the aortic valve (*C*). When the ventricular pressure falls below the atrial, the AV valve opens (*D*) and the ventricle begins to fill. Diastole ends when the ventricle again contracts and the new cycle begins.

At a heart rate of 75 beats per minute, systole will ordinarily occupy 250 to 300 msec; thus almost two-thirds of the cycle (or about 500 to 550 msec) is taken up with diastolic filling. However, with an increase in heart rate up to 180 beats per minute, which can occur in severe exercise, the length of the total cycle is reduced to about 330 msec. At this high heart rate most of the reduction is in diastolic time, which will ultimately restrict ventricular filling and limit cardiac output.

All cardiac events are normally timed according to systole and diastole of the ventricles, even though this may not always coincide with the state of activity of other parts of the heart. Figure 3.4 and most of the subsequent figures refer only to the left ventricle. It should be emphasized, however, that the events of the right side of the heart are analogous and that the right atrium and ventricle have similar timing of their electrical, mechanical, and valvular events. The primary differences in the cardiac cycle between the two sides of the heart are those relating to the lower pressures in the right ventricle and pulmonary artery.

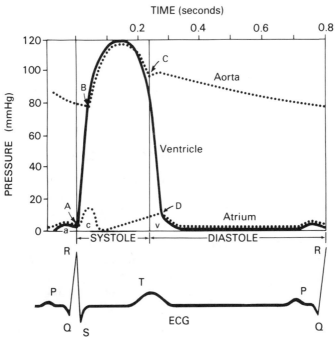

Figure 3.4. Left ventricular systole and diastole, atrial pressure waves and the electrocardiogram (ECG). *Top*, As the ventricle contracts at *A*, the mitral valve closes; as pressure increases and exceeds aortic, the aortic valve opens (*B*). Upon completion of ejection, the pressure falls below aortic and the aortic valve closes (*C*). As ventricular pressure falls below atrial, the mitral valve opens (*D*) and diastolic filling continues until the ventricle contracts again. *Bottom*, The P wave (atrial depolarization), the QRS complex (ventricular depolarization) and the T wave (ventricular repolarization) are shown. Note that depolarization inevitably precedes mechanical contraction.

Role of the Atria

From a performance standpoint, the ventricles are necessarily the central factors in the cardiac cycle; the atria, however, play a significant supporting role. The normal atrial pressure curve has three positive deflections (Fig. 3.4). Shortly after the P wave of atrial depolarization (discussed below) the atria contract with a resulting positive *a wave*, which occurs late in diastole. With the beginning of systole, the ventricular contraction causes a pressure wave to be transmitted through the thin-walled AV valves to the atria and also to the adjacent large veins resulting in the atrial *c wave*. During the last half of systole, as venous blood returns from the peripheral veins and the AV valves remain closed, atrial filling continues and atrial pressure rises with a resulting positive deflection called the *v wave*.

The atrial contraction, occurring late in ventricular diastole, aids materially in conveying blood to the ventricle and may contribute as much as 25 to 30% of the total ventricular filling. In some disease states, in which atrial contraction is absent, the heart is usually able to compensate for the loss of this atrial pump and can function reasonably well under resting conditions. However, during stress or exercise, the absence of the atrial pump may result in a serious functional impairment of cardiac output with a resultant fatigue and other signs of acute heart failure.

Electrical Events of the Cycle

In order for the cardiac muscle to contract, there must be a preceding action potential which initiates the electrical and ionic events that culminate in ventricular systole. The ECG, which is recorded at the body surface, is a graphic representation of the summed voltage changes produced by electric depolarization and repolarization of the heart. These electrical impulses begin at the sinoatrial (SA) node in the right atrium, spread over the entire heart, and initiate the contraction wave. The electrical phase of the cardiac cycle begins with excitation of the atrium (*i.e.*, atrial depolarization), denoted on the ECG by an initial upward positive deflection called the P wave (Fig. 3.4), which triggers atrial contraction.

After completion of the P wave, the ECG trace returns to the base level, *i.e.*, the isoelectric line. About 0.16 to 0.22 seconds following the onset of the P wave, a second series of negative and positive waves are seen. A negative Q wave usually precedes a positive R and a negative S wave. This QRS complex is caused by electrical depolarization of the ventricles and is quickly followed by ventricular contraction. After a short interval, a positive T wave appears which corresponds to repolarization of the ventricular muscle mass. The ECG then returns to the isoelectric line and usually there is electrical silence for the remainder of diastole. The S-T segment is an important phase of the record because it is specifically distorted in myocardial ischemia.

It should be emphasized that the action potential is the indispensable forerunner to cardiac contraction. The heart has a spontaneous, intrinsic rhythmicity and automaticity, and contraction is inevitably coupled to excitation. Electrical characteristics of the heart are considered in greater detail in Chapter 4.

Ventricular Systole

It is necessary to examine more closely some of the events associated with the cardiac cycle. Systole is often divided into three parts—an *isovolumic contraction period*, a *rapid ejection period*, and a *slower ejection period.*

Isovolumic (Isometric) Contraction Period (ICP). The ICP is the important interval between the closure of the mitral valve and the opening of the aortic valve, so called because there is no change in ventricular volume (Fig. 3.5). Several significant events occur during this period. The rate of rise of ventricular pressure (dP/dt), which is sometimes used to characterize the contractile ability of the heart (Chapter 5), is maximum during this time. In addition, during the ICP, the atrial c wave occurs and the aortic and pulmonary arterial pressures are at their lowest level. This occurs just before the opening of the aortic and pulmonary valves.

Rapid Ejection Period. The first one-third of systole is comprised of the rapid ejection period, during which about two-thirds of the ventricular volume is emptied into the aorta. Toward the end of this period, the aorta begins to distend as it absorbs the impact of the ejected blood, and the rate of rise of aortic pressure decreases. The normal end-diastolic volume (EDV) is about 120 ml and the end-systolic volume (ESV) about 40 ml. Thus the average stroke volume (SV) is about 80 ml, and the ejection fraction (EF) about 67%. A decrease in EF is a common sign of a weakened myocardium.

Slower Ejection Period. At the peak of the aortic pressure curve, the ventricles begin to relax slightly, yet blood continues to flow from the ventricle to the aorta, but at a lesser rate. This is called the slower ejection period. Near this phase, the aortic pressure actually exceeds the left ventricular pressure by a few millimeters of mercury, but outflow continues because of the inertia of the blood. This is followed by an even greater reversal of the pressure gradient, causing the flow to reverse briefly and the aortic valve to close producing the second heart sound.

Because the valves and aorta are distensible, they recoil, producing a secondary pressure wave in the aortic curve with a notch between the primary and secondary pressure curve which is referred to as the dicrotic notch. As these events occur in the left side of the heart, a similar sequence of events is occurring in the right ventricle and pulmonary artery resulting in closure of the pulmonary valve.

In practice, the term systole is often referred to as the period between the beginning of the first and the beginning of the second heart sounds although clearly one may refer to atrial systole, right ventricular systole, etc.

Ventricular Diastole

During the period between closing of the semilunar valves and the opening of the AV valves, *i.e.*, the isovolumic relaxation period (IRP), the ventricular pressure falls rapidly while the ventricular volume remains constant. When ventricular pressure falls below atrial pressure, the AV valves again open and the period of ventricular filling begins.

The ventricles become approximately two-thirds filled within the first one-third of ventricular diastole; this is referred to as the passive rapid-filling phase. In late diastole, ventricular filling is again augmented by atrial con-

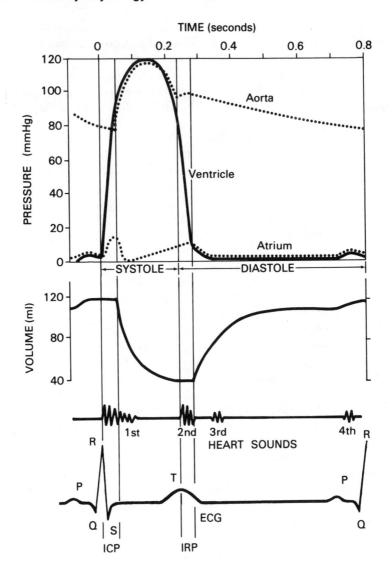

Figure 3.5. Mechanical and electrical events of the cardiac cycle showing also the ventricular volume curve and the heart sounds. Note the isovolumic contraction period (ICP) and the relaxation period (IRP) during which there is no change in ventricular volume because all valves are closed. The ventricle decreases in volume as it ejects its contents into the aorta. During the first third of systolic ejection—the rapid ejection period—the curve of emptying is steep.

traction, a period known as the active rapid-filling phase. The period between these two rapid-filling phases is sometimes called diastasis (a slower filling phase).

Heart Sounds

The two primary heart sounds are usually heard as a "lup-dup," a low-pitched first sound, followed by a quicker, higher-pitched second. The intensity of heart sounds, as heard at the chest wall, depends upon several factors: the rate of rise of ventricular pressure, the physical characteristics of the ventricles and valves, the volume contained in the heart, the position of the AV valve leaflets at the beginning of ventricular systole, and the transmission characteristics of the chest wall. The relationship of the heart sounds to other events of the cardiac cycle is shown in Figure 3.5. The major components of the heart sounds are associated with the abrupt acceleration and deceleration of blood in and near the heart, but there is not full agreement on the relative significance of valve activity and muscle vibration.

The first heart sound (S_1) is associated with the closure of the mitral and tricuspid valves at the start of the ventricular systole, and the two components can sometimes be distinguished. If so, the first component of S_1 is mitral in origin and the second component tricuspid.

The second heart sound (S_2) is usually of higher frequency and shorter duration than the first. It marks the end of ventricular systole and the beginning of diastole and is associated with the closure of the semilunar valves. It consists of two components, aortic and pulmonic. Normally, the aortic valve closes several milliseconds before the pulmonic, and the time difference is accentuated during the inspiratory phase of respiration.

This respiratory delay in closing of the pulmonary valve produces a "physiological" splitting of the second heart sound and is mainly due to the sudden decrease in intrathoracic pressure associated with inspiration. This, in turn, causes a temporary increase in venous return and an increase in right heart volume, resulting in increased right ventricular output, a temporary prolongation of ejection time, and a delay in pulmonary valve closure. At the same time, pulmonary venous return to the left heart is diminished, so that left ventricular stroke volume decreases and the aortic valve closes slightly earlier. Variations in the degree of splitting of the second heart sound occur in certain types of congenital heart disease and in cases of abnormal conduction of the electrical impulses of the heart.

A third heart sound (S_3), shown in Figure 3.5, is associated with passive rapid-filling phase. For reasons which are not clear, a physiological third sound may be present in younger individuals; however, if it occurs after the age of 40 years, it is generally considered abnormal. It may occur in fever, cardiac failure, and certain other cardiac disorders.

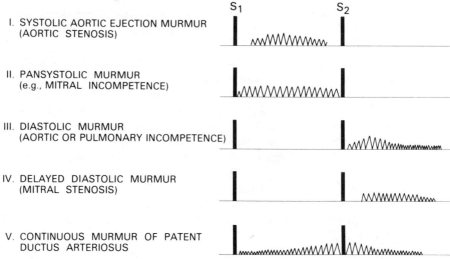

Figure 3.6. Diagrammatic representation of phonocardiograms of common systolic and diastolic murmurs. S_1 and S_2, 1st and 2nd heart sounds. (Adapted from P. Wood, *Diseases of the Heart and Circulation*, 3rd ed., Philadelphia: J.B. Lippincott, 1968.)

The fourth heart sound (S_4) is associated with the active rapid-filling phase (Fig. 3.5). While it can often be recorded by phonocardiography, it is generally not audible. When it does occur, it is usually recorded at the peak of atrial contraction and may be associated with increased atrial pressures.

Pathophysiology

Heart Murmurs

Disturbances of normal blood flow patterns in the heart and great vessels often result in abnormal sound, producing vibrations in the auditory frequency range known as murmurs. They are classified on the basis of their timing as systolic, diastolic, and continuous murmurs. If the aortic or pulmonary valve is diseased or deformed, the increased turbulence through the narrowed or distorted orifice results in the crescendo-decrescendo systolic murmur characteristic of aortic or pulmonary valve disease (Fig. 3.6*I*).

If AV valve closure is incomplete because of disease of the mitral or tricuspid valves, the valve will become incompetent and blood will regurgitate into the atrium producing a blowing "whoosh" noise following the first heart sound. If this systolic murmur persists throughout systole, as indicated in Figure 3.6 *II*, it is sometimes referred to as a pansystolic or holosystolic murmur.

Abnormal heart sounds that occur during diastole are associated either with an abnormality of AV valve opening (usually mitral) or an abnormality of semilunar valve closure (usually aortic). A murmur originating at the aortic valve and heard in early diastole may be produced by incomplete closure of the aortic valve at the end of systole. Such an abnormality could be due to fibrosis or stiffening of the valve in the open position or destruction of valve leaflets. The defect causes regurgitation of blood back into the left ventricle at the end of systole through the incompetent valve, producing the diastolic murmur of aortic regurgitation of aortic insufficiency (Fig. 3.6 *III*).

Stenosis of the mitral valve may cause abnormal heart sounds during early or late diastole (Fig. 3.6*IV*). The early component of this murmur is often initiated with an opening snap of the mitral valve; the late component may be associated with the atrial systole, just before the onset of ventricular systole, and is referred to as a "presystolic" murmur. See the following section for further description of aortic stenosis.

In addition to the preceding, certain types of murmurs may be heard throughout systole and diastole, such as the murmur of the patent ductus arteriosus (Fig 3.6*V*). This is the result of a constant movement of blood through the patent ductus, which occurs during the entire cycle and produces a heart murmur with a continuous machinery-like quality, with a waxing and waning of intensity. Blood flow is continuous through the patent ductus arteriosus during the entire cycle because of a persistent pressure gradient from the aorta to the pulmonary artery during both systole and diastole. This will not occur if there is a reversal in the pressure gradient due to severe pulmonary hypertension.

When present, the fourth heart sound usually indicates a noncompliant ventricle; this commonly occurs in ischemic heart disease, pulmonic or aortic stenosis, and pulmonary and systemic hypertension. However, it does not occur in mitral or tricuspid stenosis since the sound is also dependent upon rapid ventricular inflow.

Abnormal Intracardiac Pressures and Oxygen Saturations

In the preceding chapters, it has been pointed out that the circulation is maintained on the basis of pressure, flow and oxygen gradients and normal values in different parts of the circulatory system have been cited. There are, however, variations in the healthy population and even wider variations in disease.

In the following section approximate ranges of normal cardiac pressures and oxygen saturations are given; two examples are also presented to illustrate how deviations in these normal relationships may be produced by cardiac disorders. In later chapters the effects of other vascular diseases will be considered more fully.

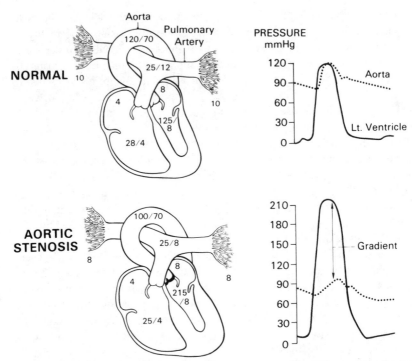

Figure 3.7. Left ventricular and aortic pressure gradients in a normal adult and in stenosis. Note in aortic stenosis the excessive left ventricular systolic pressure, the large systolic pressure gradient and the abnormally thickened left ventricle. ($\overline{X}$, mean value.) (Adapted from an original painting by F.H. Netter, *Ciba Collection of Medical Illustrations*, Vol. 5. Summit, N.J.: CIBA-Geigy Corp., 1955–1963.)

While there are phasic changes, mean right atrial pressure in the normal adult varies from about 0 to 6 mm Hg, right ventricular systolic pressure from 25 to 30 mm Hg, and diastolic pressure from 0 to 5 mm Hg. In the pulmonary artery, systolic pressure varies from about 22 to 30 mm Hg and diastolic pressure from about 9 to 12 mm Hg.

The left atrium shows pulsatile fluctuations similar to the right, but with slightly higher mean values ranging from about 4 to 10 mm Hg. Left ventricular pressure ranges from about 120 to 140 mm Hg systolic, and from 0 to 10 mm Hg diastolic. Aortic systolic pressures vary in the young adult from about 120 to 140 mm Hg, and diastolic pressures from 70 to 80 mm Hg.

Aortic stenosis is an obstruction to left ventricular ejection which produces an increased systolic pressure gradient between the left ventricle and aorta (Fig. 3.7, *bottom*). In an effort to maintain adequate flow, the left ventricular

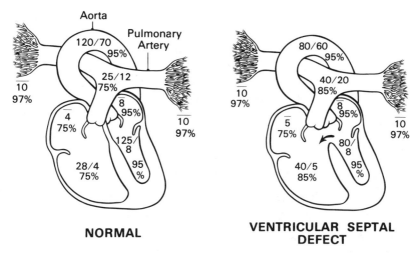

NORMAL

VENTRICULAR SEPTAL DEFECT

Figure 3.8. Intracardiac pressures and oxygen saturations in a normal adult and in ventricular septal defect. Because of the mixing of the two streams in ventricular septal defect, the left ventricular pressures are decreased and those on the right side of the heart are increased. Right ventricular and pulmonary arterial blood have a higher oxygen saturation. (Adapted from an original painting by F.H. Netter, *Ciba Collection of Medical Illustrations*, Vol. 5. Summit, N.J.: CIBA-Geigy Corp., 1955–1963.)

systolic pressure begins to rise and may increase to levels above 200 mm Hg with an aortic systolic pressure of 100 mm Hg or less. With progressive stenosis, this abnormal ventricular-aortic pressure gradient (Fig. 3.7, *bottom*) requires increased cardiac work that may result in severe left ventricular hypertrophy (Chapter 14). However, in spite of this hypertrophy, the insufficient output due to the stenosis and inadequate coronary perfusion for the enlarged ventricle may result in cardiac failure.

Oxygen Concentrations in the Cardiac Chambers. The blood oxygen content in the vena cavae, right atrium, right ventricle, and pulmonary artery is about 15 to 16 ml/dl of blood, and the oxygen saturation is normally 70 to 80%. Usually there is a slight decrease in oxygen saturation at the level of the right atrium, where blood from the coronary sinus, which has a very low oxygen content and saturation, mixes with blood from the vena cavae. On leaving the pulmonary capillary bed, the blood is usually 97 or 98% saturated, with an oxygen content of 19 to 20 ml/dl blood. Because of drainage of bronchial venous blood (from the lungs) and thebesian venous blood (from the myocardium) into the left heart, there is a small decrease in oxygen saturation in the left ventricle to about 95%. Normally, systemic arterial blood has the same oxygen content and saturation as left ventricular blood (Fig. 3.8).

In *ventricular septal defect*, a shunt of oxygenated blood occurs during systole from the left to the right ventricle through the defect, producing an abnormally high oxygen saturation in the right ventricle and frequently an abnormally high right ventricular pressure (Fig. 3.8, *right*). If not repaired, the right ventricular may become hypertrophied and the shunt may reverse to become a right-to-left shunt with cyanosis (a dusky or blue color of the skin) caused by a higher arterial blood concentration of reduced hemoglobin. The turbulence produced by blood flow through the septal defect during systole causes a systolic murmur.

Suggested Readings

Alpert NR, Hamrell BB, and Mulieri LR. Heart muscle mechanics. *Annu Rev Physiol* 41:521, 1979.

Armour JA and Randall WC. Structural basis for cardiac function. *Am J Physiol* 218:1517–1523, 1970.

Brecher GA and Galletti PM. Functional anatomy of cardiac pumping. In: *Handbook of Physiology*, Section 2: *Circulation*, edited by WF Hamilton and P Dow. Washington, D.C.: American Physiological Society 1963, Vol. II, pp 759–798.

Hurst JW (ed.). *The Heart, Arteries and Veings*, 6th ed. New York: McGraw-Hill, 1986.

Leon DF and Shaver JA (eds.). *Physiologic Principles of Heart Sounds and Murmurs*, Monograph No. 46. Dallas: American Heart Association, 1974.

Moskovitz HL, Donoso E, Gelb IJ, and Wilder RJ. *An Atlas of Hemodynamics of the Cardiovascular System*. New York: Grune & Stratton, 1963.

Rushmer RF. *Cardiovascular Dynamics*, 4th ed. Philadelphia: W.B. Saunders, 1976.

Sokolow M and McIlroy MB. *Clinical Cardiology*, 4th ed. Los Altos, Calif.: Lange Medical Publications, 1986.

Streeter DD. Gross morphology and fiber geometry of the heart. In: *Handbook of Physiology*, Secction 2: *The Cardiovascular System*, edited by RM Berne, N Sperelakis, and SR Geiger. Washington, D.C.: American Physiological Society, 1979, Vol. I, pp 61–112.

chapter **4**

Electrical Properties of the Heart

Just as an auto engine requires a well-tuned electrical system to coordinate its pistons to produce power, so the heart needs a system to coordinate contraction of its chambers; without this it is impossible for the pump to bring about the orderly sequence of atrial and ventricular systole. In this chapter, we will consider (*a*) how the contraction signal (action potential) is propagated through the heart, (*b*) the different types of action potentials and how they are generated and controlled, (*c*) how action potentials are detected for medical

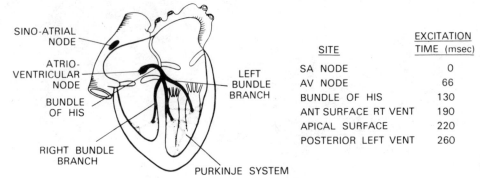

SITE	EXCITATION TIME (msec)
SA NODE	0
AV NODE	66
BUNDLE OF HIS	130
ANT SURFACE RT VENT	190
APICAL SURFACE	220
POSTERIOR LEFT VENT	260

Figure 4.1.   The conduction system of the heart. *Left*, the action potential normally originates at the sinoatrial (SA) node, travels over the atrial muscle to the atrioventricular (AV) node, and then through the bundle of His, the bundle branches, and the Purkinje system to the venticular muscle. *Right*, the time of arrival of the action potential at different parts of the heart. (Reprinted with permission from A.M. Scher and M.S. Spach, *Handbook of Physiology: Cardiovascular System*, The Heart. Bethesda, Md.: American Physiological Society, 1979, Vol. I.)

diagnostic purposes, and (*d*) a brief description of a few conduction abnormalities and some principles of their treatment.

Propagation of Cardiac Impulse

Initiation of action potentials (APs) in the various regions of the conduction system and in the regions of cardiac muscle fibers that they supply can occur spontaneously (*i.e.*, without depolarizing input from circulating humoral agents or the autonomic nervous system). The SA node, the A-V node, and the remaining specialized conduction tissue can all discharge spontaneously, that is, can initiate action potentials and serve as "pacemakers." However, the SA node ordinarily has the fastest discharge rate and, as a consequence, is the normal cardiac pacesetter or "pacemaker." The location of the different elements of this system are shown in Figure 4.1 (*left*). The impulse is conducted *via* self-propagating depolarization currents in a fashion similar to the APs in nerve fibers.

The heart has a multicellular structure but behaves like a syncytium because the individual cells communicate with their neighbors through nexuses (gap junctions) that provide the low-resistance pathway for electrogenic coupling between cells. In nodal tissue, gap junctions occupy less space and provide less resistance. This intracellular electrical resistance will decrease with a decrease in intracellular pH and may increase during a maintained increase in intracellular Ca^{2+}.

The propagation velocity in the SA node is about 0.05 m/sec and in the atrial muscle, the bundle of His, and ventricular muscle 0.8 to 1.0 m/sec. The propagation velocity in the AV node is 0.03 to 0.05 m/sec; however in the Purkinje tissue it is 5 m/sec (about 100 times greater than in the nodal systems). The impulse propagation times to the various regions are shown in Figure 4.1 (*right*). The AV node is a critical element in the system since it is the only normal avenue over which an impulse can be propagated from atrium to ventricle. An important characteristic of the AV node is its exceedingly low conduction velocity, making it responsible for the normal delay between atrial and ventricular activation. The Purkinje fibers, on the other hand, have a high conduction velocity, which facilitates coordinated contraction of the entire ventricular mass.

Action Potentials at Different Sites

Two main types of AP are generated in the heart, those characteristic of nonpacemaker tissues such as atrial muscle, Purkinje fibers, and ventricular muscle (Fig. 4.2B, C, and D) and those found in pacemaker tissues such as the SA and AV nodes (Fig. 4.2A). A typical AP of ventricular muscle (nonpacemaker tissue) (Fig. 4.2D) shows a rapid initial depolarization from about −90 mV to about +10 mV (phase 0), a quick partial repolarization phase (phase 1) and then a "plateau" voltage near zero (phase 2) which is maintained for several hundred milliseconds. This is followed by a rapid repolarization phase (phase 3) and a return to resting potential (phase 4, Fig. 4.2D).

Electrical and Ionic Aspects of the Action Potential

Resting Membrane Potentials

The negative intracellular electrical potential difference across the plasma membrane of a cardiac cell (relative to the extracellular fluid maintained at zero potential or ground) varies from about −60 to −90 mV, depending upon its location and function. This resting transmembrane potential is maintained by three factors: (*a*) the concentration (or more correctly, the "activity") gradients across the plasma membrane for specific permeable ions; (*b*) the relative permeabilities of the plasma membrane for these specific ions, and (*c*) the plasma membrane–bound, energy-consuming, Na^+-K^+ pump mechanism that extrudes Na^+ from and accumulates K^+ into the intracellular fluid. The outward-directed K^+ gradient (*i.e.*, $K^+_i > K^+_e$) and the reverse, inward-directed Na^+ and Ca^{2+} gradients (*i.e.*, $Na^+_e > Na^+_i$ and $Ca^{2+}_e > Ca^{2+}_i$) tend to move K^+ out of the cell and Na^+ and Ca^{2+} into the cell. However, under resting conditions the inside negative transmembrane potential difference is attributable primarily to the ionic gradient of the K^+ ion (due to its high permeability relative to that of other ions present in the intra-

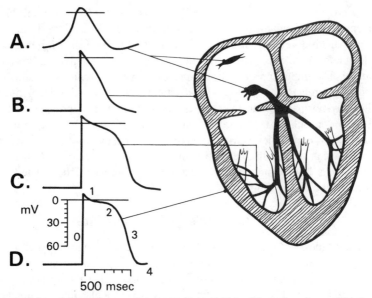

Figure 4.2.   Intracellular action potentials (AP) in different regions of the heart. The pacemaker type of potential (sinoatrial or atrioventricular node) is shown in *A*, the atrial AP in *B*, the Purkinje fiber potential in *C*, and ventricular cell AP in *D*. Zero voltage shown by horizontal lines. Note the depolarization potential and lack of plateau in the pacemaker tissue (*A*). The different phases of the AP are sometimes identified by numbers as shown in *D*. (Reprinted with permission from A.M. Scher and M.S. Spach, Cardiac depolarization and the repolarization and electrocardiogram. In: *Handbook of Physiology*, Section 2: *The Cardiovascular System*, The Heart, edited by R.M. Berne. American Physiological Society, 1979, Vol. I, p. 357.)

and extracellular fluid compartments). Thus, maintenance of the resting membrane potential as well as generation and propagation of action potentials in cardiac fibers is primarily a function of the magnitude of transmembrane gradients, selective permeabilities, and pump mechanisms for specific ions.

In the case of the resting potential, the two key membrane properties are its selective permeability to K^+ ions and the action of its Na^+-K^+ pump. The transmembrane permeability of the cardiac cell membrane to K^+ is much greater than to Na^+ or Ca^{2+}, so that the ratio of $P_{K^+}:P_{Na^+}$ is about 100:1. Since Ca^{2+} has only a negligible effect on resting potential (due to its low permeability at rest), the K^+ ion gradient dominates the ionic contribution to the resting membrane potential. This is shown by the fact that estimation of cellular transmembrane potential difference on the basis of the K^+ ion gradient alone (using the Nernst equilibrium potential equation for K^+) yields a negative value very close to the -90 mV that is actually measured across the ventricular cell membrane with a microelectrode.

Nonetheless, the net result of a finite membrane permeability for Na^+ and an inward-directed Na^+ gradient would ordinarily be a steady inward leak of Na^+ ions into the cell, with a resultant lesser negativity and eventual depolarization. This is prevented by the Na^+-K^+ pump, which transports Na^+ outward against its electrical and chemical (*i.e.*, ionic) gradient. The biochemical counterpart of the Na^+-K^+ pump is the Na^+-K^+ activated ATPase enzyme. This enzyme is part of the membrane itself and utilizes the high-energy phosphate bond energy of ATP for its active transport of Na^+ and K^+.

Pathologic conditions, such as ischemia, can reduce the ATP supply and prevent the pump from functioning, thereby leading to a loss of the ionic gradients necessary for both the resting membrane potential and the AP. If the pump is inhibited by large concentrations of digitalis (a competitive blocker of K^+ attachment to the membrane-bound Na^+-K^+ ATPase), the concentration gradients for Na^+ and K^+ will be significantly reduced as will the absolute magnitude of the resting membrane potential. The level of resting membrane potential is a critical factor in determining the rate of rise and propagation velocity of the ensuing AP; for example, the greater (more negative) the resting potential, the steeper the rise and the greater the velocity of the AP.

Action Potentials—Fast and Slow Responses

The action potentials (AP) of single cardiac cells can also be measured by insertion of a microelectrode into the interior of cells at different regions of the heart. The electronegativity of the resting cell interior as described above is characteristic of nerve, muscle, and practically all cells of the body. Any stimulus that abruptly alters the resting membrane potential beyond a critical value (threshold potential) will result in a propagated AP. The rapid depolarization at phase 0 (Fig. 4.2) is due almost exclusively to a sudden inrush of Na^+ down its concentration gradient into the cell (Fig. 4.3); there is a simultaneous, but much smaller and more gradual decrease in K^+ conductance. This permits the Na^+ ions to enter the cell faster than the K^+ ions can leave, thus reducing intracellular negativity. When the ensuing reduction in magnitude of the negative transmembrane potential across the cell passes a critical level (*i.e.*, threshold potential), which in the case of the ventricular cell is about -70 to -80 mV, an AP is generated since the intracellular electrical potential overshoots to a positive value. This initial phase of the AP is known as the "fast" response. The fast response or "spike" is followed by a rapid fall in the positive overshoot due primarily to a rapid fall in the elevated Na^+ conductance (g_{Na}) and current (I_{Na^+}) (Fig. 4.3). A rise in g_K and I_{K^+} also begins concurrently with the rise in g_{Na} but with a slower time course.

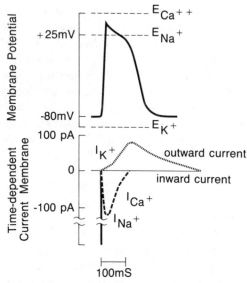

Figure 4.3. Relationship between the electrical and ionic events during an action potential (AP) in a ventricular muscle cell, showing the membrane potential (*top*) and membrane current (*bottom*). The AP activates the very rapid inward Na$^+$ current (I_{Na^+}) (*bottom*), which initiates the rapid depolarization and the AP (*top*), which, in turn quickly inactivates the I_{Na^+}. A second depolarization current, $I_{Ca^{2+}}$, now ensues, which generates the plateau phase of the AP. The entry of Ca^{2+} also triggers the contraction of the muscle. During the plateau, the outward K$^+$ current is generated, which drives the membrane potential back toward E_K and repolarizes the cell. (After Giles W. & Brown A.M. in Brown A.M. & Stubbs D. (eds.) *Medical Physiology*, Churchill Livingstone, 1983, with permission.)

In many excitable tissues (*e.g.*, nerve fiber) this rise in K$^+$ permeability restores the resting potential within a few milliseconds, but in cardiac tissue it takes several hundred milliseconds. The relation of these transient ionic currents to the change in transmembrane potential is shown in Figure 4.3. The importance of the Na$^+$ transfer during the fast response is indicated by the fact that the amplitude of the AP increases linearly with the log of the resting extracellular Na$^+$ concentration (Na$_e^+$); thus, when Na$_e^+$ is reduced from its normal value of 140 mM to about 10 to 30 mM, an action potential can no longer be generated or will be of reduced amplitude.

During the plateau (phase 2, Fig. 4.2) there is a slow inward current of Ca^{2+} ions into the cell through slow channels called the "slow response." The delay in repolarization of the cardiac cell and the resultant prolongation of the action potential is due to this slow inward Ca^{2+} current which opposes the repolarizing effect of the outward K$^+$ current (I_{K^+}). An additional and physiologically important facet of the inward Ca^{2+} current is that these Ca^{2+} ions now become available for excitation-contraction coupling, which is an essential part of the contraction process (Chapter 5). Repolarization (phase 3, Fig. 4.2) involves an increase in g_{K^+}, a decrease of $P_{Ca^{2+}}$, and an inactivation of the slow Ca^{2+} current.

Studies of these ionic currents suggest that cardiac cells are of two general physiological types, depending upon whether the fast or slow response predominates. Fast responses (*i.e.*, those in which the fast-response depolarization is prominent) are characteristic of atrial and ventricular muscle cells and Purkinje fibers; the resting membrane potential in these cells is more negative (-80 to -90 mV), the upstroke velocity of the AP is greater (100 to 500 V/sec), and the conduction velocity is more rapid than in slow cells. The pacemaker cells are located in normal SA and AV nodes. In these cells the resting potential is -40 to -70 mV, the upstroke velocity of the AP is 1 to 10 V/sec, and conduction velocity is very slow. While our knowledge of these phenomena is still incomplete, current evidence suggests that the slow inward Ca^{2+} response, which is present in all types of cardiac cells and is responsible for maintaining the plateau phase of the AP in "fast-response" cells, is the primary and perhaps the only mechanism for producing the AP in "slow-response" nodal cells.

The biochemical structure of specific ion channels within the cardiac cell membrane and the biophysical mechanisms that regulate ion channel patency are not well understood. For the electrically excitable nerve fiber membrane, the classic Hodgkin-Huxley theory postulates that action potentials are initiated by the voltage-dependent opening of "fast" membrane channels specific for Na^+ and other ions possessing similar levels of hydration and electrical charge and similar crystalline diameters. This theory further states that Na^+ channel opening (*i.e.*, activation) is, in turn, regulated by two electrically charged gates, an "m" and an "h" gate, located within the membrane channel, possibly close to its cytoplasmic side. Both gates are activated by membrane depolarization but with different time courses and in different directions. Hence, depolarization (*i.e.*, voltage activation) opens the "m" gates at a faster rate than it closes the "h" gates, leading to a transient, small, passive influx of Na^+ down an inward-directed concentration gradient. The transient Na^+ influx is reflected by the positive overshoot and spike portion of the action potential. This classic Na^+ channel–gate hypothesis has received support from the demonstration of specific membrane gating currents attributable to movement of the charged "m" gates. These currents precede the ionic currents, reflecting the transient influx of Na^+.

This channel-gating hypothesis has also been applied to explain the electrical changes that occur in the conducting pathway and cardiac muscle cells.

The absence of fast Na^+ channels and the presence of spontaneously opening, slow, Ca^{2+} channels in the pacemaker cells of the heart can explain the relatively slow time course and the automaticity of the AP in these cells. The value of the channel-gating hypothesis to explain specific ion conductance changes during AP generation in myocardial muscle cells has been enhanced significantly through demonstration of a block of the spike potential of the AP in these cells by myocardial anoxia or tetrodotoxin. The latter is a poison (derived from the puffer fish) that specifically occludes membrane fast Na^+ channels from their extracellular side.

Such blocking action can alter a nonpacemaker cell so that it will lose its fast response and be converted into a pacemaker-type cell in which the slow response (no longer overwhelmed by the fast initial Na^+ current) becomes the dominant mechanism. The conversion from a fast to a slow response is characterized by a relative reduction of resting membrane potential from a more negative value (e.g., -90 mV) to a less negative one (e.g., -60 to -70 mV).

It is also known that certain pharmacological agents such as verapamil and nifedipine, a class of drugs known as calcium antagonists, can reduce membrane Ca^{2+} conductance by blocking membrane Ca^{2+} channels. Consequently this action can partially block the slow response without altering Na^+ influx. This delays A-V conduction, decreases the firing rate of pacemaker cells, slows the heart, and tends to prevent arrhythmias. Catecholamines such as norepinephrine (NE), on the other hand, enhance the slow response and increase the firing rate of pacemaker cells. Na^+ channels are an important target for the antiarrhythmic action of local anesthetics—such as lidocaine— which are used particularly in ventricular arrhythmias. The discovery that slow-channel Ca^{2+} blockers are highly beneficial in the treatment of arrhythmias and other circulatory disorders has sparked considerable clinical interest in these drugs (Chapter 14).

Extrinsic Influences on the Heart

As previously described, the initiation of the heart beat is spontaneous and does not require a continued nervous input. This is dramatically illustrated by the transplanted heart in higher animals and humans which beats and functions reasonably well for many years in the body of the host. Nevertheless, extrinsic factors, neurohormonal, thermal, metabolic, and ionic, can and do significantly influence cardiac function. In this regard, the autonomic nervous system is particularly important, since it continually modulates the heart rate and force of contraction. These effects are mediated through the release of chemical transmitters from the endings of the autonomic nerves throughout the heart.

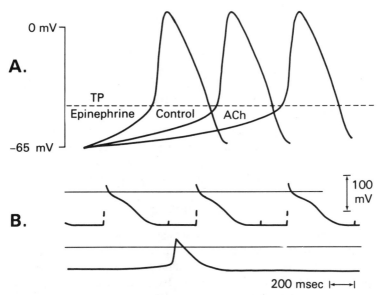

Figure 4.4.   Effects of epinephrine (E) or sympathetic stimulation, and ace-tylcholine (ACh) or vagal stimulation on heart rate (*A*) and Purkinje fiber action potentials (AP) (*B*). E increases and ACh decreases the slope of diastolic depolarization (*A*). E converts Purkinje fiber APs (*B, upper strip*) to pacemaker type (*B, lower strip*). (Reprinted with permission from E.E. Selkurt, *Physiology*, 4th ed. Boston: Little, Brown, 1976.)

Neurohumoral Effects

Vagal stimulation or acetylocholine (ACh) will (*a*) slow the heart, (*b*) decrease the strength of atrial contraction, and (*c*) cause a marked reduction in conduction velocity through the AV node. ACh, which is the primary transmitter released at the postganglionic parasympathetic nerve endings, activates the muscarinic (atropine-sensitive) receptors. The two primary effects on the cardiac cell are (*a*) activation of K^+ conductance (*via* the selective opening of K^+ channels) thus causing a hyperpolarization, a decrease in the slope of the pacemaker potential, and slowing of the heart rate, and (*b*) a decrease in the Ca^{2+} current and a "restraining effect" on the action of NE on myogenic tone, which results in a decreased contractile strength of the myocardium (Figure 4.4). Weak vagal action will prolong the A-V conduction time and slow the heart, but strong vagal action may cause a blockade of some or all of the impulses at the AV node. However, even with continued stimulation, the normal heart will, after a short interval, resume beating but at a significantly lower rate (ventricular or vagal escape).

The endogenous sympathetic transmitter is norepinephrine (NE) but epinephrine (E) has similar effects. Sympathetic stimulation or administration of NE or E will (a) activate the B_1 receptors in the heart and increase the rate (chronotropic) and force (inotropic) of cardiac contraction, (b) increase the conduction velocity through the AV node, atria, and ventricles, and (c) increase the tendency of Purkinje fibers to exhibit pacemaker activity (Fig. 4.4). The rate effect is due to an increased rate (or slope) of membrane depolarization in the SA node. The mechanism of the sympathetic effect on the heart is most likely twofold, (a) an increase in the number of open Ca^{2+} channels, which lowers the excitability threshold and speeds nodal conduction, and (b) alteration in the voltage dependence of pacemaker currents, which accelerates firing rate and favors spontaneous depolarization.

Temperature

Warming the SA node increases its spontaneous activity and its slope of diastolic depolarization, thereby speeding heart rate. There is approximately a 10 beat/min rate increase per 1°C elevation of temperature. Cooling has the reverse effect and severe cooling may arrest the heart.

Inorganic Ions

Electrolyte abnormalities, particularly of K^+ and Ca^{2+}, have important and potentially serious effects on cardiac function. Hyperkalemia (elevation of serum K^+) influences depolarization through the direct effect of increased K^+ on lowering the resting potential; the resulting decrease in the fast inward current reduces the rate of rise and amplitude of the AP and slows the conduction velocity. As a result, there is a reduction of P wave amplitude and a widening of the P-R interval and QRS complex, along with a decrease in the rate and force of contraction. The increased external K^+ concentration also accelerates repolarization, shortens the plateau phase of the AP and the QT interval, and produces characteristic tall, peaked T waves. With more severe hyperkalemia, there may be disappearance of the P waves, AV nodal block, and possibly ventricular fibrillation and sudden death.

Potassium depletion (hypokalemia) causes first an increase in the magnitude of the resting potential but with further lowering of serum K^+ (e.g., below 3mM), there will be a decrease in resting potential, with slowing of repolarization and prolongation of the AP. The result is usually a flattening of the T waves, prominent U waves, prolongation of the P-R and QT intervals, and with severe hypokalemia, a tendency toward AV block and ventricular fibrillation.

Hypercalcemia shortens the duration of the AP, increases the slow inward current, and accelerates repolarization. The characteristic ECG changes are a shortened QT interval (due to shortening of the AP) and abnormal ST segments and T waves. Hypocalcemia causes opposite changes, i.e., prolon-

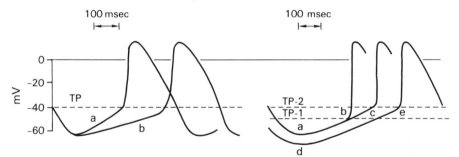

Figure 4.5. Pacemaker potentials in sinoatrial node. Illustrating the effect of diastolic depolarization slopes and potentials on heart rate. The action potential is initiated when the depolarization potential reaches threshold potential (TP). *Left*, slowing of rate of depolarization from *a* to *b* increased the time required to reach TP and lessens heart rate. *Right*, increase of level of TP from 1 to 2 or increased magnitude of resting potential from *a* to *d* also slows the discharge rate and, therefore, the heart rate. (Reprinted with permission from B.F. Hoffman and P.F. Cranefield, *Electrophysiology of the Heart.* New York: McGraw-Hill, 1960.)

gation and reduced amplitude of the AP and a prolongation of the QT interval and ST segment.

As will be described in Chapter 5, the presence of an adequate extracellular Ca^{2+} concentration is essential for normal cardiac muscle contraction. At low concentrations of intra- and extracellular Ca^{2+}, contraction will not take place. In animal experiments it can be shown that very high levels of extracellular Ca^{2+} concentration will greatly increase the strength of cardiac contraction and, if exposure is prolonged, there is less and less relaxation after each contraction until finally the heart stops in sustained calcium rigor.

Automaticity and Pacemaker Potentials

As mentioned above, the SA node, AV node, and the remaining specialized conduction tissue are all characterized as potential pacemakers, but the SA node, because of its inherently faster discharge rate, is the normal cardiac pacemaker. It was also pointed out that these pacemaker cells have slow response APs; also characteristic of this type of AP is the slow membrane depolarization during diastole. This property permits "spontaneous diastolic depolarization," *i.e.*, automaticity in the pacemaker cell (Fig. 4.2*A*) but not in the atrial or ventricular muscle cell (Fig. 4.2*B* and *D*). The magnitude and slope of these diastolic pacemaker potentials have an important influence on the heart rate.

The frequency of heart contractions may slow through (*a*) a decrease in the slope of a diastolic depolarization (Fig. 4.5, *left,a* and *b*), (*b*) a rise in

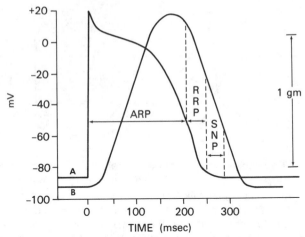

Figure 4.6. Relation between electrical and mechanical events of cardiac contraction showing the transmembrane action potential (AP) in isolated papillary muscle (*A*) and the subsequent isometric contraction curve (*B*). There is a considerable delay between the spike of the AP and the peak of the contraction. The graph also shows the refractoriness of the muscle to a subsequent stimulation. ARP, absolute refractory period; RRP, relative refractory period; and SNP, supernormal period. (Adapted from W.R. Milnor, Properties of cardiac tissue. In: *Medical Physiology*, 14th ed., edited by V.B. Mountcastle, St. Louis: C.V. Mosby, 1980.)

the threshold potential (TP-1 to TP-2 in Fig. 4.5), or (*c*) an increase in the negative magnitude of the resting potential (Fig. 4.5, *right, a* and *d*). In the case of myocardial ischemia, toxins, or other injury, an existing pacemaker may be displaced by a latent pacemaker elsewhere in the heart. There are, in any event, interactions between pacemaker regions of different inherent rhythmicities; when a frequency of excitation greater than that which is inherent to one group of cells is superseded by another group, the rate of firing of the first group is suppressed, a phenomenon known as "overdrive suppression."

Electrical and Mechanical Events of Contraction

A cell is refractory (*i.e.*, is unable to respond to a stimulus) if the stimulus arrives during depolarization or the initial phase of repolarization (*i.e.*, the voltage of the cell has not become sufficiently negative to initiate the next AP). When the intracellular voltage is more *positive* than $-50mV$, no AP can be reinitiated because of the inactivation of the Na^+ channels (*i.e.*, closure of the "h" gates as described above). Hence the cell is totally unexcitable and in its absolute refractory period (ARP, Fig. 4.6). Because the duration

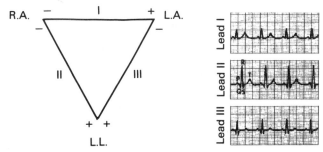

Figure 4.7. *Left,* classical ECG limb leads. *Lead I,* right arm (RA) electro-negative with respect to left arm (LA). *Lead II,* RA negative to left leg (LL) and *lead III,* LA negative to LL. *Right,* normal electrocardiogram from limb leads showing P, QRS and T waves. Wide vertical lines, 0.2 second; narrow horizontal lines, 0.1 mV.

of this prolonged refractoriness is of the same order of magnitude as the duration of contraction, the heart cannot be tetanized. As the voltage of the cell becomes more negative (during the latter part of repolarization), it requires a stronger than normal stimulus to evoke a response; this is the "relative refractory period" (RRP). Immediately following the RRP there is—particularly in the Purkinje fiber—a supernormal phase of increased excitability. The refractory period varies in different parts of the heart, being shortest in the atrium and longest in the Purkinje system and AV node. The long refractory period protects the Purkinje cell against reentry of excitation from adjacent myocardium in a retrograde manner.

Electrocardiography

In 1903, Einthoven developed the first practical device for recording cardiac potentials—a string galvanometer—which subsequently was refined into the electrocardiograph. Since the tissues of the body surrounding the heart are conductors of electricity, a small but constant fraction of the cardiac potentials may be picked up between two surface points (bipolar recording), amplified, and recorded. Such a graphic record is termed an *electrocardiogram* (ECG); if the electrodes are placed directly on the heart surface, the resulting trace is called an *electrogram.* A conventional method of electrocardiography is to record from electrodes on three extremities of the body (*e.g.* left and right arms and left leg) using the right leg electrode as ground. The arrangement of these classical "limb leads" is shown graphically in Figure 4.7 (*left*). These leads were defined by Einthoven so that the major deflections in each lead would be upright (positive) in a normal subject.

The ECG is the algebraic sum of all the myocardial APs as recorded at the surface of the body. Depolarization moving toward an active electrode produces a positive deflection and if moving away, a negative one. By convention, vertical lines are spaced at 0.04-second intervals and a paper speed of 25 mm/sec is usually employed. The vertical voltage scale is calibrated at 10 mm/mV (Fig. 4.7, *right*).

The ECG helps to determine (*a*) the extent and type of disturbance of rhythm or conduction, (*b*) the extent and location of ischemic myocardial damage, (*c*) the effect of a drug (*e.g.*, digitalis), and (*d*) the anatomical orientation of the heart.

Scalar Electrocardiography—The Normal ECG

Atrial depolarization, represented by the P wave, begins at the SA node and is conducted over the atrial muscle in all directions. There are three specialized, small bundles of atrial muscle (internodal bundles) running toward the AV node which are preferential pathways in which conduction velocity is somewhat greater. The P wave normally does not exceed 0.11 seconds—which is the time for the impulse to travel over the atrium to the AV node.

At the AV node the conduction velocity slows to about 5 cm/sec, then again speeds up to velocities of 1 m/sec in the AV bundles and to about 5 m/sec in the Purkinje system before activating the ventricular muscle to contract. The time for the passage of the AP from the atrium to the ventricular muscle is called the P-R interval (Fig. 4.8). It ordinarily ranges from 0.12 to 0.21 seconds, and over half of this period (from the end of the P wave to the Q wave) is taken up in transmission through the AV node. Prolongation of this interval is usually due to abnormal delay in the AV node, to bundle branch disease, or to metabolic effects of chronotropic drugs such as digitalis.

Ventricular depolarization begins at the left side of the interventricular septum (Q wave), spreads from the endocardial to the epicardial surface of the the the left ventricle (R wave) and finally to the right ventricle (S wave). The conduction velocity through ventricular muscle is about 0.8 to 1.0 m/sec, and the width of the QRS ordinarily does not exceed 0.06 to 0.11 second. The activation times of the different parts of the heart are shown in Figure 4.1 (*right*). Ventricular repolarization proceeds from epicardial to endocardial surface and is represented by the T wave. It normally takes 0.1 to 0.25 second.

The S-T segment is that period between the end of the QRS complex and the beginning of the T wave and represents the interval between completion of depolarization and the time when electrical recovery (repolarization) begins (Fig. 4.8). Its configuration is importantly affected by injury or ischemia of the myocardium as will be further discussed in Chapters 12 and 14. The T-P interval is an isoelectric period of quiescence whose duration varies inversely with the heart rate. The T-P interval sometimes contains a small positive deflection called the U wave, which is thought to represent the slow repolarization of papillary muscle; some cardiologists have reported that U wave

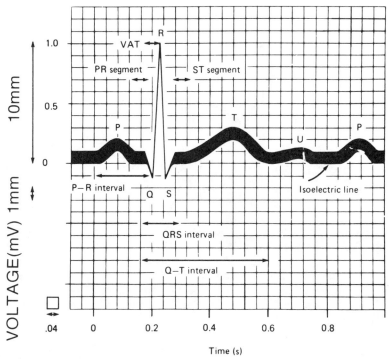

Figure 4.8. Configuration of normal human electrocardiogram showing the primary waves, intervals, segments, and ventricular activation time (VAT). The U wave is seen only occasionally and has only minor significance. (Reprinted with permission from M.J. Goldman, *Principles of Clinical Electrocardiography*, 10th ed. Los Altos, Calif.: Lange Medical Publications, 1979.)

inversion is suggestive of myocardial ischemia, but otherwise the U wave has apparently little physiological or pathological significance.

The Electrical Axis of the Heart

While the procedure described above yields a measure of the magnitude of the voltage (scalar electrocardiography), it is possible by summation to determine a resultant vector with both magnitude and direction (vectorcardiography). This is done by recording two leads simultaneously and measuring their respective voltages at the same point using the peak of the R wave. An example of such a determination of a resultant vector is shown in Figure 4.9.

The orientation of the resultant QRS axis in the frontal plane (the electrical axis) is usually inferior and leftward at an angle from 0° to +90°; this is in accord with the usual left ventricular predominance. If the angle is more positive (*i.e*, rotated more rightward), it is suggestive of right ventricular

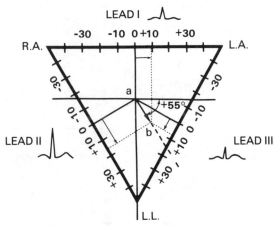

Figure 4.9. Einthoven triangle—calculation of electrical axis of the heart. Perpendiculars from the midpoint of the sides of the equilateral triangle intersect at the center of electrical activity (*a*). RA, right arm; LA, left arm; LL, left leg. If, from the midpoint, distances equivalent to the wave voltage (in this case the R wave) are laid off parallel to the respective lead, perpendiculars from these end points will intersect at a point designating the magnitude and direction of the resultant R vector (from *a* to *b*).

preponderance (right axis deviation). Change in the electrical axis of the heart can be produced by mechanical alteration of the cardiac position and also by a wide variety of cardiac and pulmonary disorders that may change the anatomical position or wall thickness of the heart.

Unipolar Leads

Bipolar leads, as described above, measure potential differences between two points on the surface of the body; however, they cannot record actual potentials at either electrode; thus waves of depolarization and repolarization at different points on the myocardium may neutralize each other and not be accurately recorded.

In 1934, Wilson introduced unipolar lead electrocardiography in which one electrode (the exploring electrode) is placed at different points on the body surface and the other, indifferent electrode, is kept at zero potential by connecting all three limbs to a central terminal through a 5000 ohm resistance. Unipolar leads are labeled V followed by a letter or number that describes the position of the exploring electrode. Because potentials so recorded may be somewhat smaller than desirable, a system of "augmented" leads is commonly used for the unipolar limb leads, for example, AVR, AVL, and AVF (Fig. 4.10, *left*).

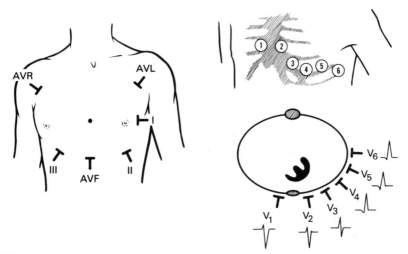

Figure 4.10. Limb leads (*left*) and precordial leads (*right*) in standard 12-lead ECG. Limb leads include leads I, II, and III and augmented limb leads with exploring electrodes on right arm (AVR), left arm (AVL), and left foot (AVF). Precordial leads V_1 to V_6 (*right*) record cardiac potentials in a transverse plane. (Reprinted with permission from R.L. DeJoseph, *Introduction to Electrocardiography: The Vectorial Approach.* East Hanover, N.J.: Sandoz, 1977.)

The Standard ECG

In the standard 12-lead ECG, six leads are recorded in the frontal plane and six in the transverse plane. The leads in the *frontal* plane, referred to as standard limb leads, are leads I, II, and III and the augmented limb leads, AVR, AVL, and AVF. These are, in effect, positive poles of a bipolar recording system "looking at" the depolarization vectors from six different positions in the frontal plane (Fig. 4.10, *left*). The other six leads are the precordial chest leads that record the depolarization vectors in the *transverse* plane, and they are numbered V_1 to V_6. They are placed in positions varying from near midsternum to left midaxillary line, as shown in Figure 4.10, *right*.

In Figure 4.10 (*right*), leads V_1 to V_6 represent summation of electrical activity of both ventricles. The QRS of the left ventricle dominates because of its thicker musculature. As the excitation spreads toward the recording electrode, the deflection is positive or upward, and as it moves away the deflection will be downward.

Arrhythmias

Arrhythmias are disturbances of rate, rhythm, or sequence of depolarization which are due to either disorders of impulse formation or impulse conduction.

Normal sinus rhythm indicates that the SA node is the pacemaker and that the rate, form, and order of excitation is within normal limits. *Sinus arrhythmia*, which is common in normal young adults and children, refers to phasic rate changes with respiration. In sinus bradycardia the rate in the adult is by definition less then 60 beats/min and in sinus tachycardia greater than 100 beats/min, but the rhythm, form, and succession of the various ECG waves are normal. The causes of arrhythmias are many and include myocardial ischemia, heart failure, blood electrolyte imbalances (especially K^+), high epinephrine levels (*e.g.*, in excitement), and certain drugs such as amphetamines, caffeine, and alcohol.

Premature Contractions and Pathological Tachycardias

It is thought that many arrhythmias arise because of an unequal transmission velocity through branches of the conduction system, with "reentry" into a proximal conduction site. The reentry theory suggests that because of ischemia or other injury there is a unidirectional block in one fiber bundle (because of partial depolarization) and a delayed or slow retrograde conduction in the previously blocked but now repolarized bundle. (Fig. 4.11*B*). The retrograde impulse from the unblocked limb may penetrate the damaged segment, reenter, and cause a premature contraction, since it has (because of the delay) reached the original pathway after the refractory period. Bidirectional block will stop the reentrant impulse (Fig. 4.11*D*). The process may become repetitive and result in tachycardia.

In addition to disordered conduction, arrhythmias may also arise because of newly developed centers of impulse formation. All cardiac tissue may, as a result of ischemia, injury, or heightened excitability, become a temporary or permanent pacemaker for the heart and thus usurp the normal pacemaker. Such sites are called "ectopic foci" and the anomalous complexes are referred to as premature systoles or extrasystoles. These abnormal impulses may be formed in the atrium outside the SA node (atrial premature beats), in the AV node (junctional premature beats), in the Purkinje fiber, or in the ventricular muscle (ventricular ectopic beats).

The ectopic beat may also be conducted in a retrograde direction and may depolarize the SA node, atria, or AV node. In this case the normal pacemaker cannot generate an impulse until repolarization is complete, so that there may be an interval between beats (a compensatory pause). During this pause there will be increased ventricular filling and an increased stroke volume in the succeeding systole. The pause and the increased stroke volume are often sensed by the patient as a "skipped beat."

Atrial premature contractions result from a nonnodal atrial pacemaker and may show an abnormal P wave; usually normal QRS and T complexes occur unless aberrant intraventricular conduction is also present (Fig. 4.12,*left*).

A   B

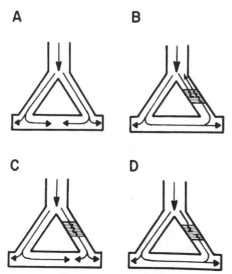

C   D

Figure 4.11. Diagram to show "reentry" pathways and possible modifications. A, Normal velocity of propagation through Purkinje bundle branches. B, Unidirectional (antegrade) block through a diseased branch with retrograde penetration of the depressed segment and impulse activation through reentry. The extrasystole may be suppressed by improved antegrade conduction (C) or development of bidirectional block (D). (Reprinted with permission from M.R. Rosen, B.F. Hoffman, and A.L. Wit, *Am Heart J* 89:526, 1975.)

Ventricular extrasystoles are usually caused by an irritable or ectopic focus within the ventricle; the QRS complex is usually abnormal (Fig. 4.12, *right*). If the ectopic focus discharges rhythmically and thus has a constant relation to the normal QRS complex, the beat is "coupled." If it occurs after every normal beat it is called "bigeminy," and if after every second normal beat "trigeminy," etc.

Paroxysmal supraventricular tachycardia occurs if the ectopic focus or the reentry circuit in the atrial tissue maintains a very high atrial rate (150 to 250 beats/min) (Fig. 4.13A, *upper*); the episodes often have a sudden onset and offset. If the rate is 250 to 300 beats/min, the disorder is called an atrial flutter. Flutter is a serious arrythmia because it often has a rapid ventricular response. Either atrial flutter or fibrillation may be followed by various degrees of heart block. In atrial flutter the rate is rapid, but coordinated contractions can occur; however, in fibrillation, contraction is not coordinated, so the muscle cannot develop sufficient power to propel blood.

It has been suggested that atrial fibrillation (Fig. 4.13A, *lower*) results from alteration of an excitation wave so that it travels around a damaged area in a circle or "circus movement." In animal experiments, the behavior of

APC   VPC

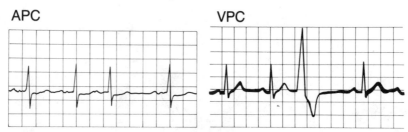

Figure 4.12.   In atrial premature contraction (*left*), the extra systole is due to an atrial premature beat that causes a deformity of the preceding T wave. In contrast, the ventricular premature contraction (*right*) is not preceded by any evidence of atrial activity. In both cases, a wide QRS premature wave follows the sinus beat. (From M.D. Alpert, *Cardiac Arrhythmias*, Chicago:Yearbook Medical Publisher, Inc., 1980 (*left*) and J.J. Gallagher in Cecil's *Textbook of Medicine*, ed. by J.B. Wyngarden and L.H. Smith, 16th Ed., Philadelphia: W.B. Saunders & Co., 1982 (*right*).)

induced atrial fibrillation is consistent with such a concept. If the ectopic focus is in the ventricle, paroxysmal ventricular tachycardia may occur (Fig. 4.13*B*, *upper*). This is a dangerous arrythmia since it frequently degenerates into ventricular fibrillation (Fib. 4.13*B*, *lower*) in which there is complete cessation of effective ventricular contraction. Ventricular fibrillation is a common cause of sudden death.

A. PAT   B. VT

AF   VF

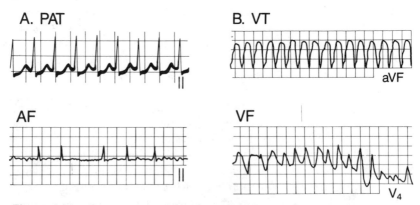

Figure 4.13.   Paroxysmal atrial tachycardia (*A, upper*) showing normal complexes; atrial fibrillation (*A, lower*) with irregular, uncoordinated atrial waves dissociated from QRS waves. Ventricular tachycardia (*B, upper*) showing rapid, abnormal QRS complexes. Ventricular fibrillation (*B, lower*) with very irregular, uncoordinated QRS complexes. (From M. Sokolow and M.B. McIlroy. *Clinical Cardiology*, 3rd Ed., Los Altros, CA: Lange Medical Publishers, 1981.)

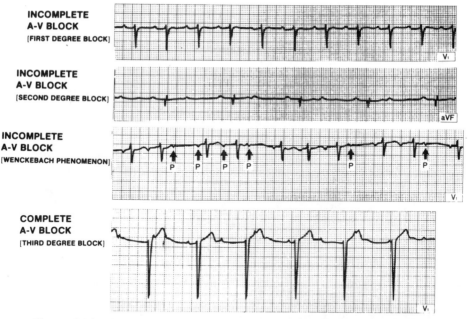

INCOMPLETE
A-V BLOCK
[FIRST DEGREE BLOCK]

INCOMPLETE
A-V BLOCK
[SECOND DEGREE BLOCK]

INCOMPLETE
A-V BLOCK
[WENCKEBACH PHENOMENON]

COMPLETE
A-V BLOCK
[THIRD DEGREE BLOCK]

Figure 4.14. Atrioventricular heart block. *Top*: Incomplete first degree block with prolonged P-R interval but otherwise normal ECG. *Second from top*: Second degree, 2:1 block, ventricle responds only to every other atrial beat. *Third from top*: Wenckebach phenomenon showing progressive AV nodal delay and finally a P wave without a following QRS. *Bottom*: Complete AV heart block; atria are activated by normal impulses from SA node but ventricular rate is slow and independent of atrial rate.

Conduction Blocks

Blockade of the conduction path may occur anywhere between the SA node and the ventricles. One of the more common is AV nodal block, of which three degrees are usually distinguished. In first degree block all the atrial impulses reach the ventricles but the P-R interval is prolonged, *i.e.*, greater than 0.2 seconds (Fig. 4.14, *top*); this is usually due to AV junctional delay.

Second degree block, in which not all P waves are followed by QRS complexes, may be of two types. In one type, Mobitz type II, the P-R interval is relatively fixed, and the ratio of transmission may be 2:1, 3:1, 4:1, etc. (Fig. 4.14, *second from top*). In partial progressive AV block, the P-R interval progressively increases, culminating in a dropped beat (Wenckebach or Mobitz type I) shown in Figure 4.14, *third from top*.

In a third degree, or complete heart block, the impulses are completely interrupted between the atria and ventricles, and the QRS complexes are dissociated from the P waves (Fig. 4.14, *bottom*). The ventricular rate is much slowed (usually 35 to 40 beats/min), so that cardiac output is inadequate. This leads to a sharp fall in arterial pressure, inadequate perfusion of the brain, cerebral ischemia, and fainting (Stokes-Adams syndrome).

Ischemic heart disease, a common cause of arrhythmias, is discussed in Chapter 14.

Treatment of Arrhythmias

While the ECG is a most valuable diagnostic tool, it should be emphasized tha it can only assess the electrical aspects of impulse generation and conduction and cannot measure cardiac contractility. A patient may have a normal ECG and yet the myocardial contractile ability may be inadequate; conversely, marked ECG abnormalities may be associated with a competent heart. In diagnosis and treatment the contractile, metabolic, and electrical aspects of cardiac function must all be considered.

A recent development in the diagnosis of arrhythmias is continuous ECG recording for a period of 24 hours. With a small tape recorder (Holter monitor) strapped to the patient's waist, an ECG may be obtained while the patient goes about normal activities. By scanning of the playbacks, the actual incidence and severity of the arrythmias over a prolonged period can be determined.

Some disturbances such as premature beats, AV block, and paroxysmal atrial tachycardia may occur without detectable structural disease of the heart. Other disorders such as second or third degree heart block, atrial flutter and fibrillation, and ventricular tachycardia are usually associated with organic disorders such as metabolic or electrolyte disturbances or with cardiovascular disease such as ischemic injury or cardiomyopathy.

The treatment of arrhythmias is highly complex and requires considerable skill and judgment; therefore, only a few general principles will be discussed in this section for the purpose of pointing out the pathophysiology involved. Aside from the effort directed toward the primary cause of the disease, therapy usually involves drugs aimed at the specific cardiac disability. Inotropic agents such as digitalis glycosides, which enhance the force-velocity relation of the myocardium (Chapter 5), are used to treat heart failure and will slow sinus tachycardia by improving cardiac output. Digitalis slows the heart rate partly through its vagal action and partly through a direct effect on the SA node and AV node; in the latter case it slows the supraventricular tachycardia by increasing the block at the AV node. Digitalis overdosage may, however, lead to advanced AV block or tachyarrhythmias.

Antiarrhythmic agents such as quinidine and procainamide are useful in disorders such as atrial fibrillation primarily because they decrease the rate of ectopic pacemaker excitation and prolong the absolute refractory period of the atrium—thus interrupting the "circus movement."

Noninvasive methods of stimulating the vagus nerve will sometimes abort attacks of paroxysmal atrial tachycardia. These methods include carotid sinus massage, the Valsalva maneuver (Chapter 13), lateral pressure on the eyeball, or the application of cool water to the face (the face immersion reflex, Chapter 13). Whenever the sinus or AV node is directly involved in the reentry circuit in a condition such as paroxysmal supraventricular tachycardia, the tachycardia may be terminated in this manner; such maneuvers cause increased vagal activity (vagotonia) and act by slowing or blocking conduction within the reentry circuit. However, when these nodes are not directly involved, the vagal maneuver may temporarily decrease the ventricular rate without affecting the atrial rate. Caution must be used during these procedures since strong vagal stimulation may induce asystole, and carotid sinus massage occasionally results in a cerebrovascular accident (stroke).

In the last several years in Europe and Japan and recently in the United States, Ca^{2+} slow-channel blocking agents such as verapamil have been used with considerable clinical success in the treatment of supraventricular arrhythmias and other cardiac disturbances. The effectiveness of these slow Ca^{2+} inhibitors in conditions such as atrial tachycardia, flutter, and fibrillation are the result of their direct electrophysiologic action (*i.e.*, the slowing of AV node conduction velocity and the blocking of reentry mechanisms). Lidocaine, which diminishes the automaticity of the His and Purkinje system, raises the threshold for ventricular fibrillation and causes bidirectional block in areas of conduction delay. It is also used in ventricular arrythmias. Through its β-adrenergic blocking action, propranolol has a primary antiarrhythmic effect. It will reduce heart rate and is used to treat certain ectopic tachycardias and premature ventricular contractions.

In some disorders of ectopic rhythm, such as atrial flutter or fibrillation, cardioversion may succeed in restoring normal rhythm. Cardioversion consists of a direct current shock applied momentarily to the chest early in systole. It temporarily depolarizes the entire heart and interrupts the circus movement of the ectopic disorder, thus permitting the sinus node pacemaker to reestablish sinus rhythm.

Artificial pacemakers are often inserted in cases of heart block, Stoke-Adams syndrome, and other conditions in which an inadequate heart rate is a threat to the patient. In this procedure a "demand-type," transvenous pacemaker is usually placed *via* the subclavian vein into the right ventricle. The demand, noncompetitive pacemaker releases an electrical signal (1 to 2 mA) at a rate of about 70 beats/min only when no intrinsic cardiac impulse is sensed by the pacemaker within a preset period. Extensive experience has demonstrated the clinical usefulness of this procedure in maintaining adequate heart rate and preventing fainting attacks.

Suggested Readings

Berne RM and Levy MN. Electrical activity of the heart. In *Physiology*, 2nd ed., edited by RM Berne and MN Levy. St. Louis: C.V. Mosby, 1988.

Carafoli E. Homeostastis of calcium in heart cells. *J Mol Cell Cardiol* 17:203–212, 1985.

Goldman JJ. *Principles of Clinical Electrocardiography*, 10th ed. Los Altos: Lange Medical Publications, 1978.

Hoffman BF and Cranefield PF. *Electrophysiology of the Heart*. New York: McGraw-Hill, 1960.

Noble D. Ionic mechanisms controlling the action potential duration and the timing of repolarization. *Japanese Heart J* 27(Supp. 3):19, 1986.

Sokolow M and McIlroy MB. *Clinical Cardiology*. Los Altos: Lange Medical Publications, 1986.

Sperelakis N. Regulation of calcium slow channels of cardiac muscle by cyclic nucleotides and phosphorylation. *J Mol Cell Cardiol* 20:Supp II, 75–105, 1988.

Trautwein W. Generation and conduction of impulses in the heart as affected by drugs. *Pharmacol Rev* 15:277, 1963.

Tsien RW and Hess P. Excitable tissues—the heart. In *Physiology of Membrane Disorders*, edited by TE Andreoli and JF Hoffman. New York: Plenum, 1986.

chapter 5

Contractile Properties of the Heart

Structural and Functional Characteristics of the Myofibril

The muscle fiber is composed of myofibrils that on microscopic section show longitudinal strands of thick myosin and thin actin filaments. The basic structural unit is the sarcomere, that portion between the Z lines (Fig. 5.1). The resting length of the sarcomere is about 1.6 to 2.4 μm. The operating range of the sarcomere for contraction is about 70 to 100% of this maximum length.

Contraction of the myocardial fiber involves a complex series of chemical and physical events that are only partially understood. The essential process consists of chemical activation by Ca^{2+} of the actin and myosin filaments and formation of the cross-bridges between fibers. As a result of this activation, the repetitive attachment and reattachment of the thin (actin) filaments to the cross-bridges of the thick myosin filaments causes a "pulling" of the actin strands toward the center of the sarcomere. The two types of filaments

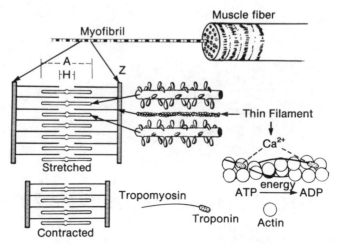

Figure 5.1. Structure of myocardial muscle cell. The myofibrils consist of overlapping thick (myosin) and thin (primarily actin) filaments with cross-bridges between them. The actin of the thin filament is closely bound to two additional proteins, tropomyosin and troponin complex. During the plateau of the action potential, CA^{2+} ions bind with troponin, which triggers the coupling of actin and myosin and the movement of the cross-bridges. Pulled by the cross-bridges, the filaments slide across each other, pulling the Z lines together and causing contraction. (Adapted from R. Rushmer, *Structure and Function of the Cardiovascular System*, Philadelphia: W.B. Saunders, 1976.)

then slide upon each other (sliding filament hypothesis) pulling the Z lines toward one another, thus shortening and contracting the muscle.

Four major proteins are concerned with the contractile process. Aside from actin and myosin, the thin filaments of the myofibrils contain at least two other proteins, *viz.*, tropomyosin, which has the function of modulating the interaction between actin and myosin, and "troponin complex" which is itself composed of three separate proteins. Troponin (bound to tropomyosin) is distributed at intervals along the actin strand (Fig. 5.1).

Excitation-Contraction Coupling

The combination of Ca^{2+} with the muscle proteins is a key factor in excitation-contraction coupling. Essentially, such coupling involves depolarization of the transverse (T) tubules and release of Ca^{2+} from storage sites within the sarcoplasmic reticulum (Fig. 5.2).

Small saclike expansions of the sarcoplasmic reticulum, called subsarcolemmal cisternae (Fig. 5.2), are located near the Z lines. The three units— the longitudinal superficial sarcoplasmic reticulum, the transverse system (T tubes), and the cisternae—are closely involved in the contraction-relaxation

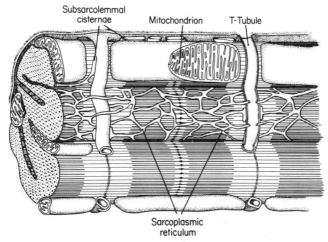

Subsarcolemmal
cisternae   Mitochondrion   T-Tubule

Sarcoplasmic
reticulum

Figure 5.2. Myofibril showing sarcoplasmic reticulum. The muscle fibril is enveloped by a cell membrane that has tubular projections (T or transverse tubules) that are open to the extracellular space. A second, completely intracellular, membrane system, the sarcoplasmic reticulum, makes close contact with the T tubules and sarcolemma. (Reprinted with permission from W. Bloom and D.W. Fawcett, *Textbook of Histology*. Philadelphia: W.B. Saunders, 1969.)

sequence. As mentioned in the previous chapter, the myocardium is a functional syncytium. The wave of excitation (the AP) spreads from one myofibril to the next with relative ease because the gap junctions between cells have a low resistance.

The ionic and electrical aspects of the cardiac action potential (AP) were described in Chapter 4. Although the exact relationship between the AP and muscle contraction is not fully understood, it is clear that depolarization of the membrane opens Ca^{2+} channels. The intracellular mobilization of Ca^{2+} in adequate quantities in its so-called activator state undoubtedly plays a pivotal role. This is shown by the fact that over the course of the contractile cycle, Ca^{2+} concentration first rises in the cell, activating contraction at the filaments, then falls again, allowing relaxation. Furthermore the resultant strength of contraction is directly correlated with the extracellular Ca^{2+} concentration.

When intracellular Ca^{2+}, concentration is low, troponin complex blocks the formation of cross-bridges between myosin and actin. As Ca^{2+} in the cell rises, this inhibition is removed and actin-myosin interaction begins. The sequence of "making and breaking" cross-bridges in quick succession "pulls" the actin filament along and causes the sarcomere to shorten.

Hydrolysis of the terminal phosphate on ATP by ATPase in the cross-bridges supplies the chemical energy required for generation of the mechanical force at each cross-bridge attachment. After the plateau phase of the AP and repolarization of the cell membrane, the intracellular Ca^{2+} is again bound to the sarcoplasmic reticulum or extruded from the cell, and the myofibril relaxes.

Thus, the AP, through its regulation of the intracellular concentration of activator Ca^{2+}, not only triggers the contraction but also influences its magnitude and duration. The force of contraction appears to depend on the number of cross-bridges formed and this number is related to the intracellular Ca^{2+} concentration. Inotropic agents may act at several possible sites.

Digitalis glycosides have been used for over 200 years in the treatment of heart failure, but until recently their mode of action has been poorly understood. It is now generally agreed that these glycosides increase the force of myocardial contraction through the action of Ca^{2+} on the excitation-contraction coupling system. Digitalis inhibits the Na^+-K^+ pump in the sarcolemmal membrane, which results in a small net increase of Na^+ ions on the intracellular side of the membrane. This excess, in turn, initiates a Na^+-Ca^{2+} exchange system, and the increased movement of Ca^{2+} into the cell during the AP is responsible for the heightened contractile force. Digitalis glycosides are capable of increasing myocardial force development by 50 to 60% and can completely reestablish cardiac function in many instances of heart failure. Catecholamines appear to increase contractile force by increasing the intracellular concentration of cyclic AMP and altering intracellular Ca^{2+} levels.

Elastic Properties of the Myocardium

Heart muscle possesses elastic as well as contractile properties. If a strip of myocardium is stretched it will develop tension disproportionate to the applied stretch. It is advantageous for conceptual purposes to separate the contractile and elastic elements of cardiac muscle. Compliance (elasticity) is an important factor in determining the resistance to diastolic inflow into the ventricle and ultimately, therefore, in determining stroke volume.

The elastic components of myocardium have been visualized by some investigators as separate parallel and series elements as shown in Figure 5.3.

The parallel element, PE (Fig. 5.3), represents the elastic behavior of resting muscle and SE the elastic behavior of contracting muscle. CE represents all the contractile elements. When muscle first contracts, shortening is rapid because the resisting load is small, but as shortening develops in isotonic contraction the SE lengthens, and with the tension increase, the velocity of contraction decreases. The force registered at the ends of the muscle will depend, therefore, not only on the contractile properties of CE, but on the elastic properties of SE and the time allowed for interaction between the lengthening of SE and shortening of CE. It should be emphasized that this concept is a theoretical one useful for analytical purposes. No anatomical analogues actually exist as purely contractile or elastic elements.

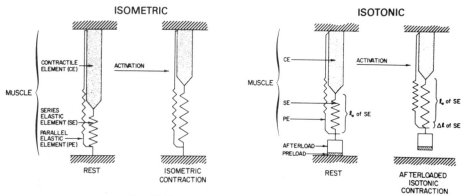

Figure 5.3. The three-component functional model of the myocardium showing the contractile component (CE), parallel elastic component (PE), and series elastic component (SE). CE and SE are in series with each other, and PE is parallel with them. The elastic elements are passive springs, and the contractile element is freely extensible. (Reprinted with permission from E.H. Sonnenblick, *Fed Proc* 21:975, 1962.)

Myocardial Contractility

How well the heart can propel blood is unquestionably a crucial determinant of circulatory performance. But which factors regulate myocardial contractility and how it can best be measured are questions that still provoke frequent sharply dissenting views among investigators. In the following, emphasis will be placed on those aspects that seem most relevant to cardiac function in the intact human.

We will consider cardiac muscle from two standpoints: first, its *intrinsic regulation, i.e.,* the basic contractile properties inherent in the muscle itself; and secondly, its *extrinsic regulation, i.e.,* its response to conditions imposed from the outside such as neural stimulation, hormones, drugs, and disease.

Intrinsic regulation involves an analysis of (*a*) myocardial response to stretching prior to contraction, *i.e.,* to added *preload stress* such as increased diastolic filling, known as the Starling effect, (*b*) the myocardial response to increased load imposed after contraction has begun, *i.e.,* to *afterload stress*, such as a rise in aortic distolic pressure, and (*c*) myocardiac response to heart rate alteration.

Intrinsic Regulation of the Myocardium

Preload Stresses—Starling's Law of the Heart

This very basic concept, originally described by Frank and Starling, states in effect that, within physiological limits, the force or tension generated by the

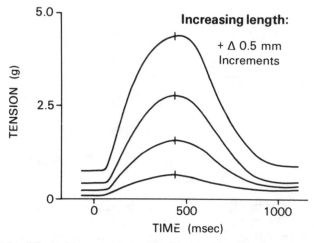

Figure 5.4. Effect of increased stretch of isolated papillary muscle on the contractile force, showing isometric contractions of the isolated muscle at different precontractile lengths while using stimuli of the same strength. Note that while the generated tension increases progressively, the time to maximal tension is constant. (Reprinted with permission from E.H. Sonnenblick, *Fed Proc* 21:975, 1962.)

contracting muscle is greater if the muscle is previously stretched. This can be shown *in vitro* by determining the peak tension developed at different precontractile lengths (Fig. 5.4).

As indicated in Figure 5.4, precontractile stretching of the muscle induced profound changes in the developed tension (which is force normalized for cross-sectional area of the muscle). This would imply that during diastole a greater influx of blood into the ventricle will cause the ensuing contraction to be more forceful. This may be thought of as a "preload" stimulus since it was applied before contraction began. It should also be noted that not only the time needed to achieve peak tension but also the relaxation time was unchanged when fiber length was unaltered.

Starling, an English physiologist, studied this phenomenon further in an isolated, canine heart-lung preparation in which he controlled the right atrial pressure (and thereby the right ventricular diastolic pressure or preload) by raising or lowering an infusion bottle connected to the vena cava. He also controlled the aortic pressure (or afterload) by means of an artificial aortic resistance. From a series of such experiments Starling showed that with increased diastolic volume, the subsequent contraction of the isolated heart did indeed result in a higher peak systolic pressure. His data also showed that if the ventricle is stretched beyond the physiological limit, the systolic pressure will then decline, indicating impending failure (Fig. 5.5).

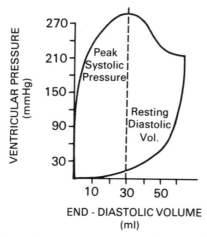

Figure 5.5. Starling volume-pressure curve of myocardial function. Classical curve indicating that within physiological limits, increased end-diastolic ventricular volume will result in increased peak ventricular pressure. Beyond the *dotted line* the ventricle is overstretched and the heart will respond to increased filling with less pressure. (Reprinted with permission from S.W. Patterson, H. Pipers, and E.H. Starling, *J Physiol* 48:465, 1914.)

Sarnoff and Mitchell found that similar relationships existed between left ventricular end-diastolic pressure (LVEDP) and LV stroke work; because the length-tension relationship of the two ventricles is usually comparable, graphs depicting *right* ventricular volume and *left* ventricular pressure—as were originally made by Starling—also show similar configurations.

This characteristic of the myocardium—also called "heterometric auto-regulation"—is an inherent, intrinsic property of the muscle fiber, which is evident in the heart fully isolated from all neural or humoral influences. It has been suggested that this property is due to the apposition—as the muscle is stretched—of more cross-bridges between the actin and myosin. It was further theorized that the "failure" part of the length-tension curve occurs because sarcomeres are stretched beyond their normal length of about 2.4 μm and that fewer cross-bridges are thereby formed between the filaments. There is, however, some recent conflicting evidence on this point so that further study of this question is needed.

The Starling effect is an important one, since it enables the heart to adapt its pumping capacity to alterations in venous return. The contractile response to altered myocardial length is particularly helpful in matching the output of the two ventricles and also in adapting to various stresses such as exercise.

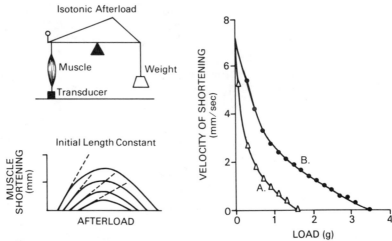

Figure 5.6. Influence of afterload on velocity and degree of shortening of the myocardium. When a muscle is permitted to shorten (isotonic contraction) against different afterloads (*top left*), the degree of shortening and initial velocity (*dashed lines*) decrease as afterload is increased (*bottom left*). *Right,* The plot of force (afterload) *vs.* initial velocity of shortening with different afterloads. At 1.6 g (*curve A*) the load is too heavy to lift, the velocity is 0, and the contraction is isometric. A greater preload (*curve B, right*), and therefore a greater initial muscle length, shifts the curve to the right, but the maximum velocity (V_{max}) is unchanged. (Reprinted with permission from E.H. Sonnenblick, *Fed Proc* 21:975, 1962.)

Afterload Stresses—Force-Velocity Curves

If a cardiac muscle strip is made to lift a load after contraction has begun (afterloading), the muscle gradually develops tension as the series elastic element (Fig. 5.3) is stretched, so that after a brief interval the muscle begins to shorten. At first the velocity of shortening is high, but as the elastic tension rises, the velocity gradually diminishes. When the afterload is increased in steps, the degree of shortening, the velocity of shortening, and the total time of contraction all decrease (Fig. 5.6, *bottom left*).

The counterpart of this in the intact human is the decreased stroke volume, decreased ejection velocity, and shortened ejection time when the aortic pressure rises (Chapter 7); the myocardial fibers need a longer time to develop the tension required to overcome the greater afterload. At the lightest load, the initial velocity of contraction is greatest; *i.e.*, the velocity varies inversely with afterload. If the velocities are plotted against afterload (Fig. 5.6, *right, curve A*), the velocity curve extrapolated to the y (velocity) axis would represent the velocity at zero load, *i.e.*, maximum velocity (V_{max}).

In the above experiment, the initial muscle length (preload) was held constant and the afterload varied. If now the preload is varied (*i.e.*, the muscle is stretched to a larger precontractile length) and the muscle is again subjected to different afterloads, a curve similar to that of Figure 5.6, *right, curve B*, will result.

It will be noted in Figure 5.6 (*right*) that the muscle with the greater preload (and thereby stretched) can overcome a larger afterload, which is in accord with Starling's law; but in addition, it is significant that V_{max} is independent of preload. Just as an increase in afterload will cause a decrease in strength, velocity, and duration of contraction of the isolated heart muscle, similarly an increase in aortic pressure will cause comparable effects in the intact ventricle (Chapter 7). However in certain instances, particularly in anesthetized animals, after an abrupt increase in aortic pressure, there may be an initial decrease followed by a temporary *elevation* of stroke work. This is not a mechanical but rather an intrinsic, inotropic response of the myocardium; it is known as the "Anrep" effect or "homeometric autoregulation" since it occurs without any change in fiber length. Existing evidence suggests that this phenomenon, which may be related to an improved myocardial blood flow, plays only a minor role in myocardial contraction in the intact human circulation.

Heart Rate Alterations

The electrical and ionic aspects of cardiac contraction and the control of the heart rate have been discussed in the preceding chapter. While this chapter is devoted primarily to myocardial contractility, that is, to the ability of the heart to produce stroke volume, perhaps the most basic measure of the performance of the heart is its ability to generate cardiac output. Since cardiac output is the product of stroke volume and heart rate, these two entities are, in this respect, of equal value.

Heart rate is of importance in two general ways, (*a*) a mechanical or indirect effect on cardiac output by virtue of the influence of rate on the length of diastole and therefore on end-diastolic volume and stroke volume, and (*b*) a direct intrinsic effect of rate on myocardial contractibility—usually termed the "interval-strength" effect. The mechanical effects of moderate heart rate changes in a healthy adult—if they occur within a normal heart rate range (60 to 170 beats/min)—will usually have only temporary and nonthreatening effects on cardiac output. However, at very rapid heart rates the time available for ventricular filling is too short, so that there is an infringement on the early ventricular filling stage (Fig. 3.5). Since the ventricles become approximately two-thirds filled during the first one-third of ventricular filling, this encroachment will result in a marked reduction in cardiac output. On the other hand, in a severe bradycardia (40 beats/min or less) the period of ventricular filling is prolonged, but since the major ventricular filling occurs early in diastole,

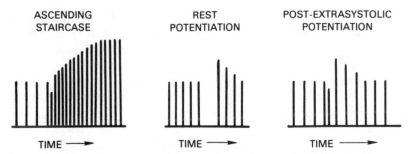

ASCENDING STAIRCASE   REST POTENTIATION   POST-EXTRASYSTOLIC POTENTIATION

TIME ⟶   TIME ⟶   TIME ⟶

Figure 5.7. Myocardial contraction: the interval-strength relation. An increase in heart rate, a prolonged beat interval, and a delay after an extrasystole all result in stronger subsequent contractions. (Reprinted with permission from E.O. Feigl, *Physiology and Biophysics*, edited by T.C. Ruch and H.D. Patton. Philadelphia: W.B. Saunders, 1974.)

the elevated stroke volume at very slow heart rates is not increased sufficiently to compensate for the reduced rate; therefore, cardiac output falls markedly. This often leads to cerebral ischemia and fainting (Stokes-Adams syndrome) as discussed in Chapter 4.

Aside from the mechanical effects of heart rate on cardiac output, there are "interval-strength" factors that can produce temporary alterations in myocardial contractility. Interval-strength relationships are complex, and only three effects will be considered here. A rapid rate increase will progressively augment cardiac contractility—this is known as the staircase or "treppe" phenomenon (Fig. 5.7, *left*).

Similarly, a longer than normal delay between beats, or a pause after an extrasystole (post-extrasystolic potentiation) will be followed by stronger contractions. These effects can be produced in isolated myocardial muscle and thus are not dependent on increased filling and are clearly intrinsic in nature. They are nonetheless amplified in the intact heart by the added mechanical effect of increased diastolic filling.

In the intact ventricle, as well as in isolated cardiac muscle, a premature depolarization results in a reduced mechanical contraction (Fig. 5.7, *right*), the magnitude of which is a function of the degree of prematurity of the extra depolarization. The next contraction then is more forceful than normal, the degree of augmentation being greater the earlier the extra depolarization is introduced. The interval-strength relation, which is of relatively minor importance in the intact human, is probably due to a time-induced alteration in Ca^{2+} availability to the muscle cell.

It is therefore evident that alteration of heart rate affects ventricular contraction in two ways. A rate alteration will clearly affect the time for diastolic filling, so that if other factors are held constant, a slowing of the rate will increase stroke volume through this mechanical effect. The degree to which

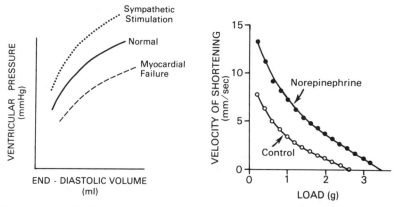

Figure 5.8.   Positive and negative inotropic effects on the ventricular volume-pressure (Starling) curve (*left*) and on the myocardial force-velocity curve (*right*). Sympathetic stimulation or administration of norepinephrine or digitalis will move the Starling curve up and to the left and the force-velocity curve up and to the right and will increase V_{max}. Myocardial ischemia, toxic agents, or heart failure will have opposite effects.

heart rate affects stroke volume depends on the degree of heart rate change. The effect of heart rate on stroke volume will be discussed further in Chapter 7. However, in addition to this factor, as described above, alteration of heart rate interval has intrinsic effects on myocardial contractility, which become evident in carefully designed, isolated heart preparations. The role of these intrinsic effects in the intact, awake animal or human (with functioning reflexes) is not yet certain.

Extrinsic Regulation of the Myocardium—Inotropic State

Outside factors that affect the inotropic state or contractility of the heart may be of three general types: (*a*) *neurohormonal effects*, due to influences of the sympathetic or parasympathetic systems or of the catecholamines; (*b*) *chemical and pharmacological effects*, for example, contractile changes due to alterations in blood K^+, Ca^{2+}, pH, or drugs such as digitalis and sympathetic "blockers"; and (*c*) *pathological effects*, for example, those due to ischemia incident to coronary occlusion or toxic effects resulting from bacteria or chemicals.

As shown in Figure 5.8 (*left*), sympathetic stimulation will produce a positive inotropic effect and move the Starling curve upward and to the left depending on the strength of stimulation. Increased contractility will also result from injection of norepinephrine, digitalis, or Ca^{2+} ions. If these same stimuli are applied either to the isolated muscle or to the intact heart, the Starling curve is moved upward and to the right and V_{max} is increased (Fig.

5.8, *right*). Therefore, in these cases a stronger myocardial contraction has resulted from an extrinsic influence as evidenced (*a*) by the shift to a higher Starling curve or (*b*) by a shift to a higher force-velocity curve with an increased V_{max}. Conversely, myocardial ischemia, toxic and anesthetic agents, hypocalcemia, hyperkalemia, or cardiac failure will result in a negative inotropic effect; these are manifested by a lower Starling curve and a lower force-velocity curve with a decreased V_{max}.

As previously described, an increase in the length of the cardiac muscle fiber or augmentation of end-diastolic volume (as occurs within an individual Starling curve) causes an increase in the ability of the contractile machinery to develop force. While this is an exceedingly important characteristic of the heart muscle that enables it to adapt itself to variations in venous return, it does not affect the inotropic state. The change in sarcomere length alters the degree of filament overlap but does not change the number of contractile sites and is not considered an alteration in contractile state. In contrast, a shift of the curves denotes an increase in the rate of activation of contractile sites, an alteration in the velocity of shortening, and a change in the basic inotropic state of the muscle.

The alteration of the inotropic state of cardiac muscle is probably related to the rate of Ca^{2+} binding to troponin. The normal serum calcium concentration (about 4.3 to 5.3 mEq/L) is about 10,000 times the level in the myocardial cells, yet a reduction of serum calcium will lessen myocardial contractility, probably because it alters calcium influx across the plasma membrane during systole.

Assessment of Cardiac Contractility

As described above, in the intact human circulation the strength of cardiac contraction may be altered in two primary ways: (*a*) by altering diastolic filling, *i.e.*, by changing precontractile muscle length, an intrinsic effect; or (*b*) by altering the inotropic state or contractility, an extrinsic effect that is usually brought about by neural or hormonal influences. For clinical as well as experimental purposes, the measurement of contractile capability of the heart is a highly important objective.

In evaluating cardiac function, a distinction should be made first of all between "performance" and "contractility." Cardiac performance refers to measurements such as stroke volume and cardiac output, which depend on contractility but are also influenced by mechanical or other extraneous factors. Contractility is the more important measurement and refers to a careful estimate, under controlled conditions, of the basic ability of the heart muscle to generate power (*i.e.*, its inotropic state). Circulatory performance such as cardiac output may, for example, be adversely affected by decreased blood volume or by an incompetent valve even though the contractile ability of the myocardium may be entirely normal. This distinction would be an important one for instance after a myocardial infarct, when it would be helpful to have a quantitative measure of the remaining myocardial contractile ability so that an estimate might be made as to whether the patient is an acceptable risk for myocardial revascularization surgery.

There are four major determinants of myocardial performance: preload, afterload, heart rate, and contractility (inotropic state). As previously noted, preload and inotropic capability are major determinants of myocardial contractile power, while afterload and heart rate (to be discussed in Chapter 7) are mainly mechanical factors that affect performance. By maintaining preload, afterload, and heart rate constant, one may determine the effect of drugs, catecholamines, or other interventions on contractility. Alternatively, one may maintain the heart rate, afterload, and extrinsic factors constant and determine the effect of preload. If one could control external factors in this fashion, ideal measures of cardiac contractility would be the determination of ventricular pressure and work at different levels of end-diastolic volume (Starling curve) or the measurement of V_{max}.

While such procedures are possible with cardiac muscle strips or isolated heart preparations, they are difficult to acheive in the intact organism. Many methods have been designed to approximate this ideal and to estimate myocardial contractility in the intact subject, but none is as yet fully satisfactory.

In clinical studies, some of the more commonly used measures of cardiac contractility are (*a*) ejection indices, (*b*) ventricular dimensions and their rate of change, (*c*) isovolumetric indices, and (*d*) systolic time intervals. Ejection indices, which are based on the effectiveness of left ventricular ejection, include aortic flow velocity, acceleration of blood in the aorta (dV/dt), and ejection fraction (the ratio of stroke volume to end-diastolic volume). Ventricular dimensions and their rate of change can be estimated by ventricular angiography, radionuclide ventriculography, and echocardiography; these techniques will be described in Chapter 7.

Isovolumetric indices are based on the pressure rise during the isovolumic contraction period (Fig. 3.5) when the ventricle is a closed chamber and is undergoing isometric contraction. One of the more commonly used of these indices is left ventricular dP/dt_{max}.

In this method, sensitive manometers are used to record the ventricular pressure curve; the tangent of the steepest point of the curve (or the peak of a wave recorded by a differentiating circuit) indicates the maximum rate of pressure change. This occurs during the isovolumic phase and is a reasonable index of the initial velocity of myocardial contraction (Fig. 5.9).

Although dP/dt_{max} will vary to some extent with preload and heart rate, it is very responsive to changes in the inotropic state and has been used clinically to characterize the contractile ability of the heart. The left ventricular dP/dt_{max}, which is normally about 1600 mm Hg/sec, tends to be less than 1200

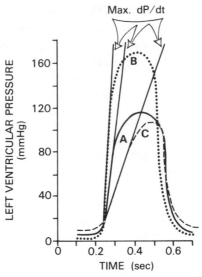

Figure 5.9. Maximum rate of rise of left ventricular pressure (peak dP/dt). Left ventricular pressure curves with the tangent at the steepest part of ascending limb designating maximum dP/dt. *A*, Control; *B*, after norepinephrine; and *C*, cardiac failure. (Reprinted with permission from R.M. Berne and M.N. Levy, *Cardiovascular Physiology*. St. Louis: C.V. Mosby, 1981, p. 81.)

mm Hg/sec in patients with disorders of the left ventricular myocardium. One of the problems with this determination is a technical one: even with high-fidelity, catheter-tip manometers, which eliminate much of the distortion of the pressure wave due to fluid transmission through the catheter, recording artifacts are still difficult to avoid. Moreover, insertion of the catheter is an invasive procedure and carries with it some risk to the patient.

Systolic time intervals (STI) have also been proposed as useful measures of cardiac contractility. STIs are based on the relative duration of the contraction and relaxation phases of the cardiac cycle and on the generalization that at a fixed heart rate the more competent ventricle will, if all other factors are held constant, eject a given stroke volume in less time (*i.e.*, have a shorter ejection period). One of the commonly used STIs is PEP/VET, the quotient of the preejection period (from the onset of the QRS complex to the beginning of the aortic pulse wave) and the ventricular ejection time (from the beginning of the aortic pulse to the incisura). In an extensive comparative analysis of 32 separate indices of cardiac contractility, Abel found that PVP time (time from the beginning of systole to peak ventricular pressure) was more sensitive to myocardial contractility and less sensitive to changes in preload, afterload, and heart rate than any of the other parameters measured.

While all of the currently available indices have certain shortcomings, they can, in many instances, yield valuable information if used in carefully defined circumstances, provided that the techniques and their limitations are understood.

Aside from the distinction between contractility and performance, there are two other generalizations that are useful in judging the function of the heart and its role in the cardiovascular system. One is the method by which the heart can increase its work output to adjust to the demand made upon it (*i.e.*, to the venous return supplied to it). Skeletal muscle when called upon to produce a greater contractile force (*i.e.*, to increase its work output) can resort to increased recruitment of additional muscle fibers. This option is not available to the myocardial syncytium, which operates as a unit. For this reason, increased or decreased work output is brought about through modulation of the contractility of the entire heart. This is done primarily by the autonomic nervous system through a balanced release of neurotransmitters, primarily norepinephrine and acetylcholine. This autonomic balancing act is particularly important when the heart needs to respond to stresses such as exercise, gravitational force such as postural change, the Valsalva maneuver, emotional trauma, or hemorrhage. To a serious stress the heart responds maximally, but its response is, of course, limited by its own supply of O_2, energy substrates, Ca^{2+}, etc.

A second generalization, which is undoubtedly evident from the previous chapters but nonetheless bears repetition, is that the heart, in spite of its central role as the all-important pump, is only one element in the circulatory system. The other key element is the peripheral circulation. As will be discussed in subsequent chapters, the heart itself cannot cope with increased cardiovascular demand. Obviously it can only pump the amount of blood brought to it and in this sense is a permissive organ. Without effective peripheral circulation the system cannot carry out the critical function of shunting blood from areas of less need to those of greater need and cannot generate the arterial pressure that is critical, for example, in maintaining cerebral blood flow. The appreciation of the role of the heart has clinical implications for diagnostic accuracy, and it also prevents administration of a readily available cardiac drug when the pathophysiological defect is elsewhere.

Oxygen Consumption and Work of the Heart

The "resting" O_2 consumption of the heart is about 8 ml/100 g/min, of which about one-fourth is for basic metabolism and the remainder provides energy for contraction. Of the total oxygen consumption, only 35 to 40% is normally due to oxidation of carbohydrates. The major cardiac energy (in postabsorptive states) is derived from noncarbohydrate sources, mainly fatty acids. The amino acid contribution is small. As with other tissues, about 95% of the energy is used to form ATP in mitochondria. The main determinants of myocardial oxygen consumption are (*a*) ventricular wall tension, (*b*) heart rate, and (*c*) velocity of myocardial shortening. Cardiac cells have a greater mitochondrial content than skeletal muscle cells, probably because they are required to contract repetitively over a lifetime and are incapable of developing a significant O_2 debt—so they need a ready source of energy. To further enhance its metabolic capability, the myocardium has a rich capillary supply, about one capillary per fiber, so that diffusion distances are short and the exchange of O_2, CO_2, and metabolites is expedited.

The main work of the heart is expended in pumping a volume of fluid against a pressure head. For this reason the external cardiac work (for the left ventricle) is usually estimated as the product of the stroke volume ejected and the mean aortic pressure during systole (stroke work). The "pressure work" may also be approximated as the product of the cardiac output and the mean arterial pressure. Since the mean pulmonary arterial pressure is about one-sixth that of the aorta and the output of the right ventricle is the same as the left, the work done per minute by the right ventricle is about one-sixth that of the left.

In addition to the potential energy in the form of pressure-volume work, kinetic energy is also generated, by virtue of the velocity imparted to the blood. Although at rest only about 2 to 4% of the useful work of the heart is in the form of kinetic energy, this fraction may increase to 20 or 25% in exercise.

Because cardiac pressure work is more demanding of oxygen than "flow work," Sarnoff and associates suggested that myocardial O_2 consumption ($M\dot{V}O_2$) might be indirectly estimated by the "tension-time index" (TTI), which is the product of the mean systolic pressure, the duration of systole, and the heart rate. In a condition such as aortic stenosis (Chapter 3), intraventricular pressure (and thus TTI and cardiac work) will be much elevated; this increased work requirement prevails in the face of a lessened aortic pressure available for coronary perfusion.

Recent exercise studies by Bruce and others in normal subjects and cardiac patients have indicated that certain indices such as the product of systolic pressure and heart rate (pressure-rate or "double product") or the systolic pressure–heart rate–systolic ejection time product ("triple product") are highly correlated with myocardial oxygen consumption ($M\dot{V}O_2$). The double product at maximal exercise can thus provide a reasonable noninvasive estimate of the limit of left ventricular capability. It should be pointed out, however, that TTI and double product estimations of coronary $M\dot{V}O_2$ do not take into account the metabolic effect of increase in wall tension which occurs in dilated hearts (Laplace's law, Chapter 1) or the alteration in contraction velocity which also has a metabolic effect as mentioned above.

Pressure-Volume Loops

The stroke work of the heart may be represented graphically by a pressure-volume diagram (Fig. 5.10). Such a diagram or "loop" represents, in a

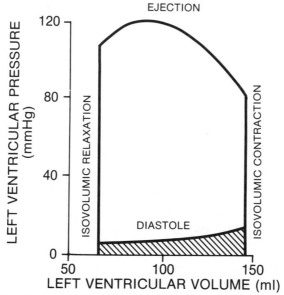

Figure 5.10.   Pressure-volume loop showing left ventricular volume and pressure changes during a single heart cycle in a normal adult at rest.

different way, the events of the cardiac cycle previously discussed in Chapter 3 and shown in Figure 3.5; in addition (since work = pressure × volume), it also represents the external stroke work expended during a single cardiac cycle. Kinetic energy is omitted.

Diastole, or ventricular filling, consists of the first or rapid filling stage, followed by the slow filling phase called diastasis, with a final contribution from atrial contraction. Note that there is only a small increase in pressure with the increase in ventricular volume. At the end of diastole, the mitral valve closes, and the period of isovolumic (isometric) contraction takes place. During ejection, ventricular pressure is greater than aortic pressure, and the myocardium shortens isotonically. At the closure of the aortic valve, isometric relaxation of the ventricle takes place. The diagonally marked area represents work done through venous filling of the ventricle. The area within the loop is the work done by the contracting heart. In certain experimental and clinical situations, pressure-volume loops of disordered hearts may be useful for analyzing the energy exchange and efficiency of the heart.

Efficiency of the Heart

Mechanical efficiency is usually estimated as the external work done divided by the energy consumed. The work may be calculated as described above and the energy by conversion of O_2 consumption (1 ml of O_2 liberates 2.06 kg-m of energy). The efficiency of the myocardium is ordinarily about 5 to 15%, although this may be considerably increased in exercise in which the cardiac output or flow component increases disproportionately to the pressure component. The remaining 85 to 95% of the energy produced is in the form of heat. Because of the metabolism-stimulating and flow-stimulating effects of temperature itself, physical work capacity is importantly influenced by the ability of the body to maintain optimum temperature. The increased blood flow to skin, which occurs in order to dissipate the excess heat, adds to cardiac work demands and, therefore, to coronary flow requirements. This may be a limiting factor in the work capacity of cardiac patients.

Suggested Readings

Abel FL and McCutcheon EP. *Cardiovascular Function: Principles and Applications.* Boston: Little, Brown, 1979, pp 197–216.

Allen DG. Cellular basis of the length-tension relation in cardiac muscle. *J Mol Cell Cardiol* 17:821–840, 1985.

Cooke R. The mechanism of muscle contraction. *CRC Rev Biochem* 21:53–118, 1986.

Galosy RA, Mitchell JH, Atkins JM, and Reisch J. Sympathetic stimulation, hemodynamic factors and indices of cardiac inotropic state. *Am J Physiol* 234:H562–H566. 1978.

Langer GA. Myocardial force development in health and disease. In: *Pathophysiology of the Heart,* edited by G Ross. New York: Masson Publishers, 1982, pp 1–39.

Mitchell JH, Wallace AG, and Skinner NS. Intrinsic effects of heart rate on left ventricular performance. *Am J Physiol* 205:41–48, 1963.

Randall WC (ed.). *Nervous Control of Cardiovascular Function.* New York: Oxford Ohio Press, 1984.

Sarnoff SJ. Myocardial contractility as described by ventricular function curves. *Physiol Rev* 35:107, 1955.

Sonnenblick E. Force-velocity relations in mammalian heart muscle. *Am J Physiol* 202:931, 1962.

Starling EH. *The Linacre Lecture on the Law of the Heart.* London: Longmans, Green & Co., 1918.

Wallace AG and Waigh RM. Excitation-contraction coupling. In: *Pathophysiology of Cardiovascular Disease,* edited by LH Smith and R Sothier. Philadelphia: W.B. Saunders and Co., 1987.

Winegrad S. Regulation of cardiac contractile proteins. *Circ Res* 55:565–574, 1984.

chapter 6

Pressure and Flow in the Arterial and Venous Systems

Aortic Pressure and Flow

As indicated in a previous chapter (Fig. 3.5), during the first third of left ventricular emptying, about two-thirds of the stroke volume is ejected into

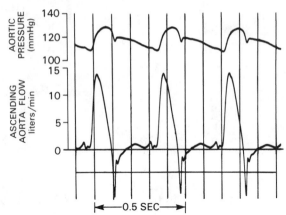

Figure 6.1. Simultaneous flow and pressure tracing in the aorta. There is a rapid ejection of blood from the left ventricle into the aorta followed by a rise in the aortic pressure. (Reprinted with permission from H.P. Peiper, *Rev Sci Instrum* **29**:965, 1958.)

the aorta. Simultaneous aortic recordings with a pressure transducer and a sensitive flowmeter illustrate this rapid emptying as a quick rise in aortic flow in early systole (Fig. 6.1). The rapid ejection is followed by a sharp fall in ejection rate. At the end of systole there is actually a small, transient reverse flow due to (*a*) an influx of blood into the coronary arteries, (*b*) a slight regurgitation of blood back into the left ventricle through the aortic valve, and (*c*) the distension of the valve as the bolus of blood is stopped from reentering the ventricle.

The pressure wave (Fig. 6.1, *top*) is the shock impulse due to the sudden ejection of blood into the aorta. This wave is transmitted through the aortic blood column and aortic wall at a velocity of about 4 to 6 m/sec which is about 20 times greater than the mean velocity imparted to the blood itself (20 to 40 cm/sec). The pressure wave has, therefore, no direct relationship to flow and could occur fully as well if there were no flow at all. Because the transmission velocity of the pulse wave is increased when the arteries become less distensible, the speed of the wave has sometimes been used as an index of arterial distensibility.

Aortic Pressure Wave

Components

Because pressure is technically easier to record than flow and since the aorta stands between the heart and the circulatory beds of the tissues, the analysis of the aortic pressure wave can yield valuable information about both central and peripheral circulatory events.

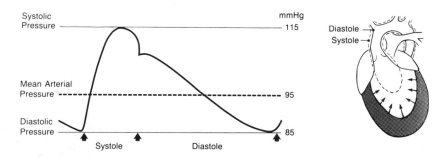

Figure 6.2. Aortic pressure curve. During systole the ejected volume distends the aorta, and aortic pressure rises. The peak pressure is known as the aortic systolic pressure. After the peak ejection, the ventricular pressure falls, and when it drops below the aortic pressure, the aortic valve closes, which is marked by the incisura, the end of systole. During diastole, the pressure continues to decline, and the aortic wall recoils, pushing the blood toward the periphery. The trough of the pressure wave is the diastolic pressure. The difference between systolic and diastolic pressure is the pulse pressure.

The ascending or anacrotic limb of a typical aortic pressure wave (shown in Fig. 6.2) is the result of the forcible ejection of the left ventricular blood into the aorta with resultant distension of the aortic wall. After it reaches its peak (*i.e.*, the systolic pressure) the ventricular pressure declines to a level below the aortic (the catacrotic limb); at this point the aortic valve closes with a small rebound wave marking the incisura and the end of ventricular systole. At a heart rate of 75 beats/min, the cycle length is 0.8 sec or 800 msec, of which about three-eighths or 0.3 sec is taken up by systole.

As described in Chapter 3, the entire left ventricular stroke volume is emptied into the aorta and its branches during systole. Actually, in the healthy adult, two-thirds of the stroke volume is ejected into the aorta during the first one-third of systole—the rapid ejection period. Part of the energy of ventricular contraction provides forward flow during systole. The remainder is used in distending the arterial tree and is stored as potential energy.

This potential energy is then released by the recoil of the arterial wall, which then propels the blood distally and provides the "diastolic runoff." This alternation of systolic and diastolic propulsion provides a more continuous (rather than pulsatile) flow to the peripheral tissues. This pressure-storing property of the aorta is sometimes called the "Wind Kessel" effect. Diastole, which occupies about five-eighths of the cardiac cycle (or about 0.5 sec), is characterized by a long, declining pressure wave due to the elastic recoil.

Meanwhile, the ventricle is relaxing and filling for the next stroke. The lowest point of the pressure wave, which occurs at the end of insovolumic ventricular contraction, is called the diastolic pressure (Fig. 6.2).

The difference between systolic and diastolic pressure is the pulse pressure. The mean aortic pressure is the average for the complete period, which is the pressure-time integral for the entire cardiac cycle. The mean pressure can be determined electronically with a polygraph recorder or by determining the area under the curve (the pressure-time product) and dividing by the length of the cycle.

The true mean pressure in an artery is less than the arithmetic average of the systolic and diastolic pressures because the lower half of the curve has a greater area than the upper half. Under ordinary conditions and at normal heart rates, the mean arterial pressure can be roughly estimated as the diastolic pressure plus one-third of the pulse pressure. At high heart rates, it approaches the diastolic plus one-half the pulse pressure. Mean pressure values are essential for certain calculations, for example, in determining pressure gradients or peripheral resistance.

Transmission

Both the pressure values and the wave configurations are altered during transmission through the peripheral arterial tree (Fig. 6.3). With increasing distance from the heart, the dicrotic notch becomes less sharp (smoothed or filtered) and dicrotic waves appear. In the descending aorta and large arteries, the systolic pressures are higher and diastolic pressures are lower (with a resultant higher pulse pressure) than in the ascending aorta (Fig. 6.3). This is due to (a) the reflection of the pulse waves from the distal vascular bed with subsequent summation at those points, and (b) resonant oscillations of the ejected bolus of blood acting on the elastic arteries.

It is important to note, however, that the mean pressure—the best single measure of effective driving pressure—is lower in the more distal arteries than at the arch of the aorta, as might be expected at a point downstream from the pressure source. However, the pressure loss in the large arteries is small because of their large radius.

With further peripheral transmission and with the progressive decrease in the arterial radii, the pulse waves are gradually dampened, particularly in the arterioles where the pressure reaches values of 40 to 60 mm Hg. The pulsatile characteristics of the pressure waves are ordinarily extinguished at the capillaries and veins. The venous pressure waves, which reappear in the large veins close to the heart, are similar to the atrial waves (Chapter 3, Fig. 3.4); they are due to backward transmission and reflect events of the right heart and not the left.

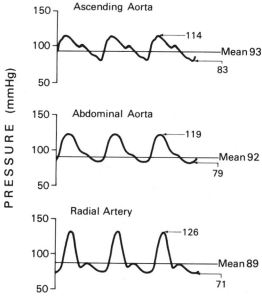

Figure 6.3. Pressure waves at different sites in the arterial tree. With transmission of the pressure wave into the distal aorta and large arteries, the systolic pressure increases and the diastolic pressure decreases, with a resultant heightening of the pulse pressure. However, the mean arterial pressure declines steadily.

Determinants of Aortic Pressure

If the cardiac output (CO) is the ratio of the driving pressure (ΔP) and the total peripheral resistance (TPR) and if we assume the vena caval pressure is approximately zero, then ΔP becomes the mean aortic pressure (MAP) and we can, as stated in Chapter 2, formulate the generalization that MAP = CO × TPR.

If the remaining factor is held constant, an increase or decrease in either cardiac output or total peripheral resistance will result in a corresponding increase or decrease in mean aortic pressure. Cardiac output may, in turn, be altered either by a change in heart rate or stroke volume, so that changes in either of these factors may affect MAP depending on the net effect on cardiac output.

An analysis of the factors influencing arterial pressure (systolic, diastolic, pulse, and mean) is important (*a*) because in the cardiovascular system, arterial pressure is the prime regulated variable, and (*b*) because clinically, disturbances of these different pressure parameters may suggest the specific nature and site of the hemodynamic disorder.

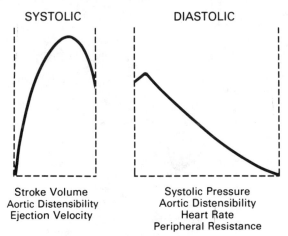

Figure 6.4.   Main determinants of aortic systolic and diastolic pressures.

Systolic and Diastolic Pressure

While mean pressure is a valuable measure, it is also possible to obtain useful information from the systolic and diastolic portions of the aortic pressure curve. The primary hemodynamic factors that produce and maintain these components of the pressure curve are shown in Figure 6.4. The relative importance of each factor has been determined mainly from circulatory models.

An increase in stroke volume will cause an increase in systolic pressure, mean pressure, and pulse pressure. A decrease in aortic distensibility (e.g., with advancing age) will result in an increase in systolic pressure; the lack of recoil will not sustain the diastolic pressure which will then fall off more rapidly, and as a consequence the pulse pressure will increase substantially. More rapid ejection will cause greater pulse pressure because of inadequate time for the aortic wall to distend in response to the ejected volume. An increased heart rate will interrupt the diastolic decline at a higher point on the curve and raise the diastolic pressure. An increased peripheral resistance will, as previously noted, raise the mean arterial pressure; the diastolic pressure and eventually the systolic pressure will also be raised, depending on the degree of change in peripheral resistance.

It should be emphasized that the above represent hemodynamic tendencies with a change in one variable. In the intact organism, the situation is often more complex, since two or more factors may coexist, and the resulting compensatory reflex responses may be superimposed. However, changes in the systolic and diastolic pressure and in the wave configuration can and do provide useful clues to important central and peripheral hemodynamic events.

Arterial Blood Pressure

Pulse Pressure

The pulse pressure is the difference between the systolic and diastolic pressures and would, of course, not exist in a constant flow system. It is due to the force imparted to the arterial blood column by left ventricular contraction, which produces a pressure increment over and above the existing diastolic arterial pressure. The pulse wave excursions, when recorded from the body surface (*e.g.*, over the radial artery at the wrist) are damped versions of the arterial pressure wave. The area of the wave will be roughly proportional to the ventricular stroke volume and the character of the wave (*e.g.*, the upstroke) will generally reflect aortic distensibility and ejection velocity, as previously described.

Palpation of the pulse at the carotid or radial artery can give general indications of (*a*) *rate and rhythm of the heart*—extrasystoles may be detected if the ejection is forceful enough to transmit the impulse to the periphery; (*b*) *pulse pressure*—often will be increased in hypertension, advanced arteriosclerosis, or aortic regurgitation; it will be decreased in deep shock in which the rapid, "thready" pulse is characteristic; (*c*) *approximate level of arterial pressure*—may be gauged by the tension required to obliterate the pulse entirely with one finger while palpating with an adjacent finger.

Normal Values

In the foregoing section, emphasis has been placed on the components of arterial pressure and the central and peripheral hemodynamic factors that may affect arterial pressure in an acute situation. There are other factors that affect arterial pressure on a long-term basis. Individuals who are more responsive to stress may show rather wide variations in arterial blood pressure. In such individuals repeated daily measurements after a brief rest period will help to determine the true normal value for that individual.

Age is an important factor. With advancing years there is a progressive tendency toward increase in both systolic and diastolic pressures (Fig. 6.5) as well as increases in peripheral vascular resistance. However, physiological age often does not parallel chronological age, and there may be wide individual differences in hemodynamic values among apparently healthy individuals. For example, Lakatta has shown that in some individuals arterial pressures do not rise with age, and many of these subjects do not have increased systemic vascular resistance. Differences in arterial pressures will depend mainly upon physical fitness, hereditary, dietary, and socio-environmental factors.

Effect of Gravity on the Circulatory System

Posture will have marked effects on vascular pressures and volumes in various parts of the body, depending on the vertical distance of the blood column

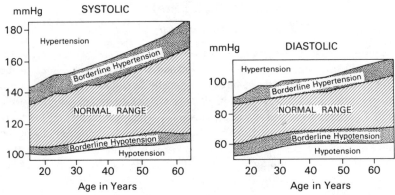

Figure 6.5. Normal range of systolic and diastolic blood pressure in different age groups. (Reprinted with permission from R.F. Rushmer, *Cardiovascular Dynamics*, 4th ed. Philadelphia: W.B. Saunders Co., 1976.)

from the heart. Upon quiet standing, the foot veins and arteries in an average adult are about 120 cm below the heart; this adds a hydrostatic pressure of 120 cm of H_2O, or about 88 mm Hg (Fig. 6.6). It is important to note that although the pressures inside the dependent vessels are increased, the driving pressure (the impetus forcing blood from the arterial side to the venous side and back toward the heart) is unchanged, that is, it is unaffected by gravity, because the increases in pressure on the arterial and venous sides are the same.

The effective driving pressure at any point propelling blood toward the heart will, therefore, be the gauge pressure (that relative to the atmosphere) minus the gravity pressure. All intravascular pressures must be so "corrected" by adding or subtracting the vertical height of the fluid column. If, for example, the gauge pressure in a foot vein of our "average" subject (referred to above) were 102 mm Hg, the effective driving pressure (ΔP) would be 14 mm Hg. However, in the upright position, the full gravity (hydrostatic) pressure would be effective laterally (*i.e.*, across the vessel walls) and would greatly increase transmural pressure and transudation of fluid through capillary walls.

In the upright position, gauge pressures in the arterial tree above the heart will be negative, and the true arterial driving pressure is obtained by *adding* the appropriate hydrostatic correction factor. However, venous pressures in the cranium are more complicated and less predictable. In the upright position, the veins inside the skull do not collapse because of their close equilibrium with cerebrospinal fluid, which is at a negative pressure, and because of the anatomical fixation of certain cranial veins (Cerebral Circulation, Chapter 11).

In order to compare vascular pressures in different individuals, it is cus-

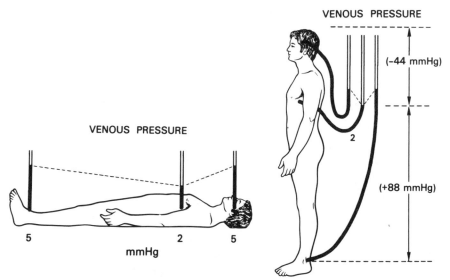

Figure 6.6.   Effect of erect position on vascular pressures in the foot and head. Pressures taken in the lower part of the body should be corrected by subtracting the pressure equivalent of the vertical distance below the heart. (Reprinted with permission from A.C. Burton, *Physiology and Biophysics of the Circulation*, 2nd ed. Chicago: Year Book Medical Publishers, 1972.)

tomary to use a common reference point. For this purpose, such pressures are commonly expressed in terms of vertical height above or below the "phlebostatic level," which passes transversely through the thorax between the anterior and posterior surfaces of the trunk at the level of the fourth intercostal space.

Volume (as well as pressure) changes will occur in the upright posture because of the height of the vertical blood column. Upon assumption of the upright position, about 500 to 700 ml (8 to 10 ml/kg) of blood is rapidly dislocated from the thorax (thoracic or central blood volume) to the lower extremities. This intravascular dislocation is very rapid and about 90% complete within one to two minutes, and results in increased volume in the lower part of the body (buttocks, pelvis, and especially the lower extremities). This is followed immediately by a progressive but slower and less marked capillary transudation into the lower extremities due to the increased hydrostatic pressure. The compensatory responses in healthy subjects tend to limit the interstitial fluid accumulation in the legs. In certain cardiac patients, however, the added hydrostatic pressure will increase net capillary transudation of fluid from capillaries causing dependent edema (Chapter 14).

These very pronounced pressure and volume changes in the circulation are largely offset in healthy individuals by several compensatory responses of the circulation—particularly (*a*) by reflex sympathetic vasoconstriction which helps maintain peripheral resistance and arterial pressure, and (*b*) by the skeletal muscle pump. The normal and abnormal responses to postural stress are further discussed in Chapter 13.

Venous System: Physical Characteristics

Pressure-Volume Relations

The basic pressure-volume properties of veins and the relative distensibility and compliance of the arterial and venous systems were discussed in Chapter 1. In this and the immediately following sections, attention will be directed to how the veins function within the circulatory system.

The study of venous hemodynamics is complicated by (*a*) the low intravascular pressure, (*b*) the intermittent nature of the flow (which varies between high velocity and absolute cessation), (*c*) the gravity effect, (*d*) the retrograde pulse transmission in the vena cavae, (*e*) the presence of valves, and (*f*) the collapsible nature of the venous wall. Thus, in many respects, venous flow patterns are more complex than those of the arteries.

As previously shown (Fig. 1.4), the veins constitute the most voluminous portion of the circulatory system. Their compliance, *i.e.*, the unit volume accommodated per unit pressure (dV/dP), is about 25 to 30 times greater than that of the arterial tree. Consequently, when blood or plasma is infused into the vascular system, these fluids, since they seek pressure equilibrium, tend to distribute themselves rather rapidly in the venous and arterial system in the same ratio (*i.e.*, about 25 to 30 times more blood migrates to the venous than to the arterial bed). Conversely, in case of hemorrhage, the loss of volume is mainly from the venous rather than the arterial system.

Venous Pressure Measurement

Venous pressures, either peripheral or central, are ordinarily determined by intravascular catheterization. Because venous pressures are low, they are usually expressed as centimeters of H_2O in a vertical manometer using a sensitive pressure transducer. The pulsatile arterial pressure is ordinarily damped out and becomes nonpulsatile at the capillary level. In the venules and large peripheral veins, the pressures remain nonpulsatile, but at the vena cavae level, pulsations again appear, reflecting contractile events on the right side of the heart. These pulsations resemble pressure wave patterns in the right atrium (Fig. 3.4). Mean pressure values on the venous side normally range from 10 to 15 mm Hg in small venules, from 4 to 8 mm Hg in peripheral veins, and from 0 to 2 mm Hg in the vena cavae. Thoracic vena caval pressure is also called "central venous pressure."

Venous Return to the Heart: Mean Circulatory Pressure

The factors influencing the return of the blood from the left ventricle through the low pressure side of the circulation and back to the heart may be generally classified as *mean circulatory pressure* and *auxiliary factors*. The mean circulatory pressure is a static pressure expressing the degree of fullness of the systemic circulation. This is a basic continuing force, sometimes called the systemic filling pressure (P_{SF}), which represents the hemodynamic gradient for the entire systemic circulation from the root of the aorta to the right atrium. Its mean value is about 7 mm Hg. The net driving pressure returning blood to the heart can then be visualized as the difference between the P_{SF} and right atrial pressure. The P_{SF} and its role in venous return is discussed further in Chapter 7.

Venous Return to the Heart: Auxiliary Factors

These do not operate continuously but assist venous return under certain circumstances. The auxiliary factors are

1. The skeletal muscle pump of the lower extremity—which assists venous return during quiet standing, walking, or running;
2. Venous valves—are present only in the extremities and are important adjuncts to the skeletal muscle pump;
3. Venomotor tone—sympathetic constriction will aid venous return, for example, during hemorrhage or other stresses; conversely, skin venodilation can materially aid the dissipation of heat from the body core to the periphery during hyperthermia;
4. Respiratory pump—can aid venous return through alteration of pulmonary volume and pressure;
5. Suction effect of cardiac contraction and relaxation.

Skeletal Muscle Pump

Upon standing, the quick migration of blood from the thorax to the lower parts of the body is a significant stress to the circulatory system, resulting in a decrease in venous return and a 20 to 25% fall in cardiac output (Chapter 13). Almost immediately, the skeletal muscles of the lower extremities begin rhythmic cycles of reflex contraction and relaxation which are responsible for the unconscious swaying motion of the body during quiet standing. During such muscle contraction the blood is squeezed centrally, and during relaxation the veins refill. This cyclical action of the antigravity muscles of the body, which milks the venous blood toward the heart, is due to the "skeletal muscle pump."

After the contraction cycle the venous valves prevent retrograde flow, and the veins fill rapidly from below during the relaxation phase of the cycle.

Competent valves are indispensable for efficient functioning of the skeletal muscle pump. During quiet standing, this rhythmic action of the skeletal muscle pump during postural sway is an important mechanism for maintaining venous return.

Standing on a thick rug creates minor instability of the lower extremities, facilitates muscle pump action, and makes standing more comfortable. Conversely, on very hard surfaces, such as cement, stimulation of the plantar surfaces of the feet (from which the skeletal muscle pump reflex originates) is inhibited and skeletal muscle pump activity is much reduced. Prolonged standing on such surfaces is fatiguing because of the continued tendency toward a decrease in cardiac output.

In order for the lower extremity muscles to serve as an effective pump during standing, it is necessary for the feet to anchor the body, so that skeletal muscles may have a counterweight against which to contract. The importance of this factor is underscored by the fact that if the body is suspended in an upright position so that the feet dangle and cannot reach the ground, the unconscious milking action of the lower extremity muscles is largely prevented. In this situation most individuals suffer marked reduction of venous return and cardiac output. A 20- to 40-minute suspension in this fashion will produce fainting and a longer exposure may be life threatening. The ancient practice of execution by crucifixion was largely based on the resultant circulatory stress from upright suspension. On the other hand, massive and widespread skeletal muscle contraction such as a grand mal epileptic seizure will cause excessive venous return with increased cardiac output and heightened arterial pressure. A similar increase in venous pressure and venous return will result from widespread sympathetic stimulation of the vascular system (Chapter 7).

While the pump is important in quiet standing, it also plays a key role in maintaining venous return during walking and running. During these activities, the muscle pump action serves to lower venous pressure in the dependent parts of the leg, facilitate venous return, and relieve venous congestion in the area. Excess blood in the extremities not only creates a deficit in circulating blood volume but in some circumstances also hampers capillary exchange and cellular nutrition of the part. The effectiveness of the muscle pump is illustrated by a marked fall in calf venous pressure with only a single step after quiet standing (Fig. 6.7A). With several steps, the muscle action will milk the blood toward the heart and maintain a lower volume and pressure in the dependent veins (Fig. 6.7B). As might be expected, the effectiveness of the muscle pump is also dependent on the rate of inflow of blood into the leg (i.e., the rate of venous filling). If the leg is kept cool (25°C), the arterial inflow is less and the return to baseline venous pressure after quiet standing will therefore be slower (Fig. 6.7Bc). At a higher skin temperature (33°C), arterial inflow to the veins is faster and the return to the higher venous volume

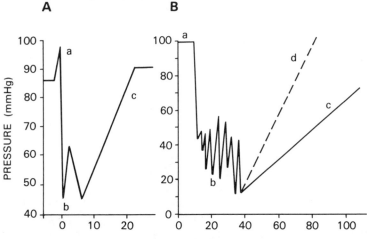

TIME (sec)

Figure 6.7. Effect of gravity and leg movement on venous pressure in the ankle. *A* shows at (*a*) a decrease of pressure of 50 mm Hg from quiet standing position to completion of first step at (*b*) and a rapid rise of pressure toward control with resumption of quiet standing at (*c*). *B,* Venous pressure at the ankle during quiet standing (*a*) and during walking (*b*). The slope of pressure return during quiet standing is relatively shallow if the skin of the foot is cool (25°C) (*c*). The rate of rise is doubled at a higher foot temperature (33°C) (*d*). (Adapted from A.A. Pollack and E.H. Wood, *J Appl Physiol* 1:649, 1948–1949; and from J.P. Henry and O. Gauer, *J Clin Invest* 29:855, 1950.)

and pressure is more rapid (Fig. 6.7*Bd*). At a still warmer skin temperature of 39°C (not shown), the venous pressure returns to the standing level in less than 10 seconds (*i.e.*, the muscle pump during quiet standing is even less efficient in milking blood centralward and in counteracting the increased venous volume and pressure in the lower extremities). This diminished effectiveness of the muscle pump at higher temperatures is instrumental in decreasing the postural tolerance of heart failure patients during hot weather. These patients already have a deficient cardiac pump and generally lessened skeletal muscle tone.

The skeletal muscle pump is, therefore, an important mechanism for counteracting the caudal sequestration of blood and maintaining venous return in the upright posture. Its importance is being increasingly recognized, and Rowell, for example, has called it the "second heart."

Venous Valves

Venous valves are very thin, transparent, cusp-like structures in the veins of the extremities, which insure unidirectional flow. The walls of the veins surrounding the valves are usually expanded into a sinus, which allows the cusps to separate fully without contraction of the walls, permitting rapid valve closure. Valves are present at about 2 to 4 cm intervals in the deep and superficial veins of the leg (even in veins of 0.08 to 0.15 mm in diameter) and are more numerous in deep than in superficial veins. Valves become scarce toward the heart, and only 24% of external iliac veins have valves. There usually are none in the common iliac vein, the abdominal vena cavae, or in the splanchnic circulation.

Varicose Veins

Varicose veins are vessels that have become distended and tortuous because of incompetent valves and/or prolonged obstruction due to pregnancy, abdominal tumor, or prolonged weight bearing. Venous valves usually become incompetent because of congenital defects or previous attacks of thrombophlebitis (inflammation of the vein). The essential defect is a chronic venous hypertension in the lower extremities due to valvular insufficiency in the superficial veins (usually the greater saphenous), the deep veins, or the communicating veins. Resting venous pressures are not abnormally high in varicose veins, but the pressure fall during walking is much less and the return to the higher pressures upon quiet standing is much faster. Varicose veins are more common in the female at a ratio of about 5:1. The defect is strongly hereditary.

In the dependent position, limbs with varicose veins contain more blood than normal because of their greater diameter, length, and distensibility. In view of this, one might anticipate an exaggerated physiologic response to the head-up position. However, this does not ordinarily occur. The lack of fainting or other reaction to the head-up position may be due to an increase in total blood volume that is often found in varicose vein patients and which may exert a partially compensating effect.

Although not a serious circulatory disorder, *per se*, varicose veins, if widespread and chronic, may predispose to circulatory problems of the lower extremities. Unlike arterial insufficiency, which usually results in ischemia and decreased flow and volume to the affected area, venous insufficiency leads to tissue congestion, edema, impairment of tissue nutrition, and painless leg ulcers that heal with great difficulty. The most serious complication of a varicosity is a thrombosis (clot) in the vein with subsequent breaking off of a clot segment and central embolization (blood stream conduction) *via* the vena cavae, and impaction into a branch of the pulmonary artery in the lungs. Small emboli are generally absorbed without difficulty but massive widespread embolization with occlusion of more than 50% of the pulmonary vascular bed may produce hypoxemia, pulmonary hypertension, shock, and death.

Venomotor Tone

The state of contraction of venous smooth muscle is a significant factor in venous return, but the effect of this muscle contraction depends on the intravascular pressure. At low pressures (0–5 mm Hg), veins take on an elliptical shape and contraction of the vascular muscle has little effect on volume; thus the venous wall movement is mainly passive. However, when venous pressures exceed 5 to 10 mm Hg, veins assume a more circular cross section and muscle fibers have increasing length and tension; in this case, venomotor activity is much more effective and a small increase in tone or contractile state can shift a large amount of blood toward the heart (Fig. 1.6).

The efferent neural control of venous smooth muscle is exclusively sympathetic and has important functional distributions (e.g., to the splanchnic and cutaneous tissues). The constriction of splanchnic veins in certain stresses (e.g., hemorrhage and shock) shifts the important reservoir of splanchnic blood into the general circulation and thus substantially aids venous return and cardiac output. Superficial veins of the extremities—especially of the skin—show sympathetic venoconstrictor responses during a deep inspiration or hyperventilation and may show contractile responses to a variety of emotional and physical stresses such as pain, fear, anger, and hemorrhage. Cutaneous vessels, including veins, play an important role in temperature regulation by constricting in cold and dilating in heat (Chapter 11). While superficial veins of the extremities respond strongly to sympathetic stimulation, deep veins of the calf and forearm respond very little and veins of skeletal muscle not at all to neural stimuli.

Respiratory Pump

This refers to the assistance given to venous return by the mechanical movements of respiration. The intrathoracic pressure is usually slightly subatmospheric and varies during quiet breathing from about − 2 to − 4 mm Hg during expiration to about − 5 to − 7 mm Hg during inspiration. As the intrathoracic pressure falls during inspiration, the intraabdominal pressure rises due to the descent of the diaphragm. These changes in pressure gradient facilitate venous return from extrathoracic veins during inspiration and diminish it during expiration.

As a result of these pressure changes, there is an increased flow and volume into the thoracic vena cavae during inspiration, which aids right ventricular filling and increases right ventricular stroke volume. However, the simultaneously increased capacity of the pulmonary vessels (during inspiration) temporarily decreases left ventricular filling and stroke volume. This process is reversed during expiration. Honig has stated that the right ventricular output changes ± 25% during respiration, but that due to the large blood volume of

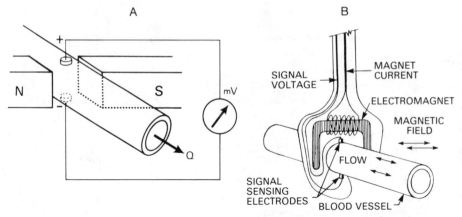

Figure 6.8.   *A*, Principle of the electromagnetic flowmeter. When a conducting fluid containing ions flows through a magnetic field, an electromagnetic force will be generated perpendicular to the field and proportional to the velocity of the fluid. (Reprinted with permission from T.C. Ruch and H.D. Patton, *Physiology and Biophysics*. Philadelphia: W.B. Saunders, 1974.) *B*, Schematic showing incorporation of the elements into a flowmeter probe.

the pulmonary reservoir, the left ventricle is far less dependent on moment-to-moment changes in venous return and its output varies only 5 to 7% during the respiratory cycle.

The above tendencies are exaggerated with heightening of the respiratory movements and the consequent increases in respiratory pressure increments. However, the effect is limited because of the likelihood of venous collapse at the point of entrance of the veins into the thorax if intravenous pressure becomes negative at that level (Chapter 7).

"Suction" Effect of Cardiac Contraction

While the P_{SF} (systemic filling pressure) is the main force driving blood toward the heart, the ventricles also contribute to venous return. During ventricular systole, when the AV valves are closed, the AV ring is drawn downward by the ventricles, enlarging the atria, thereby lowering their relative internal pressures, and thus increasing flow from the vena cavae and pulmonary veins. Current evidence further suggests that during diastole, the ventricles also exert a negative pressure by virtue of the "diastolic recoil" of their walls, particularly in hypotensive states such as circulatory shock.

Blood Flow Measurement: Methods

Because the interpretation of blood flow and blood pressure data is closely linked with how the data are obtained, a brief review will be made of the

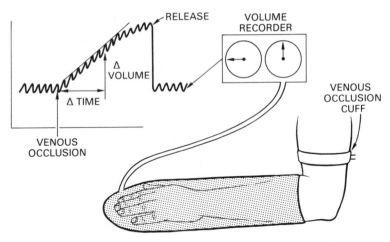

Figure 6.9. Venous occlusion plethysmograph. When the cuff is rapidly inflated to 50 mm Hg, venous outflow is prevented and for the next few seconds, the volume increase in the plethysmograph will reflect the arterial inflow. The initial slope of increased volume per unit time on the calibrated volume recorder will indicate the blood flow to the forearm in milliliters per minute.

more common methods in current use. Flow methods applicable to cardiac output, (*i.e.*, central blood flow) will be discussed in Chapter 7. Following is a brief description of the principles involved in sensing peripheral flow.

Electromagnetic Flowmeter. This invasive method is widely used in experimental studies to determine pulsatile flow in individual arteries (Fig. 6.8). A collar or probe that has two small electrodes positioned on opposite sides of the artery is placed around the blood vessel. Two small magnets in the probe produce a magnetic field across the blood vessel. When a conductor such as blood moves through this field, the electric potential developed at the electrodes is proportional to the velocity of the stream. Knowing the cross-sectional area of the vessel, the volume flow per minute can be calculated. This is an excellent method for accurate flow measurement in an isolated vessel and is particularly applicable to animal studies.

Venous Occlusion Plethysmography. This method is particularly suitable for blood flow determination in an intact limb in human subjects, for example, in the calf or forearm. By enclosing the extremity in an airtight container and sealing the skin junction, sudden temporary occlusion of the venous return with an occlusion cuff at a pressure of 50 to 60 mm Hg will permit the recording of the volume change per unit time of the limb (Fig. 6.9). Since a temporary venous occlusion will not affect arterial flow, this limb volume change will, for the first 6 to 8 seconds, faithfully record the arterial inflow to the limb. The determination can be repeated after relatively short intervals. By means of an arterial tourniquet at the wrist or ankle, the hand or foot blood flow, which is primarily skin flow, can be excluded; this will permit flow measurements on the forearm or calf alone, which consist primarily of skeletal muscle tissue. This is a convenient and useful noninvasive method in which flows to different tissues of a limb can be determined, for example, in patients with peripheral vascular disease.

Impedance Flowmeter. If band electrodes are placed about a limb (*e.g.*, the calf) and the electrodes are excited by a high-frequency (100 kHz) sinusoidal current, the observed voltage and impedance changes are dependent on the blood volume changes. From the impedance wave forms, the volume flow through the limb may be calculated. The low-amplitude, high-frequency current has no injurious effect on the tissues; the impedance method is also adaptable for noninvasive determination of cardiac output (Chapter 7, Impedance Cardiography).

Ultrasonic Flowmeter. There has been increasing interest in the use of ultrasound for a variety of biological measurements including the detection of arterial and venous flow. High frequency sound waves are directed across the vessel and reflected back from the moving erythrocytes to a sensor. There is a shift in the frequency of the sound, depending on the velocity of flow, known as the Doppler effect. By detecting the relative velocities of these sound transmissions, the volume flow in the blood vessel can be estimated knowing the cross-sectional area of the vessel. One advantage of the ultrasonic method is that the detector can be positioned on the surface of the body so that blood flow may be determined in a noninvasive manner. The adaptation of ultrasound cardiography, called echocardiography, for the determination of cardiac output, is described in the following chapter.

Nuclear Magnetic Resonance (NMR). Some atomic nuclei, such as hydrogen and phosphorus 31, have odd numbers of protons and neutrons and thus exhibit net spin and generate small magnetic fields. The alignment of the nuclei within a strong external magnetic field can be reoriented by another weak, rapidly alternating magnetic field (radio frequency) transmitted at the resonant frequency of the nuclei. There are marked differences in nuclear reorientation times in different tissues such as, fat, muscle, and blood, making it possible to produce anatomically differentiating images of these tissues. NMR imaging is now widely used in clinical medicine. The recent development of MR continuous wave (CW) technology with much faster data output permits the scanning of pulsed blood flow in a quantitative manner in human limbs. The technique is entirely noninvasive. Early studies have indicated that the method is reliable and may provide a very effective diagnostic aid in peripheral vascular disease.

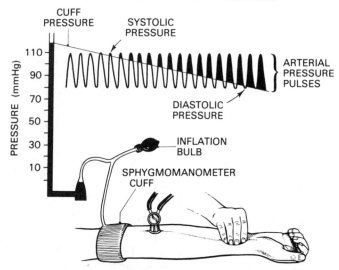

Figure 6.10.   Illustration of the auscultatory and palpatory techniques for the indirect method of measuring arterial blood pressure. The appearance and disappearance of the auscultatory sounds are illustrated. (Reprinted with permission from R.F. Rushmer. *Cardiovascular Dynamics*. Philadelphia: W.B. Saunders, 1976.)

Blood Pressure Measurement: Methods

Direct Method of Measuring Arterial Blood Pressure

This involves the placement of a needle or catheter directly into the artery. Pressure and flow studies in a pulsatile system have helped to clarify the requirements for such direct arterial pressure recording; in order to adequately register pressure fluctuations at a given heart rate, a manometer system must accurately respond to frequencies of pulsation at least seven times the frequency of the heart rate.

The strain gauge pressure transducer, which is commonly employed for such arterial pressure sensing, consists of a stiff diaphragm to which are bonded several strain gauges capable of responding rapidly to the transient pressure changes. The hydraulic system that couples the transducer to the artery by means of a catheter is an important element. To retain maximum frequency response, it should be of maximum bore and of minimum length in order to avoid excessive damping of the pressure wave.

The direct method provides the most accurate pressure data; however, it

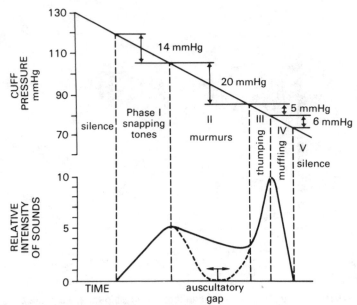

Figure 6.11. Korotkoff sounds characteristic of the auscultatory phases during measurement of blood pressure in the human. (Reprinted with permission from L.A. Geddes, *The Direct and Indirect Measurement of Blood Pressure*. Chicago: Year Book Medical Publishers, 1970.)

is invasive and, since it involves the placement of a catheter in the vessel, requires that the procedure be performed under sterile conditions.

Indirect Blood Pressure Methods

These are most commonly used because of their practicability and ease of repetition. The method depends on either (*a*) the production of Korotkoff sounds, which are mainly the result of turbulence in the stream, or (*b*) the appearance and disappearance of the palpated arterial pulse (Fig. 6.10).

The instrument used is a sphygmomanometer, which consists of an inelastic cuff that encloses a rubber bag. Inflation of the cuff to a level above systolic pressure will occlude all blood flow to and from the arm. Gradual reduction of the cuff pressure will permit a return of arterial flow as detected by the appearance of an audible tapping sound at the brachial artery below the cuff, marking the systolic pressure. Progressive decrease of the pressure will produce characteristic sound fluctuations (Fig. 6.11) until final muffling and disappearance of the sound. Muffling is the best index of diastolic pressure in children. Disappearance of the sounds is regarded as the best index of diastolic blood pressure in adults. In some individuals (especially in hypertensive patients), during the lowering of the cuff pressure, the sounds may temporarily disappear and then reappear, a possible source of error in the determination (auscultatory gap, Fig. 6.11). To avoid errors in reading, the cuff must be the correct width for the patient's arm. If it is too narrow, the pressure reading will be erroneously high; if it is too wide, the reading may be erroneously low. The width of the inflatable bladder should be 40% of the circumference of the midpoint of the limb (or 20% wider than the diameter) on which it is to be used. For the average adult arm, a bladder 12 to 14 cm wide has been found to be satisfactory.

Although the indirect method does not provide a continuous recording and is not as accurate as the direct, it is rapid and convenient. If carefully performed, this method serves adequately in most clinical circumstances.

Suggested Readings

Abel FL and McCutcheon EP. *Cardiovascular Function: Principles and Applications.* Boston: Little, Brown, 1979.

Battocletti J, Halbach RE, Salles-Cunha S, and Sances A. The NMR blood flow meter: theory and history, *Med Phys* 8:439, 1981.

Beecher HK, Fiel E, and Krogh A. The effects of walking on venous pressure at the ankle. *Scand Archives J Physiol* 73:133, 1936.

Englund N, Hallbreuk T, and Ling LG. The validity of strain gauge plethysmography. *Scand J Clin Lab Invest* 29:155, 1972.

Geddes LA. *Direct and Indirect Measurement of Blood Pressure.* Chicago: Yearbook Medical Publishers, 1970.

Geddes LA and Baker LE. *Principles of Applied Biomedical Instrumentation,* 2nd ed. New York: John Wiley & Sons, 1975.

Honig CR. *Modern Cardiovascular Physiology.* Boston: Little, Brown, pp 127–131, 1981.

Kirkendall WM, Feinleib M, Freis ED, and Mark AL. *Recommendations for Human Blood Pressure Determination by Sphygmomanometers.* Dallas: American Heart Association, 1980.

Lakatta EG. Hemodynamic adaptation to stress with advancing age. *Acta Med Scand* 711(supp):39, 1986.

Laughlin MH. Skeletal muscle blood flow. Role of the muscle pump in exercise hyperemia. *Am J Physiol* 253:H993, 1987.

Milnor WR. *Hemodynamics.* Baltimore: Williams & Wilkins, 1982.

Porth CM. *Pathophysiology,* 2nd ed. Philadelphia: Lippincott, 1986.

Rothe CF. The venous system: the physiology of the capacitance vessels. In: *Handbook of Physiology,* Section 2: *The Cardiovascular System,* edited by FM Abboud and JT Shepherd. Bethesda, Md.: American Physiological Society, 1983, Vol. III.

Rowell LB, *Human Circulation: Regulation During Physical Stress.* New York: Oxford University Press, 1986.

Shepherd JT and Van Houtte PM. *Veins and Their Control.* Philadelphia: W.B. Saunders, 1975.

Smith JJ and Ebert TJ. General response to orthostatic stress. In: *Circulatory Response to the Upright Posture,* edited by JJ Smith. Boca Raton, Fla.: CRC Press, (in press).

chapter 7

Venous Return and Cardiac Output

Undoubtedly one of the most basic cardiovascular measurements is the output of the heart. It is usually defined as the volume of blood ejected per minute by either ventricle and since the two ventricles, except in unusual circumstances, are in balance, the two outputs are essentially equal. The two prime determinants of tissue blood flow are metabolic rate and tissue mass. It is generally recognized that cardiac output increases approximately in proportion to an increase in body metabolism. This is illustrated by the fact that cardiac output is increased in fever and exercise and decreased in conditions such as sleep and hypothyroidism.

At rest, cardiac output is strongly correlated with body mass and body surface area. The latter is in more common clinical use, although there is very little experimental basis for such a preference. In the healthy resting human adult, mean cardiac output is about 80 ml/kg/min or about 3.2 L/min/ M^2 of body surface area. Thus, in an average-sized subject (70 kg), the total cardiac output would be about 5.6 L/min. Age importantly influences cardiac output. From its maximum value at age 27, cardiac output in the human decreases about 1% per year so that at age 65, it has decreased to about 60% of its value in early adulthood.

Regulation of Cardiac Output—General

In a closed, artificial, hydraulic system consisting of a pump and pipes, the output depends on the characteristics of the pump, of the system, and of the fluid. To obtain the required flow, the usual procedure is to determine the resistance and then set the pump speed at the level necessary to overcome that resistance and thus achieve the desired output. In the human circulation, however, the situation is quite different; both the pipe system and the fluid are able to change characteristics from time to time and thereby impose varying demands on the pump.

Since the main changes in cardiac output are determined by the metabolic requirements of the body and not by voluntarily switching the pump to a higher setting, it is evident that the body sets the pace and not the pump. Thus, as will be discussed later in this chapter, the heart, from a flow standpoint, plays a "permissive" role and does not regulate its own output. So in the human circulation, the heart functions as a "demand" pump and will eject only the minimum volume demanded of it.

The output of the heart therefore represents a balance between the venous return—the demand—and the ability of the heart to meet that demand. The healthy, normal heart does, however, have impressive resources at its own disposal and is well able to meet a large range of ordinary demands. On the other hand, when diseased, the heart may not be able to cope and it becomes the limiting factor in controlling the output. When its capabilities are exceeded, signs and symptoms of cardiac failure appear (Chapter 14).

For these reasons it is necessary to consider the regulation of cardiac output from two different standpoints: (*a*) *the role of systemic factors* in determining cardiac output (*i.e.*, what influences the return flow of blood to the heart) and (*b*) *the role of cardiac factors* in determining cardiac output (*i.e.*, what influences the ability of the heart to pump out the blood returned to it).

Systemic Factors Determining Cardiac Output—Venous Return Curves

In a discussion of venous flow in Chapter 6, it was pointed out that the primary factor influencing the return of blood to the heart was the force transmitted by left ventricular ejection through the arteries to the veins. This pressure gradient is sometimes called the *vis a tergo* ("force from behind").

Guyton has analyzed the forces responsible for venous return to the heart from a somewhat different perspective. He has suggested the concept of a "mean circulatory filling pressure," which is the average of the pressures in all segments of the vascular system when each of these pressures is weighted in proportion to the compliance of its respective segment. This average pressure would be a single, integrated, hydrostatic measure of the degree of filling of the circulation and would represent the force tending to propel blood toward the right atrium. He pointed out that without such a filling pressure and return force the cardiac output would be zero no matter how actively the heart pumped.

Guyton found that this single mean circulatory filling pressure of the systemic circuit could be measured in animals by suddenly arresting the heart and rapidly pumping blood from the aorta to the vena cavae until the pressures equalized. The pressure measurements must be made quickly (within about 7 seconds) before any autonomic reflexes become effective.

Determined in this manner, the mean circulatory filling pressure for the systemic system, called the *systemic filling pressure* (P_{SF}), is about 7 mm Hg in the dog and is believed to be very similar in man. The *mean pulmonary filling pressure* (P_{PF}), the comparable figure for the pulmonary circuit, is about 5 mm Hg.

Viewed in this perspective, the beating heart in the living animal has the essential function of transporting blood from the low-pressure, high-compliance venous system to the high-pressure, low-compliance arterial system. This rearrangement of volumes and pressures enables the arterial system to provide the necessary pressure head for perfusion of all the peripheral tissues. In a normal, unstressed circulation, the mean circulatory pressures would be similar to those determined in the arrested heart.

Under circumstances in which nervous and other controls are not operative, the venous return to the right atrium may be theoretically determined as the balance between the systemic filling pressure (P_{SF}), the force tending to return

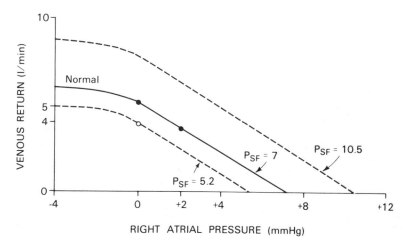

Figure 7.1. On the normal venous return curve (*solid line*), the venous return is about 5.5 L/min when the systemic filling pressure (P_{SF}) is 7 mm and the right atrial pressure (P_{RA}) about 0. If, on the normal curve, the P_{RA} is increased to about 2 mm Hg or the P_{SF} decreased to 5.2 mm Hg, the venous return would decrease to about 4 L/min. (Reprinted with permission from A.C. Guyton, *Circulatory Physiology: Cardiac Output and Its Regulation*. Philadelphia: W.B. Saunders, 1973.)

blood to the right atrium, and the right atrial pressure (P_{RA}), the opposing force. The resulting venous return at different levels of P_{SF} and P_{RA} are shown in the form of venous return curves in Figure 7.1.

In the schema of Figure 7.1, the estimated venous return can be read off the y axis at the intersecting point of the P_{RA} and P_{SF} curve. At normal values of 7 mm Hg P_{SF} and about zero for P_{RA}, the 7 mm gradient will induce a venous flow of about 5.5 L/min. In case of decreased blood volume (*e.g.*, hemorrhage) or loss of sympathetic tone, which would decrease both arterial and venous pressure, the P_{SF} will also decrease; if the P_{SF} decreases to 5.2 and P_{RA} remains at zero, the net pressure gradient is reduced to 5.2 and venous return decreases to about 4 L/min. If the P_{SF} is 7 and P_{RA} is increased to 2 mm Hg, the gradient for venous return is reduced to 5 mm Hg and the output is also reduced to about 4 L/min. Increased venous return curves (*e.g.*, the above-normal P_{SF} curve of 10.5 mm Hg in Figure 7.1) might occur with increased blood volume, increased sympathetic stimulation, or a massive contraction of skeletal muscle with excessive skeletal muscle pump action and heightened peripheral venous pressure.

It will be noted that the P_{SF} curves become flat at right atrial pressures below the zero level. This plateau is due to the collapse of veins entering the chest whenever the transmural pressure is less than zero. This stops effective flow no matter what the right atrial-P_{SF} gradient may be.

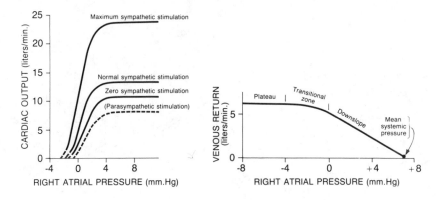

Figure 7.2. *Left, Cardiac output curve,* relating right atrial pressure and cardiac output. *Right, Normal venous return curve,* relating mean systemic pressure and right atrial pressure to venous return. (Reprinted with permission from A.C. Guyton, *Circulatory Physiology: Cardiac Output and Its Regulation.* Philadelphia: W.B. Saunders, 1973.)

While the venous return curves involve certain abstractions and include parameters that are difficult to measure, Guyton's analytic approach has been of considerable theoretical and practical assistance in understanding the basic factors concerned with venous return.

Cardiac Factors Determining Cardiac Output

Cardiac Output Curves

In Chapter 5, the classic Starling curve showed that after an increase in ventricular end-diastolic volume, the succeeding contraction will result in an increased intraventricular pressure (Fig. 5.5). This will result in an increased stroke volume and cardiac output. In this way, cardiac output can be related to right atrial pressure in the form of cardiac output curves as shown in Figure 7.2 (*left*). The up-slope of this curve is very steep, and cardiac output increases substantially with only small changes in right atrial pressure. The curves then plateau. The plateau represents the maximum cardiac pumping capacity, no matter how great the venous return.

As indicated in Figure 7.2 (*left*), at a normal level of sympathetic tone and at a normal level of right atrial pressure (*e.g.,* 0 mm Hg), the healthy heart will pump about 5 L/min. If sympathetic stimulation is increased or decreased, the cardiac output will be correspondingly increased or decreased at the same right atrial pressure—provided that the venous return is adequate. But, even very modest increases in right atrial pressure result in steep increases in cardiac output, and with a combination of 4 to 8 mm Hg of right atrial pressure and maximum sympathetic stimulation the maximum pumping capacity of the heart may increase to 20 to 25 L/min.

As pointed out by Thomsen, implicit in a "cardiac model" of circulatory regulation is the assumption that the heart always has access to an unlimited supply of venous blood, which will not be exhausted if cardiac function is enhanced. This assumption is usually invalid. For example, under normal circumstances, increases in heart rate induced by electrical pacing cause little change in cardiac output. Similarly, during cardiopulmonary bypass when the heart is replaced by a roller pump, it is not possible to arbitrarily increase pump output to any desired level. As roller pump output is increased the blood in the oxygenator reservoir is quickly depleted and pump flow cannot be further augmented unless circulating blood volume is increased. These examples indicate that the heart (or roller pump on bypass) does not normally have access to an unlimited supply of venous blood. In fact, cardiac output is often limited by the amount of blood returning to the heart from the systemic circulation, that is, the venous return (VR).

The venous return curves attempt to quantitate the venous return provided by the peripheral circulation, *i.e.*, by the mean systemic filling pressure (P_{SF}), at any given level of right atrial pressure. The cardiac output curves attempt to quantitate the output of the heart on the basis of the right atrial pressure provided by the peripheral circulation. Thus the common element is the right atrial pressure—a critical determinant of both venous return and cardiac output.

This conceptualization by Guyton also permits, for example, a combination of the venous return and cardiac output curves of Figures 7.2 left and right into single graphs (Fig. 7.3). In Figure 7.3A are shown normal venous return and cardiac output values in which these two variables are both related to right atrial pressure. The two curves intersect at a value of 5 L/min (point *a*). If the blood volume is increased by transfusion, the P_{SF} will be considerably increased as will the venous return and cardiac output (point *b*).

Sympathetic stimulation has two effects: (*a*) contraction of the peripheral vasculature, particularly of the venous bed, will increase the P_{SF} and therefore the pressure gradient for venous return, and (*b*) increase in cardiac contractile strength will move the ventricular function curve to the left (Fig. 5.8). As shown in Figure 7.3B, the venous return and cardiac output would both increase and their junction point would move from point *a* to *c*. Decreased sympathetic activity will have the reverse effect and move the cardiac output from point *a* to *b*.

It should be emphasized that the responses to stresses such as increased

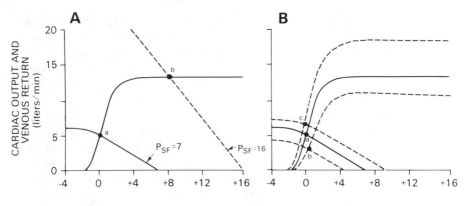

Figure 7.3. Combined venous return and cardiac output curves. *A,* A large blood transfusion increases the systemic filling pressure (P_{SF}) from 7 to 16 mm Hg and the right atrial pressure from 0 to 8 mm Hg. As a result, the venous return and cardiac output are considerably increased from point *a* to point *b*. *B,* Sympathetic stimulation increases P_{SF} through contraction of peripheral vessels (particularly veins) and so moves the venous return curve from the *solid line* to the *upper dashed line;* simultaneously it increases ventricular contractility and shifts the atrial pressure–cardiac output curve to the left. The cardiac output is, therefore, moved from point *a* to point *c.* Conversely, with sympathetic inhibition, the cardiac output might be reduced from point *a* to point *b.* (Reprinted with permission from A.C. Guyton, *Circulatory Physiology: Cardiac Output and Its Regulation.* Philadelphia: W.B. Saunders, 1973.)

blood volume, hemorrhage, and sympathetic stimulation are ordinarily damped by autonomic circulatory reflexes (Chapter 10) with a gradual return to the normal state. However, an understanding of the initial tendencies is important because they may persist for appreciable periods of time and in the diseased state may even progress.

Regulation of Stroke Volume

Since cardiac output is the product of stroke volume (SV) and heart rate (HR), cardiac output adjustments may be made by alteration of either or both of these two parameters. In the following sections the different means used by the heart to respond to the altered demands of the peripheral circulation are described.

At an HR of 70 beats/min the SV of a normal resting adult will be approximately 80 ml. The mean end-diastolic volume (EDV) at rest is variable but will normally range from about 110 to 130 ml. The ejection fraction (EF), the ratio SV/EDV, is normally about 67% in man but somewhat lower (45 to 65%) in the faster-beating canine heart; the blood remaining after ejection

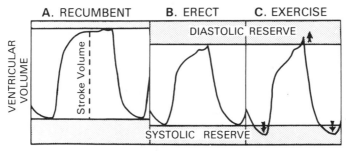

Figure 7.4.   Reserve stroke volume. Schematic representation showing ventricular volume and stroke volume (SV). Upon standing, heart rate is increased and stroke volume decreased; with exercise in the erect position, SV is increased through encroachment on both diastolic and systolic reserve. (Adapted from R.F. Rushmer, *Cardiovascular Dynamics*. Philadelphia: W.B. Saunders, 1976.)

is called the end-systolic volume (ESV). As shown in Figure 7.4, there is usually a diastolic and systolic reserve volume.

The four primary factors described in Chapter 5 as determinants of myocardial performance are also the main determinants of stroke volume; these factors are *diastolic filling (preload), inotropic state (contractility), aortic pressure (afterload),* and the *heart rate.* The first two of these factors importantly affect myocardial contraction; the last two exert mainly mechanical effects on cardiac output.

Diastolic Filling (Preload). As described in Chapter 5, the heart has an important intrinsic capability enabling it to make adjustments to changes in EDV. With increased venous return and increased filling, there is increased strength of the subsequent contraction and increased stroke volume; with decreased filling the reverse occurs.

Inotropic State. This important extrinsic factor enables the heart to contract more strongly at an equivalent diastolic volume. In the normal circulation, a positive inotropic effect is commonly mediated through sympathoadrenal discharge which will improve cardiac performance in several ways, *viz.,* ventricular contraction is more rapid (increased V_{max} and dP/dt) and is stronger. As a result the ventricles empty more completely (*i.e.,* there is a decreased ESV and increased SV) which will produce higher systolic pressures in the ventricle and aorta. Diastolic compliance, however, is not affected. If the cause of the increased inotropic state is sympathetic stimulation, there will be an associated increase in heart rate; as discussed below, the degree of stroke volume increase may be limited by the shortening of ventricular filling time incident to the rate increase. However, with sympathetic stimulation, the net result is usually an increased cardiac output. A negative inotropic effect, by vagal stimulation, will decrease heart rate and impulse conduction and diminish atrial contractility.

Aortic Pressure (Afterload). Alteration of aortic pressure will produce important effects on cardiac function because of the mechanical resistance it imposes on left ventricular emptying. Sudden aortic pressure changes will result in inverse changes in strength, velocity, and duration of left ventricular ejection and therefore of stroke volume. These effects were discussed in Chapter 5 and shown in isolated cardiac muscle in Figure 5.7. In the intact animal, there is, at the same atrial pressure, an inverse relation between aortic pressure and stroke volume when the arterial pressure is high. However, at normal mean arterial pressures (up to about 100 mm Hg), the cardiac output is relatively independent of arterial blood pressure. Even though the left ventricular stroke volume may be temporarily reduced by a moderate increase in systemic arterial pressure, the right ventricle continues to pump, which maintains the left ventricular filling pressure and end-diastolic volume. This factor, as well as the length-tension relation (Starling's law) shown in Figure 5.8, helps restore the left ventricular output at these higher arterial pressure levels.

Effect of Heart Rate on Stroke Volume. At a constant left atrial filling pressure, an increase in heart rate will decrease the diastolic filling time and, consequently, decrease the subsequent stroke volumes. However, most ventricular filling occurs during the initial rapid-filling phase. Since a modest increase in heart rate encroaches first on this late, slower-filling phase (diastisis), the effect on diastolic filling is minimized and cardiac output will increase. If other factors are held constant, the net effect of heart rate on cardiac output depends mainly on atrial filling pressure (*i.e.*, the adequacy of venous return), on the extent of the rate increase, and on the contractile or inotropic state of the ventricle.

If, while at rest, atrial filling pressures remain normal and the heart rate is progressively increased by using a pacemaker, cardiac output will rise at first, then level off, and at rates of 120 to 130 beats/min begin to decline. However, during sympathoadrenal stimulation or exercise, cardiac output will only begin to decline at rates of about 180 beats/min; this improved cardiac performance is due to a combination of increased venous return with increased atrial filling pressure and the inotropic effects mentioned above, *i.e.*, increased strength of ventricular contraction and a shortening of ventricular systole (with a relative lengthening of diastole). This better performance, however, is always contingent on an adequate atrial filling pressure and volume, that is, an adequate venous return. During exercise, the increased metabolic rate, the decreased peripheral resistance (especially in the exercising muscles), and the venoconstriction all contribute to the increased atrial filling. As a result, the increase in heart rate will be associated with an increase in cardiac output in the young adult up to rates of about 180 beats/min. With increasing age, this maximum rate will gradually decrease (Chapter 12).

Regulation of Heart Rate

While heart rate does affect stroke volume, it is a separately controlled variable that has other effects on cardiac performance. The chronotropic activity of the heart is normally determined by the rate of impulse generation in the SA node (Chapter 4). This, in turn, is influenced primarily by: (*a*) the autonomic balance between the sympathetic and vagal impulses to the node—sympathetic stimulation will increase heart rate and vagal stimulation will decrease it; (*b*) temperature and metabolic activity of the pacemaker tissue—increased temperature and metabolism will increase heart rate, reduced temperature and metabolism will have the reverse effect; and (*c*) the effect of ionic and pH changes on the heart. The latter effects are less important from a heart rate standpoint.

The autonomic balance—an important factor in cardiac control—is affected by several reflexes that influence heart rate, particularly those of the arterial and cardiopulmonary barocepters. The role of these reflexes will be discussed further in Chapter 10.

Integration of Stroke Volume and Heart Rate

As previously mentioned, an increase in thoracic vena caval and right atrial blood volume (*i.e.*, "central" blood volume and pressure) will cause an increase in the force of ventricular contraction (Starling effect) and usually an increase in heart rate. But which of these mechanisms will predominate or will both be activated? A recent reinvestigation of this question indicated that there are considerable species differences in such hemodynamic responses and that the results are strongly influenced by the state of the animal or subject.

Two generalizations have emerged from these analyses, *viz.*, (*a*) in normal human subjects, heart rate is much more important in producing major temporary adjustments in cardiac output than is stroke volume, and (*b*) the response that will ultimately be employed depends mainly on the latitude remaining to that particular response mechanism.

The latter principle is exemplified by the effect of posture on the exercise response. In the supine position, central venous pressure and end-diastolic volume are high and heart rate is relatively low; during exercise in this position, the increase in cardiac output involves a large increase in heart rate but a lesser increase in stroke volume. Experiments on normal, conscious dogs have yielded similar results (*i.e.*, the reclining animals have a high resting stroke volume and low heart rate); elevation of preload in these dogs induced mainly an increase in heart rate. However, in the same animals, a reduction of cardiac output by volume depletion was mediated almost entirely through a reduction of stroke volume. In other experiments, it was shown that after trauma, hemorrhage, anesthesia, or other stress, the heart rate is usually elevated but stroke volume is low; an infusion of blood or plasma at this stage will increase cardiac output mainly through elevation of stroke volume, with little change in heart rate.

Thus, it is evident that the cardiac response to altered venous return is an integrated one that depends mainly on the existing heart rate and stroke volume and to a lesser extent on the autonomic balance at the time. In pathological situations, such as myocardial disease, ventricular compliance may also influence the hemodynamic response to increased central venous pressure. In the conditions described thus far, the ventricular wall is assumed to have normal compliance; Figure 5.5 showed, for example, that during normal diastolic filling, left ventricular pressure increases very little (*i.e.*, the chamber walls offer little resistance to filling). However, in congestive heart failure or cardiac hypertrophy, the ventricular wall may become much less compliant and ventricular pressure will rise inordinately during diastole, thereby seriously impeding ventricular filling and cardiac output. These special cases will be discussed further in Chapter 14.

Alterations in Cardiac Output

Physiological Alterations

Exercise. The greatest change in cardiac output in normal individuals occurs during intensive exercise, with an increase in both rate and stroke volume. During exercise, the cardiac output varies linearly with oxygen consumption and may be increased 4- to 6-fold (Chapter 12).

Postural Changes. On rising from a recumbent to an upright position the cardiac output decreases about 20% because of venous pooling in the lower extremities and a decrease in effective circulating blood volume (Chapter 13).

Pregnancy. Cardiac output is increased about 10% partly because of increased body mass and partly because the blood vessels to the placenta and uterus may act as arteriovenous shunts to lower peripheral resistance; in the latter case cardiac output is then increased to maintain the blood pressure.

Pathological Alterations

Blood Volume Changes. In anemia, cardiac output is increased as a compensatory response to the circulatory hypoxia and to the decreased resistance to flow. Beriberi, a rare nutritional disease, is also characterized by anemia, a decreased peripheral resistance, and an elevated cardiac output with an increased heart rate as well as stroke volume. In hemorrhagic and traumatic shock there is a pronounced decrease in cardiac output because of decreased blood volume and lessened venous return.

Metabolic Changes. Since the metabolic rate of an organ or organism is the most important determinant of the blood flow, there are, as might be expected, marked changes in cardiac output with metabolic alterations. During fever and in hyperthyroidism, the increased output is due to the circulatory hypoxia induced by the increased oxygen demand. Studies have also shown that in normal subjects exposed to room temperatures of 30 to 33°C (87 to 92°F) at high relative humidities, cardiac output may increase by as much as 40%.

Peripheral Resistance Changes. Opening of a large systemic arteriovenous fistula, for example, in the aorta or iliac artery (peripheral shunt) or in cor pulmonale (central shunt), will result in a sudden decrease in peripheral resistance, an increase in blood volume, and a rise in cardiac output.

Cardiovascular Disease. In early hypertension the elevated blood pressure is frequently associated with an increased cardiac output; later in the disease the cardiac output decreases toward normal levels and the peripheral vascular resistance rises (Chapter 15). In congestive heart failure, in which a decreased cardiac contractility exists, the cardiac output is reduced and an inability to increase the output at ordinary work levels leads to shortness of breath and easy fatigability (Chapter 14).

Measurement of Cardiac Output

In experimental animals, cardiac output can be measured by placing an electromagnetic or ultrasonic flowmeter on the aorta or pulmonary artery for direct recording. In the human subject, the two most commonly used methods are the Fick and indicator-dilution methods. Both of these are "invasive" in the sense that they require cardiac catheterization for placement of a catheter into vessels close to the heart.

The Fick Method

The Fick principle may be used to measure blood flow through an organ or organism (cardiac output). The principle (illustrated in Fig. 7.5) is based on the measurement of the concentration of a substance entering and leaving an organ and on the total amount of the substance consumed, produced, or added. Since the total amount consumed or added will determine the concentration of the substance leaving the organ, flow may be calculated as the amount added per unit time divided by the concentration difference (Fig. 7.5).

To determine the cardiac output in the living organism, the total O_2 consumption is measured over a period of time (usually several minutes) with a respirometer, and a simultaneous determination is made of the O_2 concentration in mixed venous blood (from the pulmonary artery) and in the arterial blood. The cardiac output can then be calculated as the quotient of the oxygen consumption (ml/min) and the A-VO_2 difference (ml/L). If, for example, an adult resting subject with a heart rate of 80 beats/min had an O_2 consumption of 250 ml/min and simultaneous blood samples from the femoral artery and

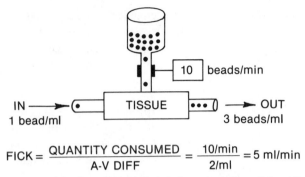

$$FICK = \frac{QUANTITY\ CONSUMED}{A\text{-}V\ DIFF} = \frac{10/min}{2/ml} = 5\ ml/min$$

Figure 7.5.   Illustration of the Fick principle for calculation of blood flow through an organ or organism. The flow equals the quantity added per unit time (beads/min) ÷ A-V difference (beads out − beads in). (Reprinted with permission from F.L. Abel and E.P. McCutcheon. *Cardiovascular Function: Principles and Applications*. Boston: Little, Brown, 1979.)

pulmonary artery (mixed venous blood) were 19.0 and 15.0 ml/O_2/100 ml respectively, the A-Vo_2 difference would be 40 ml/L and the cardiac output would be 250 ml/min ÷ 40 ml/L, or 6.25 L/min. The average stroke volume would then be 6250 ml/min ÷ 80 beats/min or 78 ml.

The Indicator-Dilution Methods

These methods require the injection of a known amount of dye or other indicator substance into the circulation and the measurement of the dilution of this material during a known period of time. The indicator must be well mixed into the blood as it is injected, should not be lost from the circulation, and must not be toxic or itself affect cardiac output.

Indocyanine green (Cardiogreen), a dye commonly used, satisfies these requirements. In practice a known amount of the dye is injected into the right heart *via* a cardiac catheter. A few seconds later the dye concentration is detected in arterial blood by withdrawing small samples of blood continuously from an arterial catheter and measuring the dye concentration with a photosensitive device called a densitometer.

The dye concentration gradually increases until it reaches a maximum, and then it begins to decline until a second rise in concentration occurs as a result of recirculation (Fig. 7.6). The down-slope of the recirculation approximates an exponential decay, so that replotting the curve with the logarithm of dye concentration as the ordinate and time as the abscissa permits the time-concentration curve for the dye on its first circulation past the point of sampling to be defined by extrapolating the down-slope. Summing the concentration of each sample and dividing by the number of samples will give the average concentration of dye (C). The product of the average dye concentration (C)

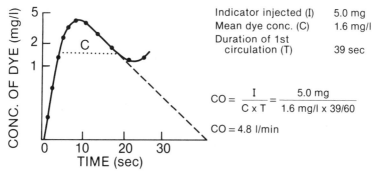

Figure 7.6. Cardiac output determination by indicator dilution. Plot of time *vs.* the logarithm of indicator dye concentration in the aorta after injection of 5 mg of indicator (*left*). The indicator disappearance time without recirculation is obtained by extrapolation. The area of the curve is represented by the product of $C \times T$ and the cardiac output is the quotient of the amount injected divided by the area of the curve.

and the time of this first passage (T) represents the area of the curve. The volume of dye-containing blood (V or CO) that must have passed the sampling site per unit time (V/T) in order to produce the curve can then be calculated by dividing the amount of dye injected (I) by the area of the curve (CT). The larger the area under the curve, the smaller the cardiac output.

A further application of this principle, called "thermodilution," is based on the injection into the right atrium of a bolus of ice-cold dextrose solution; a second catheter in the pulmonary artery with a thermistor tip provides a continuous temperature record. The degree of temperature dilution depends on the flow, and, in a manner similar to dye dilution, a temperature-time curve is inscribed which permits estimation of the cardiac output.

Noninvasive Methods for Estimation of Cardiac Output and Performance

In Chapter 3, a brief description was presented of cardiac catheterization and contrast angiography, invasive methods that are at present standard diagnostic procedures in cardiovascular medicine. There have been, in the last 10 years, increasingly intensive efforts to develop noninvasive methods for estimating cardiac output. Such efforts have been made not only because of the higher cost and added risk of invasive techniques but also because the emotional stress (which even minor invasive procedures sometimes evoke) produces its own physiological effects that may complicate the diagnostic procedure. Following are brief descriptions of three such noninvasive techniques which hold considerable promise as diagnostic aids: (*a*) echocardiography, (*b*) radionuclide imaging, and (*c*) impedance cardiography.

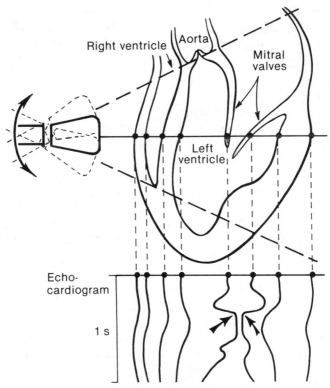

Figure 7.7. Schematic diagram of the principle of echocardiography. The ultrasonic beam is swept in an arc between apex and base. The transducer acts as both sender and receiver in rapid alternation. The distances and movements of the reflecting surfaces are recorded as a function of time. The closing of the mitral valve at the beginning of systole, for example, can be visualized. (Reprinted with permission from *Physiologie des Menschen*, edited by R.F. Schmidt and G. Thews. Berlin: Springer-Verlag, 1980.)

Echocardiography. One of the newest and potentially one of the more important noninvasive techniques for cardiovascular diagnosis is the detection of high-frequency sound waves (above 20,000 cycles/sec) created by actuating a transducer with alternating electrical current. The sound is emitted from the transducer and directed through the body. The depth and position of the echoes (reflected sonic waves) returned from the body can be detected and recorded. The movement of cardiac structures such as valves, heart wall, and pericardium can be tracked, and pathological changes can be readily followed with M (for motion) mode echocardiography. The general principle of an M mode echocardiographic scan is shown in Figure 7.7.

A major development in this field has been the introduction of real time, cross-sectional, two-dimensional (2D) echocardiography, which provides spatial anatomic information about cardiac structures. More recently a further refinement, using pulsed Doppler echocardiogrphy, permits the recording of the actual pattern and velocity of blood flow within the heart and great vessels. To determine aortic flow with pulsed Doppler, both aortic blood velocity and vessel diameter are estimated with the transducer usually placed at the suprasternal notch. Recent reports suggest more reliable results with the transducer placed in the esophagus just behind the aortic arch.

The use of two-dimensional echo and certain geometric assumptions regarding cardiac chamber configuration have permitted the estimation of ventricular end-diastolic, end-systolic, and stroke volumes. The reliability of this method is not yet certain.

Radionuclide Imaging. Another relatively noninvasive method that has come into increasing use is the visualization of the cardiac chambers with radioisotopes. The intravenous injection of a small bolus of a gamma emitter such as ^{99m}Tc pertechnetate permits rapid sequential visualization of the heart, great vessels, and pulmonary vasculature by use of an Anger scintillation camera; the image is usually recorded and stored on tape.

One of the more commonly used radionuclide techniques, "gated equilibrium radionuclide angiography," consists of injection of a ^{99m}Tc pertechnetate–labeled sample of the patient's own red blood cells to achieve an intravascular equilibrium concentration of the radioisotope in the blood stream. This label has a biologic half-life of about 4 hours. At a specific signal—usually triggered by the R wave of the ECG—precordial ventricular radioisotope density for one cardiac cycle is divided (gated) into about 20 to 28 sequential subdivisions and automatically counted by computer. The resulting left ventricular time-activity curve yields a ventricular volume record of filling and emptying which permits estimation of left ventricular end-diastolic, end-systolic, and stroke volumes, ejection fraction, and wall motion abnormalities.

An important application of this method is the determination of ejection fraction at rest and during exercise. With a healthy myocardium, the ejection fraction is usually increased during physical exercise; in case of a weakened myocardium (*e.g.*, after a myocardial infarct) the ejection fraction may be unchanged or decreased during exercise (Chapter 14).

Impedance Cardiography. This method involves the transmission of a high-frequency current across the chest. The ejection of blood into the aorta produces a characteristic impedance wave that permits calculation of the cardiac output. Four circular or spot electrodes are usually placed—two at the neck and two at the lower chest. The outer two electrodes are excited by a 100-kHz sinusoidal current and the resulting voltage monitored from the inner two electrodes (Fig. 7.8). The method is based upon the principle that if a rapid sinusoidal current is transmitted across a distensible cylindrical fluid system, the ejection of a given fluid volume into the cylinder will cause a

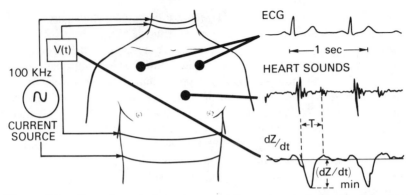

Figure 7.8. Transthoracic impedance cardiography. *Left,* Rapid sinusoidal current is transmitted through the two outer electrodes and sensed by the inner ones. *Right,* The minimum value of the first derivative of the main impedance wave (dZ/dt_{min}) and the ventricular ejection time (T) are used to calculate the stroke volume.

negative impedance wave whose area will be directly proportional to the increased cylinder volume. The stroke volume (SV) ejected into the aorta can be estimated with the formula

$$SV = r \cdot \frac{L^2}{Z_0^2} \cdot T \cdot [dZ/dt_{min}]$$

where r is the electrical resistivity of the blood; L is the linear distance between the inner (recording) electrodes; Z_0 is the baseline impedance across the chest; T is the ventricular ejection time and dZ/dt_{min} is the minimum value of the first derivative of the primary (largest) impedance wave. Recent developments in this field such as ensemble-averaging to reduce motion artefacts, the use of baseline Z_0 to follow changes in thoracic blood volume, and the ability to accurately record systolic time intervals have widened the potential usefulness of impedance cardiography as a noninvasive method for monitoring cardiac function.

Suggested Readings

Feigenbaum H. *Echocardiography,* 4th ed. Philadelphia: Lea & Febiger, 1986.

Guyton, AC. *Circulatory Physiology: Cardiac Output and Its Regulation.* Philadelphia: W.B. Saunders, 1973.

Herndon CW and Sagawa K. Combined effects of aortic and right atrial pressure on aortic flow. *Am J Physiol* 217:65, 1969.

Kubicek WG, Kottke FJ, Ramos MU, Patterson RP, Wittsoe DA, Labree JW, Remole W, Layman TE, Schoening H, and Garamella JT. The Minnesota impedance cardiograph—theory and application. *Biomed Eng* 9:410–416, 1974.

Miles DS and Gotshall RW. Impedance cardiography: non-invasive assessment of human central hemodynamics at rest and during exercise. *Exer Sport Sci Rev* 17:231–263, 1989.

Muzi M, Ebert TJ, Tristani FE, Jeutter DC, Barney JA, and Smith JJ. Determination of cardiac output using ensemble-averaged impedance cardiograms. *J Appl Physiol* 58:200–205, 1985.

Po Sit S and Vatner SF. Integrated circulatory response to volume expansion. In: *Cardiovascular Physiology IV*, International Review of Physiology, edited by AC Guyton and JE Hall. Baltimore: University Park Press, 1982, Vol. 26, pp 323–354.

Rothe CF. The venous system: the physiology of the capacitance vessels. In: *Handbook of Physiology*. Section 2: *The Cardiovascular System*, edited by FM Abboud and JT Shepherd. Bethesda: American Physiological Society, 1982, Vol III.

Scher A. Control of cardiac output. In: *Physiology and Biophysics*, edited by RC Ruch and HD Patton. Philadelphia: W.B. Saunders, 1974.

Thomsen IR. *Regulation of the Circulation*, edited by MS Dhamee. Anesthesiology Lecture Series, Medical College of Wisconsin, 1988.

Vatner SF and Boettcher DH. Regulation of cardiac output by stroke volume and heart rate in conscious dogs. *Circ Res* 42:557–561, 1978.

Zaret BL and Berger HJ. Techniques of nuclear cardiology. In: *The Heart, Arteries and Veins*, 5th ed. edited by JW Hurst. New York: McGraw-Hill, 1982, pp 1803–1843.

Zelis R, Flaim SF, Liedtke AJ, and Nellis SH. Cardiocirculatory dynamics in the normal and failing heart. *Annu Rev Physiol* 43:455–476, 1981.

chapter 8

The Microcirculation and the Lymphatic System

Anatomy of the Microcirculation

That portion of the systemic and pulmonary circulation especially adapted for exchange of water, gases, nutrients, and waste material is known as the microcirculation. It is, in a sense, the most important part of the cardiovascular system since it is here that its ultimate objective, the exchange with tissue cells, is realized. While the microcirculation is considered a closed system, its walls are much more permeable than those of any other part of the circulation.

As shown in Figure 8.1, microcirculatory vessels have an irregular course and configuration; because of their great cross-sectional area, the flow velocity is least at this point. This slowing of the stream and dispersal over a maximum

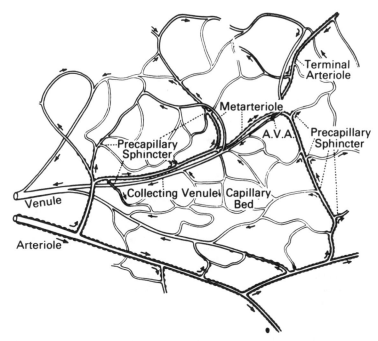

Figure 8.1. Schematic drawing of microcirculatory bed showing arterioles, metarterioles, capillaries, and venules. Note precapillary sphincters at points where capillaries branch off from the metarterioles. (Reprinted with permission from B.W. Zweifach, *Conference on High Blood Pressure*. New York: Macy Foundation, 1950.)

surface makes the microcirculation particularly suitable for exchange. It has been estimated that because of the enormous number and wide distribution of capillaries, individual tissue cells are seldom more than 40 to 80 μm from a capillary surface. Arterioles are highly muscular vessels, but metarterioles, which generally come off the arterioles at right angles, have only a single discontinuous smooth muscle layer in their walls.

The metarterioles serve to some extent as through-channels to the venules, which are much larger and have a greater capacity than the arterioles. At the point where capillaries branch off the metarterioles, a thin band of muscle (the precapillary sphincter) encircles the capillary; these sphincters serve as the main control over capillary flow. Sometimes terminal arterioles control flow into capillaries, since many beds do not have precapillary sphincters per se.

Capillaries

Capillaries of different tissues vary considerably, both anatomically and functionally. These differences are usually related to the special role of the re-

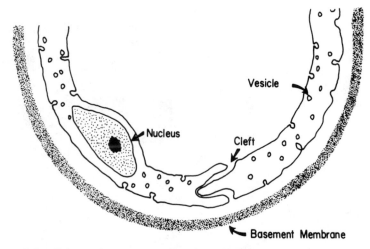

Figure 8.2.   Schematic representation of an electron micrograph of a capillary. Note the slit-pore (cleft) between the endothelial cells. (Reprinted with permission from C.A. Wiederhielm, in *Physiology and Biophysics*, edited by T.C. Ruch and H.D. Patton. Philadelphia: W.B. Saunders, 1974.)

spective tissue or organ and will be discussed further in Chapter 11 (Circulation to Special Regions). In the skin, for example, particularly of the toes, fingers, and ears, there are arteriovenous anastomoses (AVAs), which are wide-bore, direct channels between the arterioles and venules. Unlike capillaries of other organs, the AVAs are under neurogenic control; their shunting capabilities enable them to reduce heat loss through the skin during cold exposure.

The true capillaries are the most important functional units of the micro-circulation. They are short, narrow tubes, about 7 to 10 μm in diameter, with a wall consisting of a single layer of endothelial cells and a basement membrane; they have no smooth muscle (Fig. 8.2). However recent work has shown that at least 5% of endothelial cell protein consists of actin and myosin and that these cells have "stress" materials (contractile materials) in their cytostructure, so it is very likely that these cells have contractile properties. It is also likely that these contractile filaments regulate hydraulic conductivity across venules.

But, perhaps an even more important property of endothelial cells is their role as a sensor and intermediary of microvascular motility in larger vessels (arteries and arterioles).

Between adjacent endothelial cells are slit-like pores or clefts that range from about 50 to 90 Å in width but which are frequently constricted at one point to about 40 Å. The cytoplasm of the endothelial cells usually contains pinocytotic vesicles that are believed to play a role in transport processes across the cell. Although there are a wide variety of capillary structures among

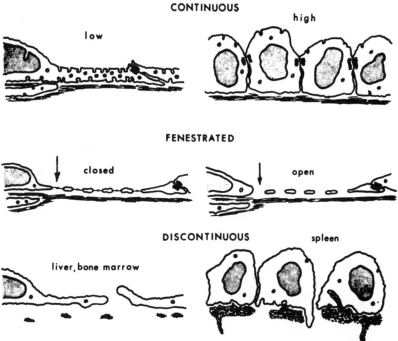

Figure 8.3. Continuous, fenestrated, and discontinuous types of capillary wall as shown by schematics of electron micrographs. The classification is based on the completeness of the endothelial layer and in general parallels the extent of the physical barrier to filtration. (Reprinted with permission from G. Majno, in *Handbook of Physiology*, Section 2: *Circulation*, edited by W.F. Hamilton and P. Dow. Washington, D.C.: American Physiological Society, 1965, Vol. III.)

the different tissues, three main types have been distinguished by electron microscopy on the basis of the continuity of their filtration barriers; these have been labeled continuous, fenestrated, and discontinuous types.

Continuous Capillaries

These are capillaries with no recognizable intercellular openings; one subgroup with a "low" or flattened cellular type is seen mainly in muscle, nerve, and adipose tissue; a second subgroup with a "high" or cuboidal epithelial structure is more common in lymph nodes and the thymus gland (Fig. 8.3, *top*).

Fenestrated Capillaries

This type of capillary (Fig. 8.3, *center*) has small gaps that are either "closed" as in endocrine glands and intestinal villi or "open" as in renal glomeruli.

These gaps usually range from 800 to 1000 Å and are, therefore, about 15 to 20 times wider than those of the continuous capillaries.

Discontinuous Capillaries

This type of capillary (Fig. 8.3, *bottom*) has an endothelium with large intercellular gaps; these vessels are usually referred to as sinusoids and are typical of liver, bone marrow, and spleen. It should be pointed out that the so-called tight junctions of the continuous capillaries are sufficiently wide to permit rapid diffusion of small molecular substances. There is no barrier to diffusion of gases. The other two types of capillaries with larger gaps have much greater permeability, so that in the sinusoids, large proteins and even cells can pass. Thus, to a large extent the transfer of substances between the capillaries and interstitial fluid can be correlated with these anatomical differences in capillary structure. Due to the lipid solubility of gases and the high surface area to volume ratio of microvessels, considerable exchange of O_2, CO_2 and other gases can occur across small arterioles and venules as well.

Regulation of the Microcirculation

As mentioned in Chapter 1, the mean intravascular pressures in the capillary range from about 25 to 30 mm Hg at the arteriolar end to about 8 to 10 mm Hg at the venular end. Flow through the arterioles and metarterioles is controlled mainly by the sympathetic vasoconstrictors on the basis of circulatory reflexes as will be described in Chapters 9 and 10.

Flow through the capillaries, however, is not under neural control. Rather it is regulated by the arteries, arterioles, and precapillary sphincters, which are, in turn, influenced by the local metabolic state of the tissue—a process called autoregulation (Chapter 9).

Research during the last 10 years has considerably altered our concepts of the relative roles of central and local regulation of the microcirculation. It is now evident that the microvasculature has a paramount role—through metabolic and myogenic autoregulation—in controlling its own circulation. It is also now evident that the endothelial cells play a pivotal role in this local regulation by virtue of (*a*) their own contractile properties, (*b*) their role as sensors of parenchymal ischemia and flow variations, and (*c*) their role as intermediaries of impulses to other endothelial cells and the vascular smooth muscle of the microcirculation.

The result is that in case of increased activity of parenchymal cells (*e.g.*, skeletal muscle) there is an "ascending vasodilation" that coordinates increased flow to the part. This increased flow is contributed not only by "true capillaries" but also by terminal and small arterioles and venules in the area.

The exact manner in which the signal is propagated to the upstream vessels is not yet certain.

Thus, flow through individual capillary areas can be adjusted to meet both the local demands of the tissues and the overall control of the circulation. Rate of flow through individual capillary beds can vary considerably. In skeletal muscle, for example, only about 5 to 10% of the capillaries are open at rest; however, with increased metabolic activity, the microvasculature dilates widely. As O_2 needs are satisfied, the vessels again constrict.

Transcapillary Exchange

Movement across the capillary wall is influenced by several factors; (a) the size, shape, and molecular characteristics (e.g., lipid solubility) of the substance being transported, (b) the balance of hydrostatic and colloid osmotic forces across the membrane, (c) the capillary surface available for exchange, and (d) the physical characteristics of the capillary membrane.

The continuous type of capillary is often found in muscle, connective tissue, the pulmonary circulation, and brain. Consequently the filtration coefficient (i.e., the rate of filtration per unit pressure difference of the fluids) is relatively low in these tissues. In the renal glomerulus and intestinal mucosa, which have fenestrated capillaries, the filtration rate is moderate to high. In the hepatic sinusoids and spleen with discontinuous or practically "open" capillaries, molecules of all sizes pass readily; these tissues "leak" the greatest amounts of protein and have the highest interstitial plasma protein concentrations.

There are two general methods—diffusion and filtration—by which substances pass through capillary walls, depending mainly on their lipid solubility. These are discussed in the following sections.

Diffusion

This is the most important transcapillary exchange mechanism. It may take place through the intercellular slit-like pores or through the cell membrane of the endothelial cell itself. Lipid-soluble materials such as oxygen, carbon dioxide, and certain anesthetic agents diffuse rapidly with little hindrance through the lipoprotein membrane of the endothelial cell membrane. Water-soluble substances on the other hand are limited to diffusion through the intercellular slit-pores, in which case the molecular movement is aided by the physical process of filtration.

Filtration-Absorption

Starling described the exchange of fluid across the capillary wall on the basis of the hydrostatic and osmotic pressures on each side of the membrane (law

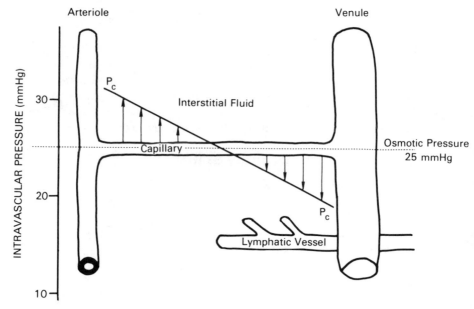

Figure 8.4.   Schematic diagram showing filtration and reabsorption along an average capillary. P_c is the capillary hydrostatic pressure, which decreases progressively from the arteriolar to the venular side. The relation of P_c to capillary osmotic pressure causes filtration on the arteriolar side and reabsorption on the venular side. (Adapted from E.M. Landis and J.R. Pappenheimer, in *Handbook of Physiology*, Section 2: *Circulation*, edited by W.F. Hamilton and P. Dow. Washington, D.C.: American Physiological Society, 1963, Vol. III.)

of the capillary). Later, Landis provided specific pressure measurements to verify this concept. He measured hydrostatic pressures of about 32 and 15 mm Hg in the arteriolar and venular end of a capillary respectively and plasma osmotic pressures due to plasma proteins (oncotic pressures) of about 25 mm Hg. According to the Starling-Landis concept, the resultant pressure gradient along the capillary governs transport across the capillary (Fig. 8.4).

At the arterial end, an excess of hydrostatic over osmotic pressure tends to promote filtration (movement into the tissue), and at the venous end an excess of osmotic over hydrostatic pressure tends to promote reabsorption. In the intermediate region there is a gradual decline in filtration and a beginning of reabsorption. It should be noted that the areas under the triangles are approximately equal, indicating that filtration and absorption are also balanced and about equal. Further studies have indicated that the total amount of water filtered through the capillaries of the body is about 20 liters per day; of this amount, about 16 to 18 liters are reabsorbed into the capillaries; the remaining 2 to 4 liters per day are removed by the lymphatic system and returned to the circulation. In reality, some capillaries may be filtering along their whole length while others may be absorbing. Thus, all capillaries may not be acting exactly as the model capillaries described in the text. Rather, the net filtration and absorption reflects the activity of a population of capillaries.

Although Figure 8.4 refers only to capillary hydrostatic (P_c) and plasma oncotic (π_p) pressures, the interstitial hydrostatic (P_i) and interstitial osmotic pressures (π_i) must also be considered. While P_i and π_i are both quite low compared to the respective P_c and π_p values, the interstitial pressures may, in pathological circumstances, increase and become significant factors in transcapillary fluid exchange as described later in this chapter. Therefore, a more accurate definition of transcapillary forces would be the balance between the net transmural hydrostatic pressure ($P_c - P_i$) and the net transmural oncotic pressure ($\pi_p - \pi_i$).

Two-thirds or more of the oncotic effect of the 7 g/dl of plasma proteins is due to albumin. Because of their large molecular size only a small percentage of plasma protein diffuses across the capillary wall in most tissues. However, as previously mentioned, in the sinusoids the plasma proteins move more easily into the interstitial fluid, so that π_i begins to approach π_p.

Capillary Permeability

As previously stated, the transport of material across the capillary wall depends not only on diffusion and on the balance of pressures across the capillary but also on the structure and porosity of the capillary wall and the nature of the material being transported. For water-soluble substances that are transported primarily *via* the slit-pores, a single mathematical expression can be used to describe the movement across the capillary wall

$$F = (P)(S)[(P_c - P_i) - (\pi_p - \pi_i)]$$

where F is the net movement of fluid, P is the specific permeability of the capillary, and S is the capillary surface area perfused. S depends mainly on the number of capillaries open to flow, P_c and P_i are the hydrostatic pressures in the capillary and interstitial fluid, and π_p and π_i are the osmotic pressure values in the plasma and interstitial fluid respectively. The right side of the equation is a restatement of the balance of hydrostatic and osmotic forces previously described. Note that if F is positive there will be an outward transport of fluid from the capillary, and if negative, an inward one.

In Table 8.1 are listed the specific permeabilities of a few common substances as well as their molecular weights and sizes. As will be noted, in the continuous or tight capillary that prevails in muscle, the permeability ranges from high values for the smaller molecules to practical impermeability for the larger protein molecules. This is consistent with the concept that the movement of these substances across the capillary barrier is essentially a passive one, primarily dependent upon physical forces. The permeability factor may be affected by hypoxia, drugs, and certain pathological conditions.

Table 8.1.
Permeability of Mammalian Muscle Capillaries to Some Water-Soluble Molecules

Substance	Molecular Weight	Approximate Molecular Radius (Å)	Specific Permeability*
H_2O	18	1.5	28
NaCl	58	2.3	15
Urea	60	2.6	14
Glucose	180	3.7	6
Sucrose	342	4.8	4
Inulin	5,500	12–15	0.3
Myoglobin	17,000	19	0.1
Serum albumin	67,000	36	0.001

*Expressed as mol/sec/cm^2 of membrane per mol/concentration difference $\times$ 10^5. (From E.M. Landis and J.R. Pappenheimer, in *Handbook of Physiology*, Section 2: *Circulation*, edited by W.F. Hamilton and P. Dow. Washington, D.C.: American Physiological Society, 1963, Vol. II.)

Lymphatic System

The lymphatics comprise a type of secondary interstitial drainage system supplementing venular drainage. Lymphatics are porous, thin-walled vessels resembling capillaries. From closed, blind ends lying in the interstitial space, lymph channels drain centrally and are occasionally interrupted by lymph nodes. Inside the nodes the vessels break up into numerous sinuses, lined by lymphoid cells, which reunite into efferent lymph channels. Ultimately, all the lymphatic vessels empty into two main trunks, the thoracic duct (on the left) and the right lymphatic duct. These drain into the junctions of the subclavian and internal jugular veins on their respective sides. The primary function of the lymphatic system is to clear the interstitial spaces of excess fluid, protein, lipids, and foreign materials.

Lymph resembles interstitial tissue fluid with which it is in close equilibrium. Its composition is similar to plasma except that its average protein concentration is lower (*i.e.*, about 2 g/dl). The highest protein concentration is that of hepatic lymph, which has a range of about 5 to 6 g/dl. Pressure in the lymphatics is similar to that of interstitial fluid and fluctuates from about −3 mm Hg to +5 mm Hg. Guyton and his colleagues have reported that interstitial pressure normally is about −6 mm Hg. These investigators believe that this negative pressure is important to maintain relatively dry tissue spaces, so that diffusion distances between capillaries and cells are optimally short.

Lymph flow is relatively sluggish, and total flow in man is about 2 to 4 L/day. This flow is increased by muscular activity or massage, increased volume pressure, hyperemia, or inflammation. Lymphatic vessels are highly permeable and are capable of picking up large particles (*e.g.*, dying blood cells, carbon, bacteria, and foreign particles). Intestinal lymphatics (lacteals) pick up large lipid globules such as chylomicra after a fat meal.

Edema

Edema is the accumulation of excess fluid in the interstitial spaces of the body. Clinical edema usually develops in dependent areas such as the feet and becomes more evident in tissues in which expansion is limited (*e.g.*, around the eyes). Edema may be produced in several ways as described below.

General Increase in Venous Pressure

As is shown in Figure 8.4 and also in Figure 8.5A, when there is a normal balance of filtration and reabsorption forces, there will be no accumulation of interstitial fluid. However, if the pressure is consistently increased in the veins, it will also rise in the venules and eventually in the arterial end of the capillary. This will result in an increase in filtration and in the accumulation of interstitial fluid, illustrated by the net force tending to move fluid out of the capillary (Fig. 8.5B). This condition occurs most commonly in congestive heart failure with elevation of right ventricular end-diastolic pressure, venous congestion, and a resultant dependent edema (discussed further in Chapter 14).

Hypoproteinemia

If the plasma protein concentration decreases to a low level, the plasma oncotic pressure will also fall so that the capillary hydrostatic pressure overbalances the oncotic pressure, with a resultant tendency for fluid accumulation in the tissue spaces. The loss of plasma protein—primarily albumin—occurs most commonly in nephrosis (in which large amounts of albumin are continuously lost in the urine), in nutritional edema (in which there is inadequate protein in the diet), and with severe burns (in which the capillaries are damaged).

Lymphatic Obstruction

If the small amount of protein that continually "leaks" through the capillary walls and is normally returned *via* the lymph cannot be reabsorbed, it will accumulate in the tissue until it reaches a significant concentration and prevents the return of fluid into the venular end of the capillary. This occurs rarely but when seen is usually due to a tropical parasitic disease called "filariasis"; the larvae (microfilaria) gradually obstruct the lymphatic vessels. The edema may become so excessive that a leg may swell to two or three times its normal size—hence the clinical term "elephantiasis" for this type of massive edema.

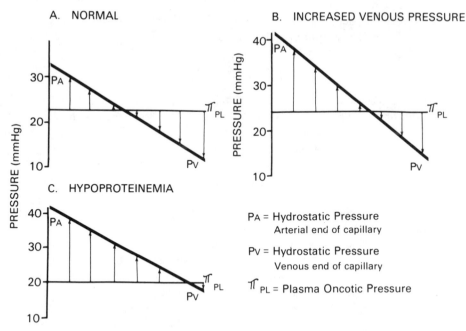

Figure 8.5. Effect of variations in hydrostatic and colloid osmotic pressures on fluid filtration-reabsorption balance. *A*, Normal balance of capillary hydrostatic and plasma oncotic pressures; *B*, elevation of venular and capillary pressures with excessive filtration and increased interstitial fluid; *C*, decreased plasma protein and plasma oncotic pressure, with excessive capillary filtration and tendency toward edema.

Local Edema

Localized edema may occur in an organ or region if there is extensive venous obstruction with elevation of venous and capillary pressures (*e.g.*, a widespread venous thrombosis).

Suggested Readings

Daniel TO and Ives HE. Endothelial control of vascular function. *NIPS* 4:139–142, 1989.
Duling BR, Hogan RD, Langlilli BL *et al.* Vasomotor control: functional hypermia and beyond. *Fed Proc* 46:251–263, 1987.
Folkmann J. Angiogenesis: what makes blood vessels grow? *NIPS* 1:199–202, 1986.
Furchgott RF and VanHoutte PM. Endothelium-derives relaxing and contracting factors. *FASEB J* 3:2007–2018, 1989.
Gore RW and McDonagh PF. Fluid exchange across single capillaries. *Annu Rev Physiol* 42:337–357, 1980.
Guyton AC, Granger HJ, and Taylor AE. Interstitial fluid pressure. *Physiol Rev* 51:527, 1971.
Haddy FJ, Scott JB, and Grega GJ. Peripheral circulation: fluid transfer across the microvascular

membrane, In: *Cardiovascular Physiology II*, International Review of Physiology, edited by AC Guyton. Baltimore: University Park Press, 1976, Vol. 9.

Hudlicka, O. Capillary growth: role of mechanical factors. *NIPS* 3:117–120, 1988.

Intaglietta M and Johnson PC. *Principles of Capillary Exchange in Peripheral Circulation*, edited by PC Johnson. New York: John Wiley & Sons, 1978.

Landis EM and Pappenheimer JR. Exchange of substances through the capillary walls, In: *Handbook of Physiology*, Section 2: *Circulation*, edited by WF Hamilton and P Dow. Washington, D.C.: American Physiological Society, 1963, Vol. II.

Lombard JH, Hinojosa-Laborde C, and Cowley AW. Hemodynamics and microcirculatory alteration in reduced renal mass hypertension. *Hypertension* 13:128–138, 1989.

Majno G. Ultrastructure of vascular membrane. In: *Handbook of Physiology*, Section 2: *Circulation*, edited by WF Hamilton and P Dow. Washington, D.C.: American Physiological Society, 1965, Vol. III.

Renkin, EM. Some consequences of capillary permeability to macromolecules: Starling hypothesis reconsidered. *Am J Physiol* 250:H706–10, 1986.

chapter 9

The Peripheral Circulation and Its Regulation

Normal Distribution of Blood Flow

How blood flow is distributed to the various organs is obviously of considerable importance; total flow is limited and it must be disposed only in amounts needed when and where it is needed. If, in a 70-kg adult, a cardiac output of 5400 ml/min were partitioned evenly on a weight basis, the mean flow would be about 7.7 ml/min/100 g of tissue. However, the actual flow distribution is quite uneven. Figure 9.1 shows average values for tissue blood flow and oxygen consumption in the normal adult human at rest.

As the top bar graph shows, three tissues, liver (hepatosplanchnic region), kidney, and skeletal muscle receive about two-thirds of the total flow. If the

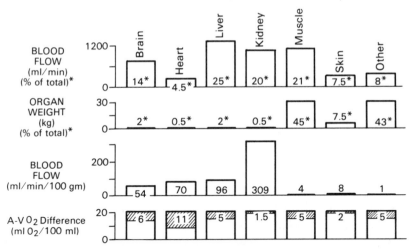

Figure 9.1. Blood flow, organ weight, vascularity (blood flow per unit weight), and A-V oxygen extraction of main organs in normal adult at rest. Body weight, 70 kg; cardiac output, 5400 ml/min; mean vascularity, 7.7 ml/min/100 g; mean A-V$_{O_2}$ difference, 5 ml O_2 per dl. (Liver flow includes that of the intestinal and other organs draining into the portal vein and therefore actually refers to hepatosplanchnic flow.)

organ flows are divided by the respective organ weights, the blood flow per unit weight or "vascularity" (Fig. 9.1, 3rd graph) is obtained. As described in Chapter 2, when comparing relative flow or peripheral resistance values, it is necessary to consider the weight or surface area of the respective organ or organism.

Four organs, *viz.*, kidney, liver, heart, and brain, all have a high flow/unit weight because of a relatively low vascular resistance/unit weight; in contrast, *resting* skeletal muscle and the relatively avascular tissues such as skin, bone, cartilage, fat, and connective tissue (which are grouped under "other") have a low blood flow/unit weight because of their relatively high vascular resistance.

Just as the flow distribution to the different organs is uneven, so is the flow distribution *within* organs (*e.g.*, in the heart, kidneys, and brain) as will be discussed in Chapter 11. Since these intraorgan flow characteristics have functional significance, regional blood flow determinations have become increasingly important.

The kidneys, being primarily clearance organs, obviously need a very large flow to carry out their function; their close proximity through short arterial vessels to the high aortic pressure and their innate vascularity contribute to the high resting flow. The renal clearance function is associated with only a modest oxygen demand so that the flow is mainly "nonnutritional." As a consequence, the renal A-V oxygen difference is small (1.5 ml of $O_2/100$ ml of blood). Therefore, in spite of the very large flow, the estimated oxygen consumption of the kidneys, about 4.6 ml/min/100 g (3.09×1.5), is less than that of the liver (4.8) or heart (7.7) (Fig. 9.1).

That fraction of the arterial O_2 content taken up in the tissues is usually termed the O_2 extraction ratio. If the arterial O_2 content were 20 ml/dl, the O_2 extraction for resting skeletal muscle (Fig. 9.1) would be 0.25 and for myocardium 0.55. The remaining fraction of unextracted oxygen represents an important reserve.

In certain stress situations, both the total flow and flow distribution shown in Figure 9.1 (*top graph*) would be considerably altered. For example, during severe exercise, cardiac output can increase 4 to 6 times; furthermore, the percentage of total flow received by skeletal muscle would increase to about 90% because of a marked decrease in vascular resistance in the dilated muscle vessels (Chapter 12). Since, in addition to the increased fractional flow to muscle, there will also be an increase in the O_2 extraction ratio, the total O_2 consumption of skeletal muscle can, in severe exercise, increase 15 to 20 times over the resting level.

Range of Flow Responses in Different Organs

Changes in vessel caliber may occur passively in response to transmural pressure changes or through active contraction (vasoconstriction) or relaxation (vasodilation) of its circular smooth muscle. Such activity will, in the small arteries and arterioles, mainly influence peripheral resistance, but in the small veins and venules, the primary effect is on the capacitance of the peripheral bed.

Vessel caliber may change over a wide range. Vasoconstriction of small arterial vessels may be so intense that flow practically ceases. On the other hand, if all constrictor nerves are cut and the vessels maximally dilated by pharmacological agents, flow may increase 2- or 3-fold in the brain and liver, 5-fold in the myocardium, and over 20-fold in skeletal muscle (Fig. 9.2).In contrast to this, renal vessels can only increase their flow about 16%. Such large flow alterations in certain tissues are possible because of the fourth power effect of the radius on flow (Chapter 2).

Principles of Flow Regulation

Given its inherent vascular architecture, altered flow demands might be met either by a change in the arterial perfusion pressure or by adjustment of vessel caliber. From the organism's standpoint, it is most efficient to keep arterial pressure relatively constant in order to insure adequate coronary and cerebral flow and to meet the peripheral demands through adjustment of individual resistances. In effect this is what normally occurs. The primary objective of

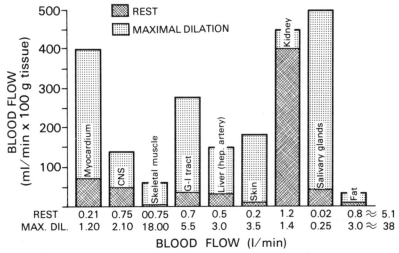

Figure 9.2.   Regional blood flow at rest (*shaded areas*) and at maximal dilation (*stippled areas*) per organ and per 100 g tissue. (Reprinted with permission from S. Mellander and B. Johansson, *Pharmacol Rev* 20:117, 1968.)

this chapter is to consider how this is brought about. The adjustment of vessel caliber is accomplished by two general mechanisms, central regulation and local regulation.

Central Regulation of Flow. This may be either *neural control*, which is carried out almost entirely by the autonomic nervous system, primarily *via* sympathetic nerves, or *humoral control*, that is, through bloodborne agents that may be (*a*) organic substances such as 5-hydroxytryptamine or angiotensin, (*b*) blood gases O_2 or CO_2, or (*c*) ions such as Ca^{2+} or K^+.

Local Regulation of Flow. This is carried out either through biological agents, so called local hormones such as prostaglandins, bradykinin, or histamine, or through inorganic agents such as O_2 or CO_2 or H^+, which are vasoactive, parenchymal metabolites derived in the individual tissues, and which act directly on nearby vascular beds. The flow alterations are due mainly to effects on the precapillary or postcapillary vessels.

In considering the regulation of blood flow to an organ or organism, an important distinction must be made between short-and long-term circulatory adjustments (*i.e.*, those made rapidly over minutes or hours in contrast to those that occur over days and weeks. The mechanisms involved in these two processes are quite different. In the following sections, the short-term adaptations will be considered first and in greater detail.

In the final section of the chapter, long-term regulation of flow will be discussed in general. In succeeding chapters, vascular luminal adjustments of greater duration, which apply to specific situations, will be described at some length. These will include circulatory changes that develop during physical training and those incident to aging (Chapter 12) and circulatory adjustments that occur in pathological circumstances such as ischemic heart disease and congestive failure (Chapter 14) as well as in hypertension and shock (Chapter 15).

Central Regulation of Flow

Neural Control of Flow

Autonomic Transmitters and Receptors

The autonomic nervous system (ANS), which includes the thoracolumbar (sympathetic) outflow and the craniosacral (parasympathetic) outflow, is responsible for integrating and modulating the functions of all the autonomous organs of the body, including the cardiovascular system. Neural transmission along the ANS is done in the usual fashion, by means of self-propagating action potentials; transmission across synapses and across junctions with other tissues is *via* rather unique and specific chemical agents known as neurohumoral transmitters. These transmitters combine with receptors on the effector cells to activate the end-organ.

There are two primary transmitters involved in the ANS: (*a*) acetylcholine (ACh), released at all autonomic ganglia, at parasympathetic nerve endings, and at voluntary neuromuscular junctions, and (*b*) norepinephrine (NE), released at most sympathetic cholinergic endings (*e.g.*, at sweat glands) and the cholinergic vasodilators in skeletal muscle. At these endings ACh is released. Epinephrine (E) is liberated (along with a small fraction of NE) by the adrenal medulla into the blood.

Endogenously active sympathomimetic amines (NE, E, dopamine) are known as catecholamines. An outline of the synthesis of these compounds is given in a simplified diagram in Figure 9.3.NE, derived in a series of steps from tyrosine, is for the most part synthesized locally by the adrenergic nerve terminal. About 80% of the NE released by the nerve action potential is removed *via* an active reuptake process into the neuron for reuse. The remainder either diffuses into the surrounding tissue or blood or is metabolically degraded. The importance of the uptake process lies in the consequent availability (or not) of the NE for continued combination with the effector cell, and so it is a determinant of the strength and duration of the NE effect. Since the transmitter originates within the body, it is termed endogenous. The NE secreted by the nerve cell remains active for only a few seconds but the E secreted by the adrenal medulla can remain active for several minutes.

If the transmitter (*e.g.*, NE or ACh) is injected (exogenous source) and reaches the receptors *via* the blood stream, the effect will be similar to that of neurally released NE or ACh—a ''sympathomimetic'' or ''parasympatho-

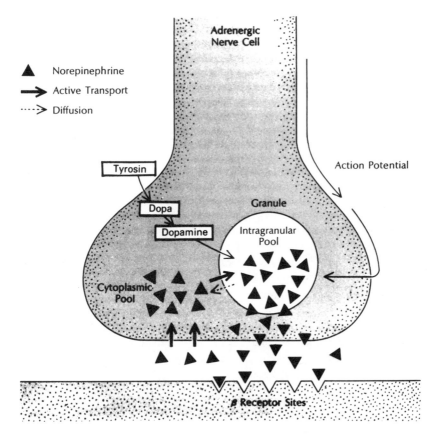

Figure 9.3. Schema showing local synthesis and release of norepinephrine (NE) in the heart. Ninety per cent of the cardiac NE is synthesized locally. The NE is stored, either in the granules or in the cytoplasm, and is released by the action potential. It then leaves the nerve cell, attaches to the myocardial β-receptor site and stimulates myocardial contraction. (Reprinted with permission from E. Braunwald, *The Myocardium: Failure and Infarction*. New York: HP Publishing Co., 1974.)

mimetic'' effect will be produced. But whether generated by neural or humoral means, autonomic effects on the various end-organs are diverse and complex. A significant (and initially baffling) discovery was that specific chemicals could prevent or competitively "block" certain autonomic effects (but not others) and thus render the transmitter temporarily ineffective at these effector sites.

In 1948, Ahlquist proposed that divergent sympathetic responses were due to the existence of two different types of "receptors" at the various anatomical sites, which responded differently to the transmitters. These he called "α" and "β" receptors. Because exogenously administered NE or neurally released NE produces a strong vasoconstriction of the blood vessels of skin, kidney, splanchnic area, and skeletal muscle (*i.e.*, a "pure" vasoconstriction), he assumed that such receptors were abundant at these sites. At other sites (*e.g.*, in vessels of the brain and heart), NE produces limited or no constriction, since at these locations such receptors are scarce. These were called α-receptors and the action an α-constrictor action. Although NE is the primary endogenous agonist (activator) of α-receptors in the human and most mammals, E also has strong α-stimulating effects.

Specific agents such as phenoxybenzamine (Dibenzyline) or phentolamine (Regitine) will antagonize or block α (but not β) receptors and thus, depending on the dose, will minimize or prevent the α-vasoconstriction. The rapid and effective increase in peripheral vascular resistance produced by reflex sympathetic α-constriction is an important defense mechanism against a blood pressure fall (*e.g.*, during hemorrhage). An animal previously injected with a strong α-blocking dose of phenoxybenzamine will have a much lower resistance to hemorrhage than a control animal.

β-Receptors are most prevalent in the heart, in blood vessels of skeletal muscles, and in bronchiolar smooth muscle. They are activated by epinephrine at low doses or by one of its synthetic analogues, isoproterenol (Isuprel). When occupied by the transmitter, β-receptors initiate (*a*) increased heart rate and contractile strength of the myocardium and (*b*) vasodilation of skeletal muscle blood vessels. β-Receptors (but not α) can be blocked by propranolol (Inderal). Propranolol is used in the treatment of certain types of hypertension and can assist in controlling blood pressure by reducing the inotropic activity of the ventricle.

As mentioned above, there are postganglionic sympathetic cholinergic nerve endings located in vessels of skeletal muscle. These endings, rather paradoxically, release ACh, which binds "cholinergic" (or more specifically "muscarinic") receptors and causes vasodilation. This effect, which can be blocked by the primary muscarinic blocking agent, atropine, is thought to be involved in certain emotional responses such as fright or rage.

Some investigators have also reported the existence of "dopaminergic" receptors. Dopamine, which is only one of the intermediate compounds in the synthetic pathway of NE, has a vasodilator effect on renal, splanchnic, and coronary vascular beds, an action that can be blocked by specific antagonists (*e.g.*, haloperidol).

It has been shown that in congestive heart failure, there is a depletion of myocardial catecholamines, with consequent reduction of inotropic capability. The depletion is probably due to the marked reduction of tyrosine hydroxylase, the rate-limiting enzyme in the conversion of tyrosine to DOPA.

As is evident from the above, certain tissues, by virtue of having different kinds of receptors, are capable of different types of vascular response if the proper stimuli are provided. This is particularly true of skeletal muscle. Figure 9.4 illustrates the effects of successive blockade of different receptors on skeletal muscle blood flow. Skeletal muscle, because it comprises about 45% of the body bulk and has unusual constrictor and dilator capabilities, represents an enormous pool of vascular resistance.

Parasympathetic control of blood flow (to be discussed later in this chapter) is much more limited than that of the sympathetic system.

Autonomic neurotransmitters and receptors are currently the focus of intensive investigation, and recent studies have revealed that there are many substances and complex interrelationships involved at neuroeffector junctions. There are, for example, two subtypes of β-receptors—β_1 and β_2. These vary not only in their sensitivity to NE and E but also in the chronotropic and inotropic responses they invoke in different species. In addition, two types of α-receptors have been proposed, α_1 and α_2. α_1-Receptors are found primarily postsynaptically in vascular smooth muscle; they apparently mediate vasoconstrictor responses to NE. α_2-Receptors are mainly located presynaptically and can inhibit the release of NE from the sympathetic nerve terminals. Thus, NE can inhibit its own release. α_2-Receptors are abundant in the CNS and may be important in the central control of blood pressure. Recent studies have further shown that in addition to NE itself, certain agents such as ATP, prostaglandins, and histamine can also act presynaptically to inhibit NE release at the nerve terminals. In contrast, other agents such as angiotensin II can facilitate NE release.

The physiological significance of these complex interactions is not yet clear. The expectation that such developments will eventually lead to progressively greater ability to control regional vasculature with specific autonomic agents has spurred unprecedented efforts to develop more specific and effective agents for the treatment of cardiac and peripheral circulatory disorders.

Sympathetic System—Circulatory Effects

Descending fibers from the cardiac and vasomotor centers of the medulla synapse with cells of the intermediolateral cell column of the spinal cord; preganglionic fibers from the cord travel *via* the anterior spinal roots to the thoracolumbar sympathetic chain (Fig. 9.5). Descending impulses from the cerebral cortex and hypothalamus may also, by way of these spinal pathways, induce sympathetic vascular responses.

The postganglionic sympathetic fibers from the cervical and upper four thoracic sympathetic ganglia supply the heart and the entire peripheral circulation. The cardiac sympathetics are widely distributed to the SA and

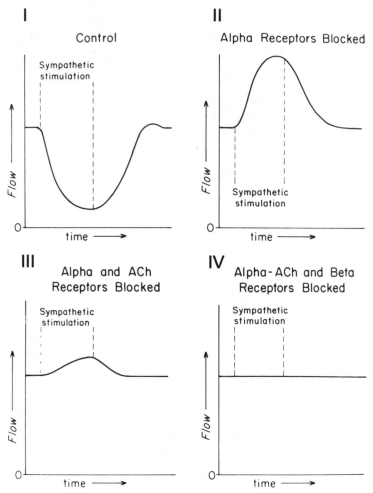

Figure 9.4. Results of stimulation of sympathetic nerves on blood flow in skeletal muscle. *I*, A strong vasoconstriction is present due to α-receptor action; *II*, after α-blockade, a sympathetic vasodilator effect is unmasked; *III*, after atropine the main vasodilator action in *II* is shown to be due to sympathetic cholinergic action. In *IV* the smaller, residual vasodilator action (β-effect) is abolished with a β-blocker. (Reprinted with permission from T.C. Ruch and H.D. Patton, *Physiology and Biophysics*. Philadelphia: W.B. Saunders, 1974.)

AV nodes and to the myocardium. Stimulation of these fibers activates β-adrenergic receptors and causes increases in rate and conduction velocity in the heart and increased myocardial contractility. The effects of sympathetic stimulation on the electrical and contractile events of the heart are

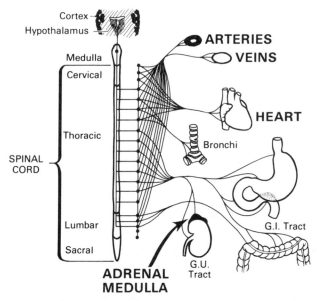

Figure 9.5. Sympathetic pathways to the heart and vasculature.

discussed in Chapters 4 and 5, respectively. The remainder of this chapter will be concerned primarily with sympathetic effects on the peripheral circulation.

Other sympathetic postganglionic fibers join the somatic and other autonomic nerves to reach practically all arteries and veins of the body. Upon stimulation, these fibers activate α-adrenergic receptors to produce a general vasoconstriction which is particularly marked in the skin, skeletal muscle, and splanchnic and renal vascular beds. Reports have indicated that sympathetic stimulation may also activate peripheral β-adrenergic receptors, which will tend to produce vasodilation, particularly in skeletal muscle. The importance of this response, however, is in dispute. In any event, the β-adrenergic dilator tendency in muscle is overshadowed by the much stronger α-constrictor action.

Preganglionic sympathetic fibers supply the adrenal medulla where they control the release of E and NE into the bloodstream.

Sympathetic stimulation will produce other important, noncirculatory effects (*e.g.*, relaxation of smooth muscle of the respiratory bronchioles, gastrointestinal tract, and urinary tract and lessened secretion of sweat and lacrimal glands). Sympathetic stimulation also increases hepatic and muscle glycogenolysis and induces hyperglycemia; these metabolic effects assist in energy maintenance during prolonged stress such as physical exercise.

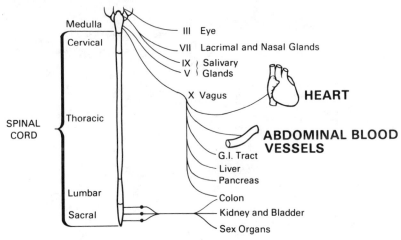

Figure 9.6.   Parasympathetic pathways to the heart and vasculature.

Parasympathetic System—Circulatory Effects

Preganglionic fibers of the craniosacral division of the ANS arise either in motor nuclei of the brain stem and exit with the cranial nerves, or in the sacral division of the spinal cord (Fig. 9.6).

The vagus (tenth) cranial nerve supplies the heart. These fibers are distributed to the cardiac pacemakers, conducting tissue, and to the myocardium, particularly that of the atrium. Vagal innervation to the SA node and AV junctional region is particularly important. Vagal stimulation activates cholinergic (muscarinic) receptors in the heart, which exert strong inhibitory effects by slowing heart rate and AV conduction velocity (Chapter 4) and by decreasing cardiac contractility, primarily of the atria (Chapter 5). As described later in this chapter, parasympathetic vasodilator fibers have been reported in vascular beds of the brain, myocardium, salivary glands, sex organs, and possibly intestine.

Preganglionic fibers of this division run to—or almost to—the innervated organs before synapsing, so that parasympathetic effects tend to be more discrete and specific than sympathetic effects. Aside from its cardiovascular action, parasympathetic stimulation also induces contraction of nonvascular smooth muscle of bronchioles, gut, and bladder; contraction of the pupil of the eye (miosis), and increased secretion of certain exocrine glands.

Vasoconstriction

Sympathetic vasoconstrictor impulses arise in the vasomotor center of the medulla (*a*) as a result of intrinsic or extrinsic reflexes from various parts of the body or (*b*) as descending impulses from the higher centers of the brain.

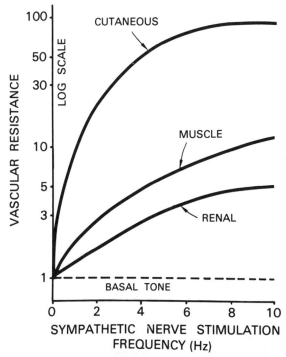

Figure 9.7. Relative responsiveness of skin, muscle, and kidney vessels to vasoconstriction. Skin vessels show a greater increase in vascular resistance at equivalent stimulation frequencies. (Reprinted with permission from T.C. Ruch and H.D. Patton, *Physiology and Biophysics*. Philadelphia: W.B. Saunders, 1974.)

The origin and nature of these two pathways will be discussed in Chapter 10. But however activated, sympathetic impulses will—as described above—promptly and almost simultaneously cause general constriction of the small arteries and veins.

However, all regions are not equally sensitive to constrictor impulses. Skin and muscle arteries show greater constriction at equivalent stimulation frequencies than do renal arteries (Fig. 9.7). The sensitivity of the vascular muscle is also influenced by metabolites, so that during physical exercise, sympathetic stimulation will produce a much lesser degree of constriction in skeletal muscle vessels than it will at rest.

In addition to the action of arterial vasoconstriction on peripheral flow, there is an important effect on the transcapillary pressure gradient and therefore on plasma volume. Hydrostatic pressure distal to the point of arterial constriction will be reduced; as a consequence there will be less filtration from and more reabsorption of tissue fluid into the capillaries (Chapter 8). In circulatory shock, for example, the increased vasoconstriction will notably increase the circulating plasma volume.

Fluid replacement is, however, a somewhat slower process than the vasomotor action itself. Although vasoconstriction is well advanced within 2 to 3 minutes after the onset of hypotension, the influx of fluid into the capillaries only begins after several minutes but continues for some hours afterward.

An important part of the sympathetic vascular response is *venoconstriction*, which can significantly decrease venous capacitance and shift blood toward the heart, thus aiding venous return. At low impulse frequencies in the sympathetic vasoconstrictor nerves (*e.g.*, to skeletal muscle), the venoconstrictors (the capacitance vessels) respond more fully to decrease venous capacitance and move blood toward the heart. However, the decrease in lumen size and the consequent increase in vascular resistance is significantly greater in the precapillary (resistance) vessels than in the capacitance vessels. It is the greater increase in precapillary resistance (*i.e.*, the greater ratio of precapillary to postcapillary resistance increase) which brings about the fall in mean capillary hydrostatic pressure and the reabsorption of tissue fluid into the capillary in response to sympathetic vasoconstriction.

Vascular beds differ in their relative contribution to the resistance/capacitance balance. As mentioned previously, skeletal muscle, because of its bulk, is a large contributor to peripheral resistance. On the other hand, constriction of the splanchnic bed results in a substantial reduction of splanchnic venous capacitance and thus can be a significant factor in assisting venous return.

In summary, it should be noted that generalized vasoconstriction will usually have three vascular effects: (*a*) arteriolar constriction, which will increase vascular resistance, heighten the central arterial pressure, and decrease flow to the constricted beds; (*b*) a reduction of capillary hydrostatic pressure with a resultant net increase in plasma volume; and (*c*) venoconstriction, which will reduce the caliber of the capacitance vessels and assist venous return.

Vasodilation

While vasoconstriction results primarily from sympathetic stimulation of α-receptors, vasodilation is more complex and may be induced in several different ways:

Inhibition of the Vasoconstrictor Center of the Medulla. This type of vasodilation may be the most common pathway, and some investigators have questioned the existence of a true medullary vasodilator center.

Sympathetic Cholinergic (Muscarinic) Vasodilators. As previously mentioned, small arterial vessels in skeletal muscle are unique because they are innervated by sympathetic cholinergic vasodilator fibers that can be blocked by atropine. These receptors are activated only in unusual circumstances such as the "defense reaction" (Chapter 10).

β-Sympathetic Vasodilators. These receptors seem to be present primarily in skeletal muscle. When unmasked by α-blockade, they respond with a mild, relatively transitory, vasodilation.

Parasympathetic Vasodilators. The activation of glossopharyngeal fibers to submaxillary salivary glands can evoke glandular secretions that ultimately result in the release of a neurohormone, bradykinin, that has a strong local vasodilator effect. In addition, sacral vasodilators to genital erectile tissue are important in reproduction. However, the arterioles of most other organs do not have parasympathetic innervation.

Vascular Tone and the Abolition of Tone

Basal tone is the low-level, continuous, active tension that exists in the vascular smooth muscle when it is at rest or under "basal" conditions. Even when deprived of all extrinsic neural or humoral influences, a measure of basal tone remains, due to the inherent action of the smooth muscle cells themselves (*i.e.*, the myogenic component of tone).

If the sympathetic constrictor fibers are intact, a somewhat higher level of continuous contractile activity is present due to low-frequency efferent impulses from the vasoconstrictor center of the medulla. Vasoconstrictor tone is not equal in the different tissues; it is highest in skeletal muscle, skin, and splanchnic vessels and least in vessels of the brain, myocardium, and kidney. The degree of basal tone of neurogenic origin can be determined in experimental animals by severing the vasoconstrictor fibers and measuring the change in blood flow and peripheral resistance.

Vascular tone is important in the continuous maintenance of arterial pressure. In the case of severance of the spinal cord, there will be a flaccid paralysis of all somatic motor elements below the transection (paraplegia); in addition, the sympathetic preganglionic vasoconstrictors will be interrupted, and vasoconstrictor vascular tone to the entire body mass below the lesion will be lost. This usually results in a drastic fall in arterial pressure to levels of 60 to 80 mm Hg (spinal shock) due to (*a*) the abrupt reduction of peripheral resistance, (*b*) the loss of venoconstriction, and (*c*) the loss of skeletal-muscle pump action. A similar, though temporary and less severe, fall in blood pressure, results upon administration of an α-adrenergic blocking agent such as phenoxybenzamine.

The higher the cord lesion, the more serious is the vascular disability. If the section is above the sixth thoracic segment, a condition of orthostatic hypotension usually exists; this means that a patient tilted to any type of head-up position will be unable to compensate for the gravity effect on the circulation by invoking the usual baroceptor reflexes (Chapter 13). The relatively

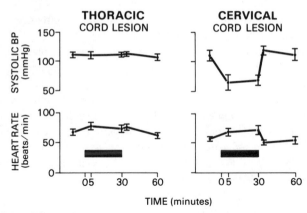

Figure 9.8. Effect of paraplegia on vascular responses to a posture change. *Black bars* indicate change from supine to sitting position. Patient with cervical cord lesion shows orthostatic fall in arterial pressure compared to patient with lower thoracic section. (Reprinted with permission from R.H. Johnson and J.M.K. Spalding, *Disorders of the Autonomic Nervous System*. Philadelphia: F.A. Davis, 1974.)

inadequate orthostatic response of a patient with a cervical cord lesion compared to a patient with a lower thoracic cord lesion is illustrated in Figure 9.8.

Several days after spinal transection, vascular constriction begins a slow recovery, perhaps because of heightening of myogenic tone or the gradual establishment of spinal vascular reflexes. There also begins within a few days a denervation sensitivity of the vasculature involved. The vessels become abnormally sensitive to circulating or injected catecholamines so that local ischemia may develop. This phenomenon is usually more severe if the postganglionic (rather than preganglionic) fibers are interrupted. This effect is probably due to an increase in the number of receptors because of loss of tonic impulses of the smooth muscle.

Humoral Control of Flow

Probably the most important humoral agents influencing flow are the *circulating catecholamines*. These may be (*a*) endogenous, that is, derived from the adrenal medulla or from excess catecholamines released at neural endings; or (*b*) exogenous (*e.g.*, administered intravascularly). In either case, the cardiovascular effects will be similar to those of sympathetic neural action. In severe exercise, circulatory shock, or other forms of stress, the plasma concentration of catecholamines (epinephrine and norepinephrine) will increase markedly and reinforce the circulatory effects of sympathetic stimulation. However, the humoral catecholamines normally have only minor cardiovascular effects compared to those resulting from neural stimulation. Norepinephrine, the primary catecholamine, has a pure vasoconstrictor action in most beds. Epinephrine at low doses causes vasodilation through β-receptor stimulation, but at high doses its α-constrictor effect overshadows the β-dilator action, particularly in skeletal muscle. The metabolic effects of sympathetic stimulation are due primarily to epinephrine.

Other humoral vasoactive substances circulating in the bloodstream include angiotensin II (the most potent vasoconstrictor in the body), vasopressin, serotonin (5-hydroxytryptamine), and several prostaglandins. Except for the effect of prostaglandins on the renal circulation (discussed in Chapter 11), the physiological role of these substances in normal cardiovascular regulation is not yet certain.

Local Regulation of Flow

Functional Hyperemia

When tissues become metabolically more active (*e.g.*, during exercise or if their temperature is raised), the microcirculatory vessels dilate and flow increases, a process known as active hyperemia. The mechanism of this effect is not certain but is thought to be a vasodilator action of accumulated metabolites such as CO_2, lactic acid, or adenosine on the terminal arterioles or precapillary sphincters. The "metabolic" theory is strengthened by the fact that during severe exercise, when skeletal muscle metabolism is at its peak and metabolic products such as CO_2, lactic acid, etc., accumulate in the tissues, blood flow is very high.

Other metabolites such as K^+ and H^+ as well as decreased Po_2 and increased osmolality have also been proposed as primary dilator agents. There is increasing evidence that the responsible metabolites may vary with the tissue involved. In the hypoxic myocardium, for example, adenosine and some of its related compounds have been implicated as the active agents. In the salivary gland, bradykinin, and in the kidney, prostaglandins are known to have strong local vascular effects.

As described in Chapter 8, there is convincing evidence that the endothelial cells play an important role in regulating local blood flow, partly through their own contractile properties and partly through their role in mediating the vasodilation and vasoconstriction of the microvasculature. Just how the endothelial cells bring about this effect is not well understood; however, Fridovich *et al.* have recently extracted a substance produced by the endothelium in response to a variety of stimuli. This agent, called endothelium-derived relaxing factor (EDRF), will produce relaxation of the vessel walls of the microvasculature and disaggregation of platelets. EDRF may be one of the locally produced agents that help to match the blood flow and metabolic state of tissue.

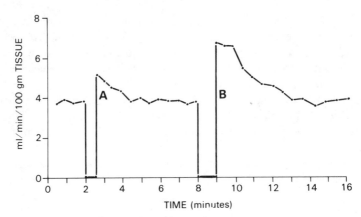

Figure 9.9. Reactive hyperemia. *A*, Temporary increase in blood flow to forearm after 30-second occlusion. After 60-second occlusion, *B*, the reactive flow is of greater magnitude and duration.

Reactive Hyperemia

If blood flow to a tissue is arrested by arterial occlusion for a period of a few seconds to several minutes, the flow upon release will exceed the control flow for a short period before returning to preocclusion levels. This excess afterflow is known as "reactive hyperemia" and, as indicated in Figure 9.9, the resulting degree and duration of the overshoot are roughly proportional to the duration of the occlusion (*i.e.*, to the metabolic debt incurred).

Tissues differ in their reactive hyperemic response; heart and brain show large responses, skeletal muscle intermediate, and liver, lung, and skin the least. The cause of the increased flow is not clear but the relation between the length of occlusion and degree of hyperemia suggests that either oxygen lack in the tissues or the accumulation of metabolites is responsible. Reactive hyperemia will result after ischemia (partial or full occlusion of arterial supply) or hypoxia (reduced P_{O_2} in the tissue).

Autoregulation

If individual organs are perfused with blood at different pressures so that flow-pressure relations can be studied, the initial response in almost all cases resembles *curve A*, Figure 9.10. In some tissues, particularly kidney, brain, and heart, the flow will change within 30 to 60 seconds to an "autoregulatory" adaptation such as *curve B* (Fig. 9.10), in which there is a tendency to maintain the local blood flow relatively constant in the face of a changing perfusion pressure. Some tissues such as skin and lung show minimal autoregulation.

Curve A is a passive type of curve, and its exponential nature is due mainly to the constantly increasing diameter that occurs in a flexible tube subjected

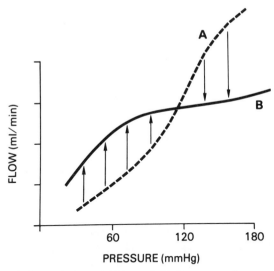

Figure 9.10. Autoregulation of kidney. Initial pressure-flow response curve (*A*) changes to plateau-type curve (*B*) within 30 to 60 seconds.

to increasing transmural pressure (Chapter 2). During autoregulation (*curve B*), the higher flows are achieved at low pressure by relaxation of the vascular muscle, and the lower flows at higher pressures by constriction. The net result—the maintenance of a relatively consistent flow—is particularly advantageous to vital organs such as brain and heart; in the case of hypotension or failing circulation, local flow will increase. In the case of higher pressure, excess flow will be reduced.

Those organs with the smallest neurogenic tone (brain, heart, and kidney) show the highest autoregulatory ability. Conversely, tissues with the highest resting vascular tone (*e.g.*, skin) have the least autoregulatory ability. Although the ability to autoregulate is affected to some extent by neural and humoral influences such as vasoconstrictor tone and the pH of the blood, the autoregulatory response is largely intrinsic and occurs when tissues are fully denervated and isolated. Autoregulation is, therefore, essentially a local phenomenon mediated *via* changes in active tone in the small blood vessels.

Different explanations have been advanced for autoregulation. One of these, the myogenic theory, suggests that increased perfusion pressure increases the muscle tension in the vessel wall, stimulating it to contract, and thus reducing flow. With reduction in perfusion pressure, there is relaxation of the smooth muscle of the wall and an increase in vessel caliber. This theory proposes, therefore, that distension or relaxation of the muscle is the self-regulating mediator.

Other investigators believe that autoregulation is associated with the state

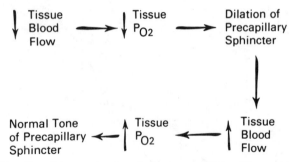

Figure 9.11. Possible mechanism for autoregulation of tissue blood flow involving effect of altered P_{O_2} on precapillary sphincter tone.

of oxygenation of the tissue; a decrease in flow will produce a decrease in local tissue P_{O_2} and an increase in tissue P_{CO_2} and other metabolites related to O_2 supply. The decreased P_{O_2} or accumulation of vasoactive metabolites would theoretically relax the arterioles and the flow would rise again. With restored flow, the P_{O_2} and P_{CO_2} levels of vasoactive metabolites in tissue are returned toward normal, as shown in Figure 9.11. Regardless of the validity of any specific theory, it seems very likely that tissue flow is regulated in a manner similar to the negative feedback mechanism shown in Figure 9.11.

Long-Term Regulation of Flow

The previous portions of this chapter relate to rapid adjustments of the circulation. But what are the responses if demands for additional flow are built up more gradually? If, for example, the main arterial supply to a part of the body such as skin or muscle is gradually occluded, the pressure and flow in the distal vessel will be reduced. What is the response of the tissue to such a situation? In tissues with adequate collateral circulation (*e.g.*, skeletal muscle), collateral vessels will dilate over the ensuing days and weeks so that total arterial flow to the part will gradually be restored to near normal levels. Thus the local circulatory demand has in some way instigated an increased blood supply. This type of adaptation is, however, severely restricted in tissues such as brain or kidney, in which collateral vessels are minimal or absent. In such cases an infarct (area of necrosis) is likely as a result of vascular occlusion with degeneration, loss of function, and replacement fibrosis occurring in at least a portion of the involved area. The question of myocardial infarct is discussed in Chapter 14.

On the other hand, if arterial pressure and flow to a part is excessive, (*e.g.*, in arteries above the level at which partial occlusion of the abdominal aorta has been produced in an experimental animal), the flow to tissues above the occlusion level will at first be excessive because of the hypertension in this portion of the arterial tree. Gradually, however, the flow to the involved regions will return to normal by virtue of gradually increased constriction of the arteries and arterioles in the area. Thus, if blood flow is artificially increased or decreased, it will, if left alone, tend to gradually return to previous control levels. Similar circulatory responses occur with alterations of oxygen supply. Prolonged hypoxia will stimulate increased flow and in embryonic or fetal tissue will promote the generation of new blood vessels.

It appears, therefore, that the relation of flow to tissue metabolism is the dominant factor in the long-term regulation of blood flow. It seems likely that the mechanism of this effect is either *via* oxygen demand or through an oxygen-linked metabolite. But how oxygen lack actually brings about increased flow or vascular architectural expansion is not certain. However, recent studies on angiogenesis (growth of new blood vessels) in tumor growths as well as in normal myocardium, skeletal muscle, and fibrous tissue have thrown light on this interesting subject. The growth and regression of capillaries governs both growth and involution of tissues and angiogenic peptides; angiogenic steroids serve as an elaborate control system for capillary growth.

It was discovered that heparin potentiates angiogenesis by enhancing the motion of endothelial cells and by increasing the effect of certain endothelial growth factors. This function is independent of the anticoagulant action of heparin. Certain heparin-bound growth factors such as endothelial cell growth factor (ECGF) and fibroblast growth factor (FGF)—as well as other peptides—seem to induce vascular growth either by inducing directional locomotion of endothelial cells or by mobilizing other macrophages or parenchymal cells to release other stimulators of endothelial locomotion and proliferation. It has also been found that certain steroids (which lack glucocorticoid or mineralocorticoid activity) will inhibit angiogenesis in the presence of heparin.

There is also evidence that increased mechanical load on the blood vessel wall will stimulate the synthesis of connective tissue and contractile proteins as well as cell growth in the heart and other tissues. But while the increased physical stretch and tension of vasodilation on the growth potential of vascular cells may be a factor, it is known that the vascular cells of younger tissue are more responsive to the growth stimuli of hypoxia and ischemia than are those of older tissue. While the study of angiogenesis is in its infancy, it has in less than two decades grown into a major field of science with important ramifications for the study of embryology, senescence, cancer, and many other pathological conditions.

Selected Readings

Damore PA and Thompson RW. Mechanisms of angiogenesis. *Annu Rev Physiol* 49:453–464, 1987.

Duling BR, *et al.* Vasomotor control: functional hyperemia and beyond. *Fed Proc* 46:251–263, 1987.

Folkman J. Angiogenesis: what makes blood vessels grow. *NIPS* 1:199–202, 1986.

Fridovich I, *et al*. Endothelium-derived relaxing factor. *NIPS* 2:61–64, 1987.

Hoffman BB and Lefkowitz RJ. Adrenergic receptors in the heart. *Annu Rev Physiol* 44:475–484, 1982.

Johnson PC. Principles of peripheral circulatory control. In: *Peripheral Circulation*, edited by PC Johnson. New York: John Wiley & Sons, 1978.

Johnson RH and Spalding JMK. *Disorders of the Autonomic Nervous System*. Philadelphia: F.A. Davis, 1974.

Mellander S and Johansson B. Control of resistance, exchange and capacitance functions in the peripheral circulation. *Phamacol Rev* 20:117–196, 1968.

Randall WC. *Nervous Control of Cardiovascular Function*. New York: Oxford University Press, 1984.

Rothe CF. Reflex control of veins and vascular capacitance. *Physiol Rev* 63:1281, 1983.

Rowell LD. *Human Circulation During Physical Stress*. London: Oxford University Press, 1986.

Shepherd JT and Mancia G. Reflex control of the human cardiovascular system. *Rev Physiol Biochem Pharm* 105:1, 1986.

chapter 10

Regulation of Arterial Blood Pressure

Arterial Pressure Regulation—General Principles

The two prime objectives of circulatory regulation are (*a*) the maintenance of an adequate and relatively constant arterial pressure and (*b*) a sufficient control of blood flow through local tissues to insure adequate metabolism, capillary exchange, and temperature balance. Blood flow was discussed in Chapter 9. The important topic of arterial pressure control is considered in this chapter.

The method by which arterial pressure is regulated depends upon whether short-term or long-term adaptation is required. Short-term adjustments (over minutes and hours) are intended to correct temporary imbalances of pressure such as those caused by postural change, hemorrhage, or other acute stresses. But whatever the cause of the circulatory disturbance, the reaction is a combination of (a) adaptation of the local blood vessels to the altered volumes and pressures (e.g., autoregulation) and (b) rapid autonomic neural responses, intended to return the arterial pressure toward normal.

On the other hand, long-term arterial pressure adaptation (weeks and months) is usually accomplished through changes in extracellular fluid and blood volume, microcirculatory architecture, and renal mechanisms. The latter are strongly influenced by neurohumoral factors that control water and sodium excretion by the kidney.

Arterial blood pressure is probably the most important controlled variable in the circulation. We know from the general hemodynamic equation discussed in Chapter 2 that blood pressure is, in effect, the mathematical product of cardiac output and peripheral resistance. The cardiovascular centers of the medulla, which are the primary acute circulatory controls, regulate the arterial pressure mainly through adjustment of these two variables. However, the medullary cardiovascular centers are themselves influenced by impulses from higher neural centers and by multiple sensors throughout the body. Some of these sensors are located within the vascular system and give rise to intrinsic reflexes; other sensors are located elsewhere in the body and give rise to extrinsic reflexes. Thus, the arterial pressure, acting through classical feedback mechanisms, is both a controlled and a controlling variable as shown in Figure 10.1.

Cardiovascular Centers of the Medulla

The medulla oblangata is the site of the most critical cardiovascular control centers in the body. Investigators have found that several key physiological functions, such as the coordination of circulatory and respiratory control as well as important synaptic relays from higher centers to spinal cord sympathetic elements, are carried out by neuronal elements of the ventrolateral medulla.

However, the main nervous control of the circulation resides in several functionally diverse areas or "centers" in the dorsal reticular matter of the medulla and lower pons. These are collectively known as cardiovascular (CV) centers, and together with the respiratory center, with which they have close neural connection, they constitute the "vital nervous centers" whose integrity is absolutely essential for survival of the organism.

There are two major divisions of the cardiovascular control area, cardiac and vasomotor, which are concerned with the neural control of the heart and peripheral blood vessels, respectively. These two areas are not well defined

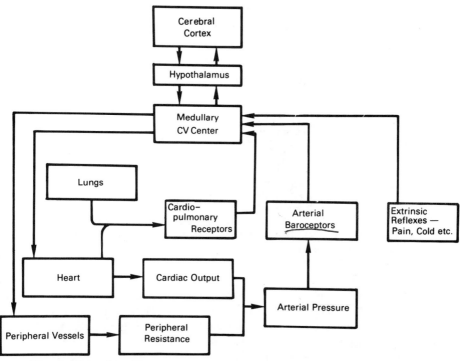

Figure 10.1.   Simplified schema showing primary pathways for short-term regulation of arterial blood pressure.

and there is both anatomical and functional overlap between them. Careful animal experiments involving surgical transection as well as microelectrode stimulation and functional mapping have indicated that both the cardiac and vasomotor areas have, in turn, further subdivisions with specialized functions.

One of the clearest entities in the cardiac area is a ''cardioinhibitory center'' located in the nucleus ambiguus and dorsal nucleus of the vagus nerve. Vagal efferents from these sites carry impulses that act primarily to decrease heart rate and to a lesser degree the contractility of the atria. The existence of a corollary sympathetic ''cardiostimulatory center'' in the lateral medulla has been reported, but its identity as a discrete center is less certain.

The ''vasomotor center'' of the medulla consists, in most species, of a lateral ''vasoconstrictor area'' whose neurons descend in the spinal cord and synapse with cells of the intermediolateral cell column. Their preganglionic fibers are responsible for the widespread sympathetic vasoconstriction described in Chapter 9. The ''vasodilator area'' is more questionable, and it is probable that vasodilation is mainly due to inhibition of the vasoconstrictor center.

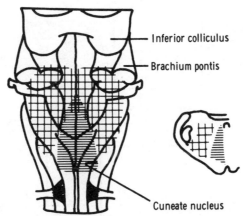

Inferior colliculus

Brachium pontis

Cuneate nucleus

Figure 10.2. Location of pressor (*crosshatched*) and depressor (*horizontally lined*) areas in the brain stem of the cat. (Reprinted with permission from J. Alexander, *Neurophysiology* 9:205, 1946).

The close proximity of these centers to each other and their tendency to function in a coordinated fashion in the interests of arterial pressure control have led to the characterization of the lateral and superior portions of the CV center area as the "pressor area," and the more medial as the "depressor area" (Fig. 10.2). In most species, stimulation of the pressor area will induce both an increase in cardiac rate and contractility and a generalized increase in peripheral resistance, while depressor area stimulation usually elicits the converse. The "vasoconstrictor," "cardiostimulatory," and "cardioinhibitory" areas are tonically active (*i.e.*, they emit, event at rest, a constant low level of efferent impulses, so that cutting of these efferent fibers will eliminate vasoconstrictor, cardiac stimulatory, and cardioinhibitory effects on the respective target organs).

The various CV centers usually function reciprocally, that is, when vagal slowing is initiated by the cardioinhibitory center, there is simultaneously reduced activity of the cardiostimulatory center.

Intrinsic Reflexes of the Cardiovascular System

"Intrinsic" reflexes, those that arise from within the circulatory system itself, are usually distinguished from "extrinsic" reflexes, those originating in other systems or organs. The intrinsic reflexes, by far the more important in the short-term regulation of blood pressure, are for the most part activated by special receptors. These receptors are usually sensitive to pressure or to special chemical stimuli. Those sensitive to pressure are termed stretch receptors, baroceptors, or mechanoreceptors. The "chemoreceptors" of the vascular

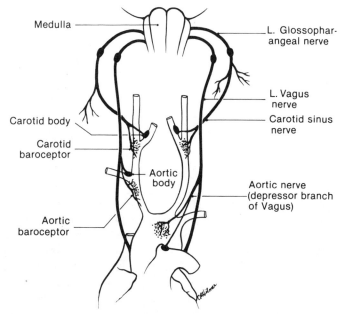

Figure 10.3. Diagrammatic sketch showing the central connections of the aortic and carotid sinus baroceptors.

system are primarily concerned with respiratory regulation but may in certain circumstances play a secondary role in circulatory control.

Much of the understanding of intrinsic reflexes of the cardiovascular system, as well as of the roles of higher centers, has necessarily been obtained from animal research—which is indispensable in this type of investigation. Just as there are differences between animals, cardiovascular control in the human varies to some extent even from that of higher mammals. In our treatment of control mechanisms in this—as well as in other chapters—our descriptions will refer to human responses, as nearly as we can determine them from the present state of animal and human research.

Arterial Baroceptors

Afferent fibers from specialized pressure-sensitive endings in the walls of the aortic arch and internal carotid arteries travel *via* the aortic and carotid sinus nerves, join the vagus and glossopharyngeal nerves respectively, and make connections with the CV centers of the medulla. Impulses from the carotid and aortic chemoreceptors, which are near their respective baroceptor endings, travel over the same afferent nerves (Fig. 10.3).

Stretching of these baroceptor endings generates action potentials in the afferent nerves (Fig. 10.3), whose frequency is approximately proportional

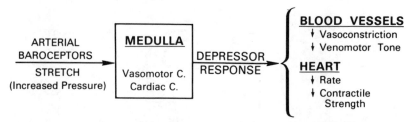

Figure 10.4. Hemodynamic response to arterial baroceptor stimulation.

to the pressure change in the artery. This means that *increased* arterial pressure at the baroceptor site will increase the frequency of afferent impulses in the aortic and carotid sinus nerves. This stimulus results in greater activity in the medullary depressor area and inhibition of the pressor area, so that heart rate and myocardial contractility are *decreased* and vasoconstrictor and venoconstrictor tone are *lessened* (Fig. 10.4). Increased blood pressure, therefore, leads to reflex action aimed at reducing the pressure back toward normal levels (depressor reflex). If baroceptor stretch is decreased, the afferent impulse frequency is decreased, and the reverse response occurs (pressor reflex). Thus, in common with most reflexes that stabilize a controlled variable, arterial baroceptors (ABs) involve negative feedback.

The high-pressure baroceptors respond to absolute stretch (*i.e.*, to changes in both mean arterial transmural pressure and pulse pressure) but even more strongly to the rate of change of pressure, dP/dt. The baroceptor response is greatest in the physiological range of blood pressure (80 to 150 mm Hg), and there is evidence that the carotid baroceptors are somewhat more sensitive than the aortic (Fig. 10.5).

Current evidence suggests that, in the human, the arterial baroceptors (ABs) have a primary influence on the reflex control of cardiac rate and contractility but probably a secondary one on the control of total vascular resistance. AB vasoconstriction control is particularly marked in mesenteric arteries and in venoconstrictor control of the splanchnic bed, which is important in influencing venous return to the heart. Evidence also indicates that during the pressor response, there is an increased release of renin in the kidney, a greater tubular reabsorption of Na^+, and a tendency toward expansion of the plasma volume; these effects are mediated by the ABs.

As indicated in Figure 10.5, at higher arterial pressure levels, the ABs are less sensitive to any given pressure increment, probably because of the lower compliance of the arterial wall at higher degrees of stretch. Arterial baroceptors normally respond more actively to a decrease in pressure than to an increase (*i.e.*, they are more effective in combating acute hypotension than acute hypertension).

An important property of arterial baroceptors is their ability to adapt to

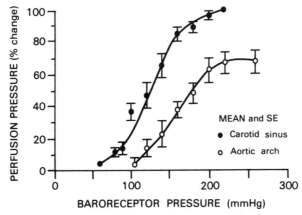

Figure 10.5. Baroceptor sensitivity at different arterial pressure levels in the dog. At equivalent pressures the carotid baroceptors were more sensitive than the aortic receptors. (Reprinted with permission from D.E. Donald and A.J. Edis, *J Physiol* 215:521, 1971.)

permanent or semipermanent alterations in arterial pressure. Even in acute hypertension (6 hours or less) and in exercise, the ABs continue to function but are ''reset'' at a higher level, which then becomes the baseline for further baroceptor response. Reports indicate that the baroceptors will also reset to a lower level in the case of hypotension. These ''resets'' are reversible if the baseline pressure changes.

Methods have been developed for measuring the sensitivity of the arterial baroceptor response by (*a*) inducing mild, temporary alterations in arterial pressure through administration of pharmacologic vasoconstrictors or vasodilators or (*b*) applying positive or negative pressure to the area of the neck over the carotid sinus receptors. The rapidity and degree of the heart-rate response to the transmural pressure change is a measure of the sensitivity of the reflex. Such experiments have shown a decreased responsiveness of ABs with advancing age, hypertension, and coronary artery disease. It has been suggested that arteriosclerotic changes and decreased compliance of the arterial walls are responsible for the decreased sensitivity of the receptors in these conditions.

Sundloff and Wallin have reported a further manifestation of the arterial baroreflex. They found increasing and decreasing bursts of efferent sympathetic nerve impulses to the limbs immediately following and synchronous with the fall and rise of the aortic pressure wave. There was a strong negative correlation between the diastolic level of aortic pressure and the frequency of the immediately following sympathetic nerve impulses to the peripheral vascular bed. There was, however, no correlation between mean burst incidence and static blood pressure levels. These findings suggest another (closely

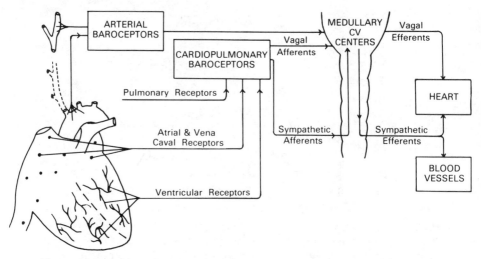

Figure 10.6.   Arterial and cardiopulmonary baroceptors and their central connections.

related) type of arterial baroreflex, which does not sense static levels of mean and pulse pressures (as described above) but provides a rapid, dynamic, beat-by-beat adjustment of peripheral resistance on the basis of the immediately preceding diastolic pressure. This reflex apparently supplements the regular arterial baroreflex but has the same objective—stabilization of the arterial blood pressure.

In general, the strength of the baroceptor reflex decrees that in most short-term situations, there is a reciprocal relationship between arterial blood pressure and heart rate. However, this does not universally hold. For example, during static (isometric) exercise, systolic and diastolic blood pressures and heart rate all increase progressively (Chapter 12). In the diving (face immersion) reflex, there is a sharp decrease in both arterial pressure and heart rate (Chapter 13), and during the ''defense reaction'' (described later in this chapter) there is a pronounced increase in arterial pressure as well as heart rate. It is likely that supramedullary centers, which are involved in all three of these instances, are responsible for the sudden but temporary inhibition of the baroreflexes.

Cardiopulmonary Reflexes

Cardiopulmonary receptors are intrathoracic sensors, most of which are located at low-pressure sites in the walls of the heart, great vessels, and lungs. These receptors are usually classified on the basis of location: (*a*) atrial and vena caval, (*b*) ventricular, and (*c*) pulmonary (Fig. 10.6).

Atrial and Vena Caval Receptors

These are low-pressure mechanoreceptors whose impulses travel mainly *via* large, myelinated (fast-conducting) and small, unmyelinated (slow-conducting) vagal afferent fibers. Three different varieties of these atrial receptors have been recognized: type A, which fire only during atrial systole; type B, which fire only during atrial filling; and an intermediate group, which fire during both atrial systole and filling.

Cardiac reflexes—particularly those arising from atrial and vena caval receptors—are currently a very active focus of research. Our basic understanding of reflexes is mainly derived from animal studies involving the dissection of nerves to their receptor origins, balloon distensions of heart chambers at graded volumes and pressures, and electrical stimulation of afferent nerves at different frequencies and intensities. The physiological consequences of such manipulations are noted both in the presence and absence of competing influences (*e.g.*, the arterial baroceptor reflexes). The results of such basic experiments are then compared with studies in human subjects and patients in which cardiopulmonary receptor stimulation is altered (*e.g.*, by changes in central blood volume). While there are some differences of opinion on the scope and function of these reflexes, the following is a brief outline of the views advanced by most investigators on the probable role of cardiopulmonary (CP) receptors.

Heart Rate Effects. The most widely known of these is the *Bainbridge reflex*, which refers to the tachycardia that is sometimes produced by increased filling of the atrium or atriocaval region, for example, by large intravenous infusions of blood or saline. The afferent pathway is *via* large myelinated fibers of the vagus nerve, and the efferents are primarily in the sympathetic fibers to the SA node. Although this reflex has long been observed in a number of species, the heart rate response to atrial filling in man is complicated by other simultaneous circulatory responses, so that in the intact human this reflex probably plays a secondary role.

Blood Pressure and Renal Effects. There is now considerable evidence that stimulation of CP mechanoreceptors, whose afferents travel mainly *via* unmyelinated vagal fibers, trigger a widespread complex of circulatory effects that alter arterial pressure, heart rate, and renal function. Recent studies suggest that these CP impulses originate not only in the atria but also in the ventricles and lungs.

Shepherd, Donald, and other investigators noted that an increase in central blood volume and pressure (*e.g.*, through large intravenous fluid infusions, prolonged bed rest, or the zero-gravity state) will increase the firing of these CP receptors. This, in turn, will result in a decrease in sympathetic vasoconstriction of skeletal muscle and renal and mesenteric arterioles, an increase in splanchnic venous capacitance, and a diminution in heart rate (*i.e.*, a depressor response). This decrease in sympathetic activity is accompanied by a lesser release of renin by the kidneys, a decreased Na^+ reabsorption from the renal tubules, and a diuresis with a resultant tendency toward a diminution in plasma volume.

Corollary studies have shown that a decrease in central blood volume (*e.g.*, in head-up tilt or hemorrhage) or the cutting of afferent vagal fibers from CP receptors in an experimental animal result in a sympathetic vasoconstriction of skeletal muscle and renal and mesenteric arterioles, a decrease in splanchnic venous capacitance, and an increase in heart rate—a pressor response. This sympathetic hyperactivity is accompanied by increased release of renin by the kidneys, greater Na^+ reabsorption from the tubules, antidiuresis, and a tendency toward an increase in plasma volume.

In other words, these CP receptors, under normal resting conditions, appear to exert a tonic inhibitory effect on sympathetic vasoconstriction and cardioacceleration. A lessening of this receptor stimulation, through a decrease in central blood volume or through cutting of these afferent nerves, "unloads" the receptors and thereby decreases their firing rate. This invokes a sympathetic pressor effect *via* the vasomotor and cardiac centers of the medulla as well as an antidiuretic effect. It should be noted that the heart-rate changes accompanying the reflex induced by these receptors are directionally opposite to those resulting from the Bainbridge reflex.

CP receptors are capable of adapting to a continued increase in atrial pressure by resetting. It has been shown, for example, that in experimental congestive heart failure in dogs, in which the atria are distended, the atrial receptors gradually adapt, and the diuretic reflex is attenuated. This adaptation is reversed if the heart failure is relieved.

From the preceding, it will be noted that the characteristics, effects, and general functions of this CP receptor response are similar to those of the arterial baroceptor reflex. It is evident (*a*) that the low- and high-pressure mechanoreceptors act in concert in an effort to buffer arterial pressure changes, (*b*) that both have cardiovascular and renal manifestations, and (*c*) that both can adapt to a sustained alteration in baroceptor stretch by resetting.

However, there are also certain differences between those reflexes: (*a*) the CP reflexes react to lesser pressure changes—nonhypotensive hemorrhage, for example, will induce prompt CP responses, since these receptors act at low-pressure atrial sites that are affected earlier by the hypotension; (*b*) CP receptors (at least in man) have stronger reflex vasoconstrictor effects on skeletal muscle arteries, while ABs induce stronger splanchnic vasoconstriction and apparently greater effects on heart rate; and (*c*) the plasma volume effects of CP receptors are more pronounced, and the role of CP endings as "volume receptors" appears to be a very significant one.

The mechanism of the renal effects is at present not fully understood. Plasma volume regulation involves complex interrelationships between circulatory reflexes, CNS osmoreceptors, and several endocrine systems. Current evidence indicates that the atrial CP mechanoreceptors mediate their plasma volume effects primarily through regulating renal sympathetic nerve activity, the renin-angiotensin-aldosterone (RAA) system, arginine vasopressin (AVP), and atrial natriuretic factor (ANF). However, because (compared to autonomic neurogenic reflexes) they are slower acting, they play a relatively minor role in early and rapid hemodynamic adjustments to circulatory stress. The main effector sites of these neurohormones are the renal tubules. These mechanisms are further discussed in Chapter 11 (Renal Circulation). The role of these reflexes in hypotensive stresses is discussed in Chapter 13 (Response to Hemorrhage) and in Chapter 14 (Congestive Heart Failure).

Investigators have reported that mechanoreceptors may be stimulated by either stretch or contraction of the muscle with which they are in contact, depending on the orientation of the receptors. It is believed, for example, that increased atrial muscle contraction is the mechanism for the diuresis seen in certain clinical and experimental pathological conditions, such as paroxysmal atrial tachycardia or atrial fibrillation, in which there is unusual contractile activity of the atrial wall. This effect does not occur in ordinary sinus tachycardia since there is no undue stimulation of the receptors in this case.

Ventricular Receptors

When stimulated by increased stretch or by strong ventricular contraction, afferent impulses from ventricular receptors (traveling mainly *via* unmyelinated or slow-conducting vagal fibers) reach the medulla and elicit a bradycardia and vasodilation (*i.e.*, a *depressor* response).

A peculiar characteristic of these receptors is that a very similar, hypotensive response is produced by injection into the heart or coronary circulation of a specific chemical agent called veratrine (an alkaloid extract from lilacs). This unusual chemoreceptor response is known as the *Bezold-Jarisch reflex*. This reflex may also be triggered by intracoronary injections of other chemicals such as nicotine, bradykinin, histamine, or digitalis. A similar response can be elicited by the injection of a contrast medium during coronary angiography and by the accumulation of metabolites under certain pathological conditions. The hypotensive reaction in cardiogenic shock produced by coronary occlusion may be partly due to activation of these ventricular receptors (Chapter 14).

The above-described responses to stimulation of ventricular receptors are the result of afferent impulses that travel *via* the vagus nerves. Ventricular distension in experimental animals will also stimulate sympathetic afferent endings in the ventricle, which will invoke strong arterial *pressor* responses as well as alterations in respiration. The functional significance of these sympathetic ventricular CP reflexes is not clear at present.

Pulmonary Receptors

A variety of reflexes arising from the lung are known to be important in the control of respiration, but their circulatory significance in man is still uncertain. However, pulmonary congestion, which occurs during severe exercise or increased pulmonary venous pressure, may activate juxtapulmonary receptors (so-called J receptors) and induce reflex tachycardia and dyspnea (difficulty in breathing).

It should be pointed out that most of our information on CP reflexes has been derived from animal experiments. While these have contributed immeasurably to our knowledge, species differences in these types of reflexes are often significant. Thus, the full role of these reflexes in the human is still not known.

Arterial Chemoreceptors

These special endings, located in the carotid and aortic bodies (near the carotid sinus and aortic arch receptors), respond to a reduction in arterial P_{O_2}, an increase in P_{CO_2}, or an increase in arterial H^+ concentration, with hyperventilation, sympathetic vasoconstriction (mainly in skeletal muscle), and bradycardia (vagal). While the main purpose of the arterial chemoreceptor reflex is to stimulate respiratory minute volume, its secondary circulatory effects appear to be aimed at increasing oxygen delivery to the brain and heart through general peripheral vasoconstriction and increased arterial pressure. The chemoreceptor reflex becomes a protective factor in certain pathophysiological situations such as the hypoxia of altitude (low arterial P_{O_2}) and circulatory shock (peripheral ischemia). The special role of the chemoreceptors in the diving (face immersion) response is discussed in Chapter 13.

Summary—Intrinsic Reflexes of the Circulatory System

Our present knowledge, while admittedly incomplete, does permit a few generalizations regarding circulatory reflexes:

1. The intrinsic reflexes of the arterial and cardiopulmonary baroceptors are, by far, the most important instruments of the circulatory system in maintaining arterial pressure—and thereby adequate flow to the brain and heart—during short-term circulatory stresses.

2. Aside from neutralizing abnormal arterial pressure alterations, these two intrinsic reflex systems also dampen out the numerous pressure fluctuations that occur during normal daily activities. Studies have shown that even during resting and basal states, dogs with denervated baroceptors tended to show very wide swings in arterial pressure and a striking inability to maintain a constant pressure level. Undoubtedly, this stabilization of ar-

terial pressure by the sympathetic reflex systems lessens flow fluctuations to important organs such as the brain and heart.

3. The arterial (high-pressure) baroreflexes seem to play the major role in controlling cardiac rate and contractility, renal and mesenteric arterial resistance, and splanchnic venoconstriction.

4. The cardiopulmonary baroreflexes (all low pressure except for those of the left ventricle), while not yet as well defined as the arterial baroceptors, have a significant role in cardiovascular regulation. They elicit circulatory responses that generally supplement and modulate the arterial baroceptor reflexes, the common objective being the stability of arterial blood pressure. Grassi and others have reported that these reflexes play the major role in mobilizing peripheral vascular resistance in the human response to short-term circulatory stress (e.g., postural change).

5. The baroceptors, particularly the cardiopulmonary, serve also as "volume" receptors that mediate their responses through neurohumoral agents and play important roles in maintaining longer-term blood-volume and water-balance control.

Extrinsic Reflexes of the Cardiovascular System

Certain stimuli originating outside the circulation may invoke cardiovascular responses via somatic afferent pathways. The central connections are not well known and the responses are usually less consistent than those of the intrinsic reflexes described above. Extrinsic reflexes play a relatively minor role in normal circumstances but play important and protective roles in certain types of environmental stress and circulatory disease. Below some of the more common extrinsic reflexes are discussed.

Pain

Pain produces a somewhat variable hemodynamic response. Mild to moderate pain usually elicits increased arterial pressure and tachycardia. Severe pain, as might be experienced by undue stretching of the gall bladder, intestine, or ureter or deep trauma to a bone or joint, may induce bradycardia, hypotension, and sometimes circulatory collapse and fainting. Overly rapid evacuation of a markedly distended hollow organ may also cause reflex hypotension and sometimes circulatory collapse. This reflex is responsible for the clinical admonition that if pressure in overdistended organs such as the stomach or urinary bladder is relieved by intubation or catheterization, the decompression should be done slowly. Pain accompanying myocardial ischemia is discussed in Chapter 15.

Cold

Somatic afferent fibers from cutaneous thermosensitive endings travel to the hypothalamus and reflexly induce cutaneous vasoconstriction and piloerection

(erection of hair). Intense local cold, for example, by immersion of one hand to the wrist in ice water for 1 minute (the *"cold pressor" test*) will result in an increase in arterial pressure through stimulation of both pain and cold receptors.

It has been reported that in some patients with coronary heart disease, the cold pressor test increases coronary artery resistance, decreases coronary blood flow, and sometimes precipitates angina (chest pain) of cardiac origin; these changes did not occur in normal subjects (Fig. 10.7). The cause of angina is not certain but may be due to either reflex coronary vasoconstriction or a relative myocardial ischemia due to the increased aortic afterload.

Special Somatic Reflexes

Strong somatic afferent stimulation may cause circulatory responses, particularly of the depressor type. *Rapid angular acceleration* (rotation or spinning of the body on its own axis) will, for example, induce excessive afferent stimulation from the labyrinth of the inner ear and may cause nausea, vomiting, and a depressor reflex. The *oculocardiac reflex* refers to bradycardia and hypotension induced by lateral pressure on the eyeball; the latter reflex, by virtue of its efferent vagal path, is sometimes effective in aborting attacks of cardiac arrhythmias such as atrial fibrillation (Chapter 5).

Higher Center Influences

CNS Ischemic Response

Apart from the baroceptor responses induced by a fall in blood pressure, severe hypotension, such as occurs in circulatory shock, will result in a profound, generalized vasoconstriction. Since the mechanism of this powerful reflex is probably hypoxia or ischemia of the brain stem, it is known as the "CNS ischemic response." It apparently represents a "last ditch" effort to maintain adequate perfusion of the CV medullary centers and is activated only when the arterial pressure is reduced to levels of about 50 to 70 mm Hg.

A similar mechanism is thought to be operative in the "Cushing reflex," which is marked hypertension following acute elevation of cerebrospinal fluid (CSF) pressure. In this instance the flow of blood to the brain stem is decreased by the external pressure of CSF fluid on the blood vessels, thus activating the CNS ischemic response. The arterial blood pressure rises progressively in an effort to exceed the CSF pressure and maintain adequate blood flow to the brain.

Role of the Hypothalamus

The hypothalamus, as a midway point between the cerebral cortex and the medulla, provides a level of integration for a number of essential cardiovascular activities. Animal experiments have shown that from a functional stand-

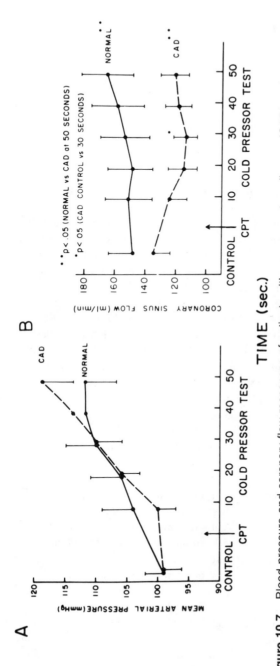

Figure 10.7. Blood pressure and coronary flow responses of patients with coronary artery disease (CAD) and normal subjects to the cold pressor test. *A* indicates similar arterial pressure response in the two groups, and *B*, a decrease in coronary flow in the patients. *Arrow* indicates start of 50-second cold pressor test. (Reprinted with permission from G.H. Mudge, W. Grossman, R.M. Mills, M. Lesch, and E. Braunwald, *N Engl J Med* 295:1333, 1976.)

point the hypothalamic circulatory control is located in the rostral parasympathetic and caudal sympathetic centers. Stimulation of the former causes vagal activation and sympatho-inhibition, and stimulation of the latter, the reverse response. The work of Hilton and others indicates that these centers are necessary for the mediation of the baroceptor reflexes.

In addition, the hypothalamus plays a key role in coordinating responses to *emotion, exercise,* and *temperature change.* Experimental animals with lesions in the ventromedial hypothalamus will, upon relatively slight provocation, react with intense rage associated with high blood pressure, sweating, and pupillary dilation. The hypothalamus plays a key role in determining the circulatory and other autonomic responses that accompany swings of mood and emotion.

The efficient and effective performance of *physical exercise* or work requires a close integration of the circulation and metabolism. That this is done by the hypothalamus is suggested by the fact that stimulation of the fields of Forel will, in the dog, produce a series of autonomic reactions closely resembling those that accompany physical exercise; these include highly coordinated responses of dilation of skeletal muscle vessels, constriction of nonmuscle beds, and release of plasma catecholamines into the blood (Chapter 12, Physical Exercise).

The control center for *temperature regulation,* located in the preoptic region of the anterior hypothalamus, plays a key role in balancing heat production and loss. When the body (or the hypothalamus) is heated, sympathetic vasoconstrictor impulse traffic is decreased, vascular smooth muscles are relaxed, the cutaneous arteriovenous anastomoses (AVAs) of exposed areas are opened, and sweating occurs; all of these are essential to the preservation of heat balance. With cold the reverse response occurs in order to reduce heat loss (Chapter 11, Cutaneous Circulation).

Corticohypothalamic Patterns—Defense Reaction

From a circulatory standpoint, one of the more important behavior patterns involving the cerebral cortex and the hypothalamus is the ''defense reaction.'' It has been shown that stimulation of a localized area in the ventral hypothalamus of the cat will produce circulatory reactions very similar to those invoked by the presence of actual danger or threat of danger to the animal. These reactions include sympathetic cholinergic vasodilation of skeletal muscle (to permit immediate maximum muscular effort), generalized sympathetic vasoconstriction and elevation of arterial pressure, increased plasma catecholamines, and increased rate and contractility of the heart. These changes, similar to those mentioned as preparation for muscular exercise, instantly prepare the animal for full-scale ''fight or flight'' reaction.

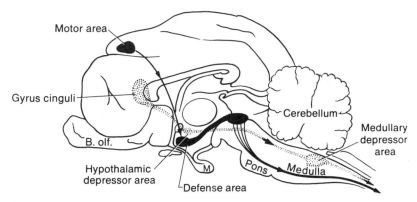

Figure 10.8.   Illustration of the cortical and spinal connections of the defense center and "depressor area" of the hypothalamus. (Reprinted with permission from B. Folkow and E. Neil, *Circulation*. London: Oxford University Press, 1971.)

It has also been observed that stimulation of another hypothalamic site, the depressor area, located very near the defense center, calls forth a strong sympathetic inhibition involving hypotension and bradycardia. This sympathoinhibition resembles the "playing dead" reaction used by certain animals as a protective measure and is thought to be involved in psychogenic fainting. It has been suggested that in the face of overpowering stress, the cortico-hypothalamic depressor response may offer, in addition to fight or flight, a third option, fainting and oblivion (Chapter 13, Fainting). The pathways involved in the defense reaction and the depressor reaction are shown in Figure 10.8.

Integrated CNS Control of the Circulation

The previous sections of this chapter have described specific control centers of the brain and important reflex patterns that govern the responses of the circulatory system to short-term environmental stresses. It has been stated, for example, that the medullary cardiovascular centers are indispensable and vital elements in circulatory control. These concepts are correct according to our present understanding.

There is, however, increasing evidence that in the constant interplay of these responses in the daily lives of higher animals and humans, the individual centers, particularly those of the medulla, are not the autonomous controlling forces they were once considered to be. As Hilton and others have pointed out, it now appears more than likely that a highly integrated cardio-respiratory-metabolic control is exercised by a hypothalamic-medullary complex.

While earlier views emphasized the primacy of the simple reflex patterns and medullary center controls, with higher center activity mainly in emergency situations, current evidence points to a more continuous regulation by the integrated "hypothalamic-medullary complex." This "complex" integrates the afferent reflex information at several different levels. In this integration process, certain hypothalamic systems appear of particular importance, for example, the defense center and its baroceptor inputs and the temperature control center. In addition, there is increasing awareness of the importance of psychological factors in determining circulatory performance. Aside from the defense center responses to fear and rage, the cardiovascular system is undoubtedly influenced to a considerable degree by the cerebral cortex in response to more subtle forms of psychological stress. This is a large but still relatively undefined area for future research.

Finally, it should be recalled that entirely aside from nervous and humoral control mechanisms, individual organs and tissues have a considerable degree of circulatory autonomy. As previously described, the myocardium, for example, is capable of very significant intrinsic heterometric adjustments (Chapter 5), and individual organs are capable of highly important circulatory autoregulation (Chapter 9). All of these are independent of nervous control.

Long-Term Regulation of Arterial Blood Pressure

The previous portions of this chapter have been concerned with relatively short-term regulation of blood pressure. Guyton has advanced the concept that long-term control has a very different basis, namely the blood volume–urinary output balance, which in turn, is influenced by neurohumoral and other factors. As indicated in Figure 10.9, an increase in arterial pressure, ⓛ, causes increased fluid output through the kidneys, a reduction in extracellular fluid volume, ③, blood volume, ④, and venous return, ⑥. The subsequent decrease in cardiac output will act to reduce the arterial pressure.

The continuous and overriding nature of this mechanism is due to two important factors: (a) only very small changes in body fluid volume are required to produce marked changes in arterial pressure, and (b) the kidney–body fluid control system has infinite gain. The latter implies that if atherosclerosis or some other process heightened renal vascular resistance, the arterial pressure would rise to whatever degree required to generate the necessary urinary output.

In Chapter 9, evidence was presented that both short- and long-term blood flow regulation are dictated by the metabolic needs of the tissue and, in the case of cardiac output, of the body as a whole. Thus the heart does not control its own output but merely pumps—within its capability—whatever blood is brought to it.

Guyton's interesting concept has the further implication that cardiac output and arterial pressure are separate entities, controlled by different mechanisms, and, in a sense, independent variables. Thus, an elevated blood pressure may

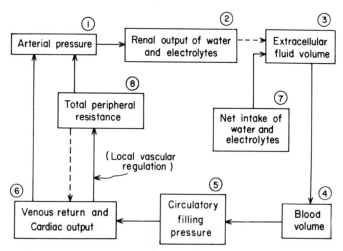

Figure 10.9.   Renal–body fluid mechanism for long-term regulation of arterial blood pressure. (Reprinted with permission from A.C. Guyton, *Textbook of Medical Physiology*, 5th ed. Philadelphia: W.B. Saunders, 1976.)

be initiated by the need for ample perfusion through a renal bed in order to maintain urinary output. On the other hand, the hypertension may endure because of the increased peripheral resistance needed for the tissues to autoregulate their flow at an acceptably low level. Guyton's theory offers at present one of the more plausible explanations for long-term circulatory regulation of blood pressure.

Cowley and his colleagues have further investigated this relation between body fluid volumes and arterial pressure. They found that after acute expansion of blood volume in experimental animals, cardiac output is increased but arterial pressure changes are blunted by hemodynamic adjustments. However, with chronic blood volume expansion, both peripheral resistance and arterial pressure rise substantially. Thus the results of acute and chronic blood volume expansion are very different. These studies are further discussed in Chapter 15 in relation to the pathogenesis of essential hypertension.

Suggested Readings

Brown AM. Cardiac reflexes. In: *Handbook of Physiology*, Section 2: *The Cardiovascular System*, edited by RM Berne, N Sperelakis, and SR Geiger. Bethesda: American Physiological Society, 1979, Vol. I.

Cowley AW, Barber WJ, Lombard JH, Osborn JL, and Liard JF. Relationship between body fluid volumes and arterial pressure. *Fed Proc* 45:2864–2870, 1986.

Cowley AW Jr, Liard JF, and Guyton AC. Role of the baroreceptor reflex in daily control of arterial blood pressure and other variables in dogs. *Circ Res* 32:564–576, 1973.

Donald DE and Shepherd JT. Autonomic regulation of the peripheral circulation. *Annu Rev Physiol* 42:429–439, 1980.

Estrin JA, Emery RW, Leonard JJ, Nicoloff DM, Swayze CR, Buckley JJ and Fox IJ. The Bezold reflex: a special case of the left ventricular reflex. *Proc Natl Acad Sci USA* 76:4146–4150, 1979.

Fox IJ, Gerasch DA, and Leonard JJ. Left ventricular mechanoreceptors: a haemodynamic study. *J Physiol (Lond)* 273:405–425, 1977.

Grassi G, Gavazzi C, Cesura AM, *et al*. Changes in response to reflex modulation of sympathetic tone by cardiopulmonary receptors. *Clin Sci* 68:503–510, 1985.

Guyton AC. Essential cardiovascular regulation—the control linkages between bodily needs and circulatory function. In: *Developments in Cardiovascular Medicine*, edited by CJ Dickinson and J Marks. Baltimore: University Park Press, 1978, pp 265–302.

Hilton SM and Spyer KM. Central nervous regulation of vascular resistance. *Annu Rev Physiol* 42:399–411, 1980.

Kostreva DR, Hess GL, Zuperku EJ, Neumark J, Coon RL, and Kampine JP. Cardiac responses to stimulation of thoracic afferents in the primate and canine. *Am J Physiol* 231:1279–1284, 1976.

Millhorn DE and Eldridge FL. Role of ventrolateral medulla in regulation of respiratory and cardiovascular systems. *J Appl Physiol* 61 (4):1249–1263, 1986.

Randall WC. *Nervous Control of Cardiovascular Function*. New York: Oxford University Press, 1984.

Ramirez AJ, Bertinieri G, Belli L, *et al*. Control of blood pressure and heart rate by arterial and cardiopulmonary baroceptors in the cat. *J Hypertension* 3:327–335, 1985.

Rowell LB. *Human Circulation—Regulation During Physical Stress*. New York: Oxford University Press, 1986.

Seagard JL, Pederson HJ, Kostreva DR, Van Horn DL, Cusick JF, and Kampine JP. Ultrastructural identification of afferent nerves of cardiac origin in thoracic sympathetic nerves in the dog. *Am J Anat* 153:217–232, 1979.

Shepherd JT and Mancia G. Reflex control of the human cardiovascular system. *Rev Physiol Biochem Pharmacol* 105:1–99, 1986.

Sundloff G and Wallin BG. Human muscle nerve sympathetic activity at rest. Relationship to blood pressure and age. *J Physiol* 274:621–637, 1978.

Uvnas B. Central cardiovascular control. In: *Handbook of Physiology*, Section 1: *Neurophysiology*, edited by J Field. Baltimore: Williams & Wilkins, 1960, Vol. II, pp 1131–1162.

Zucker IH and Gilmore JP. Atrial receptor modulation of renal function in heart failure. In: *Disturbances in Neurogenic Control of the Circulation*, edited by FM Abboud, HA Fozzard, JP Gilmore and DJ Reis. Bethesda, Md: American Physiological Society, 1981, pp 1–16.

chapter 11

Circulation to Special Regions

Cerebral Circulation

Anatomy

The main arteries to the cerebrum—the anterior, middle, and posterior cerebral—come off the circle of Willis, which in turn is derived from the basilar and internal carotid arteries. Branches of the vertebrals and proximal basilar artery supply the cerebellum and base of the brain (Fig. 11.1).

The blood vessels traverse the subarachnoid space before penetrating the brain substance. Venous drainage is *via* the superficial venous intradural sinuses of the cranium, which empty primarily into the internal jugular vein. The anatomical fixation of the dural sinuses to the skull, as well as the balance of intravenous and cerebrospinal fluid pressures (described below) prevent the collapse of the intracranial veins when subjected to negative transmural pressure upon standing.

Cerebrospinal Fluid

The cerebrospinal fluid (CSF), which in an adult has a total volume of about 100 to 160 ml, is formed in the choroid plexuses of the four ventricles at a rate of 400 to 600 ml/day; it circulates freely between the ventricles and cisterns of the brain, the subarachnoid space, and the central canal of the spinal cord (Fig. 11.2). Originating as a plasma filtrate, it becomes CSF through facilitated diffusion, active transport, and secretion, the last being an energy-requiring process of the choroidal epithelium (Fig. 11.2B). It differs from blood serum mainly in its very low protein content (20 to 40 mg/100 ml) compared to that of serum (5500 to 8000 mg/100 ml). Protein content of CSF is, however, diagnostically useful, since it is increased in multiple sclerosis, spinal canal blockade, and brain tumors.

CSF is usually obtained *via* lumbar puncture (Fig. 11.2C). It has a normal

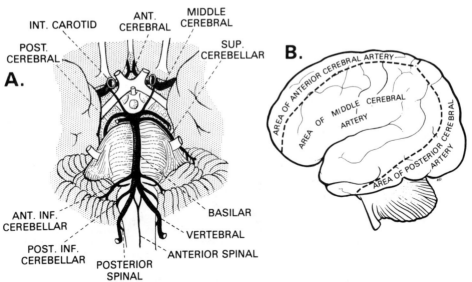

Figure 11.1.   Arterial supply to the brain. *A*, Arterial circle of Willis at base of the brain is formed by the basilar and internal carotid arteries. *B*, Approximate area of distribution of the three main arteries to the cerebral hemispheres. (Reprinted with permission from E. Gardner, *Fundamentals of Neurology*. Philadelphia: W.B. Saunders, 1963.)

pressure of 120 to 180 mm H_2O), which represents a balance between its rate of formation and absorption back into the bloodstream. Reabsorption is mainly *via* arachnoidal villi that invaginate the dural sinuses (Fig. 11.2*A*). Interference with reabsorption will elevate both CSF and intracranial pressure (ICP) as shown, for example, by the pressure increase that occurs during lumbar puncture if both internal jugular veins are compressed. Similarly, a block of arachnoidal villi by infection, a severe head injury, or a tumor may result in a progressive accumulation of CSF and an increase in ICP. ICP and CSF pressures are similar, provided there is no interference with pressure transmission within the cranium and that proper corrections are made for the gravity effect (discussed later in this section).

In an infant, the cranial bones, which have unfused junctions (sutures), may be forced apart by such pressures so that the head may reach enormous size (hydrocephalus) with resultant brain compression, mental retardation and, if not arrested, death.

Acute elevation of CSF pressure will tend to reduce the cerebral blood flow; however, increased CSF pressure will activate the CNS ischemic reflex (Chapter 10) and arterial pressure will rise linearly to stay above CSF pressure (Cushing reflex). The heart rate then usually slows through baroceptor action;

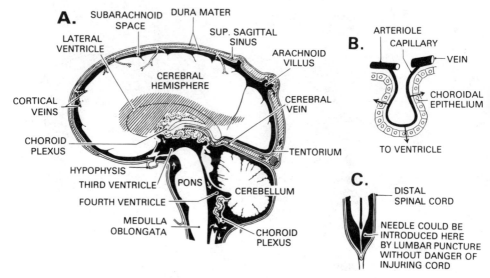

Figure 11.2. Circulation of cerebrospinal fluid (CSF). A, Median section of the brain with projection of one lateral ventricle (*oblique lines*), the 3rd and 4th ventricles, central canal of the cord, and subarachnoid space. CSF is formed from blood plasma and choroidal epithelium, *B*; passes into the ventricles and ultimately drains into the dural sinuses *via* the arachnoidal villi, A. (Reprinted with permission from E. Gardner, *Fundamentals of Neurology*. Philadelphia: W.B. Saunders, 1963.)

high pressure in the presence of bradycardia is suggestive of elevated CSF pressure. The rise in arterial pressure, along with the autoregulatory capacity of the cerebral vessels, will compensate, but only partially, for the increased resistance to flow induced by the heightened ICP. If cerebral autoregulation is maintained, ICP may reach pressures of 50 to 60 mm Hg before CBF is reduced sufficiently to produce ischemia; above this ICP level, blood flow may be drastically reduced, and coma and death may follow quickly. Patients with severe head injury often have impaired autoregulation, and cerebral flow may fall to critical levels when the ICP reaches only 20 to 30 mm Hg.

Because the brain literally "floats" in CSF, its effective weight *in situ* is reduced from about 1400 g to less than 50 g. This affords cushioning against trauma and reduces the risk of shearing or tearing of the brain tissue from its connections to extracranial tissues as they traverse the various foramina of the skull. Brain injuries may occur upon sudden rotational acceleration of the head (*e.g.*, from a blow to the side of the jaw) or severe linear acceleration, which, because of brain inertia, may cause damage at the point opposite the impact (countrecoup).

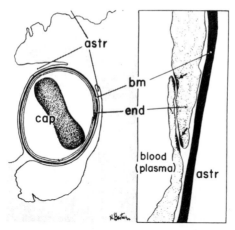

Figure 11.3. Microscopic view of a brain capillary containing an erythrocyte and almost surrounded by the perivascular feet of an astrocyte (*astr*). The capillary membrane consists of endothelial cells (*end*) (with a tight junction) and a continuous basement membrane (*bm*). (Reprinted with permission from H.D. Patton, J.W. Sundsten, W.E. Crill, and P.D. Swanson, *Introduction to Basic Neurology*. Philadelphia: W.B. Saunders, 1976.)

Blood-Brain Barrier

The capillaries of the brain because of their selective permeability are frequently referred to as a "blood-brain barrier." Most proteins and high molecular weight compounds, dyes, inulin, sucrose, mannitol, and catecholamines pass with difficulty or not at all. However, some clinically important precursors of neurotransmitters (*e.g.*, L-tryptophan and L-dopa) can penetrate the blood-brain barrier and are useful in treating neurological disorders. The relative impermeability to heavy metals and certain antibiotics poses therapeutic problems in the treatment of brain infections. On the other hand, anesthetics (volatile and nonvolatile), ethanol, CO_2, O_2, urea, and all lipids pass rapidly through brain capillaries. The barrier is partly morphological, that is, associated with its "tight" endothelial junctions and basement membrane structure (Fig. 11.3). The permeability barrier is in part also due to nonmorphological factors (*i.e.*, different diffusion rates and transport mechanisms across these capillaries). While the microstrucure of the choroid plexus is unlike that of the brain capillary, the former has a similar permeability barrier, so that some investigators refer to a blood-CSF barrier as well as a blood-brain barrier. The similar composition of brain interstitial fluid and CSF would tend to support such a concept.

The limited permeability of brain capillaries is diagnostically useful, for

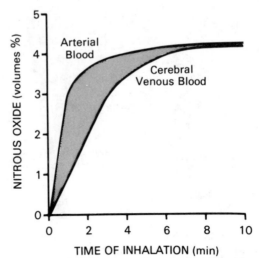

Figure 11.4. Inert gas method for measuring cerebral blood flow (Kety-Schmidt method). N_2O concentrations in arterial and cerebral venous blood while breathing a 15% N_2O gas mixture for 10 minutes. (Reprinted with permission from S.S. Kety and C.F. Schmidt, *J Clin Invest* 27:476, 1948.)

example, in "brain scans" in which a radioactive material such as technetium (^{99}Tc) adsorbed onto a protein molecule is injected intravenously. This substance, which would ordinarily not penetrate the brain, may show up as a darkened area on a gamma screen if the permeability mechanism is damaged by a tumor or infarct.

Measurement of Cerebral Blood Flow

The widely used "inert gas" method involves inhalation of a subanesthetic dose of an indicator such as nitrous oxide (N_2O) with periodic measurement of arterial and venous (internal jugular) concentrations until equilibrium (at about 10 minutes). At this point the arterial and venous N_2O concentrations are equal and that in brain tissue is about equivalent to the 10-minute venous blood sample concentration (Fig. 11.4).

Using the Fick equation (Chapter 7), the cerebral blood flow (CBF) is calculated as follows:

$$\text{CBF (ml/100 g brain tissue/min)} = \frac{100 \times N_2O \text{ uptake}}{(A-V) N_2O \text{ concentration}}$$

so that

$$\text{CBF (ml/100 g brain tissue/min)} = \frac{100 \times V_{10} \times S}{\int_0^{10}(A-V) \, dt}$$

in which

$$V_{10} = \text{venous } N_2O \text{ conc at } 10 \text{ min}$$

and

$$S = \text{partition coefficient of } N_2O \text{ in blood and brain, which equals one.}$$

Normal Values for CBF in Man. In the normal adult brain, which weighs 1400 to 1500 g, CBF is 50 to 60 ml/100 g brain tissue/min, so that total brain flow is about 750 ml/min or 15% of the total cardiac output. The white matter (neuroglia) receives about one-half of the average figure, but flow to the more vascular gray matter (neurons) is about two times the average.

There are a number of problems in the study of cerebral circulation. The difficulty stems from (*a*) the complex architecture of the brain, (*b*) the fact that regulatory mechanisms that govern cerebral and noncerebral tissues in the head are different and must be separated, and (*c*) the fact that the metabolic rate of brain tissue is heterogenous (*i.e.*, flow to gray and white matter varies widely). However, recent developments in methodology, such as the use of radionuclide-labeled microspheres, positron-emission tomography, and radioautography, have greatly enhanced the study of cerebral blood flow.

Previous data have indicated that brain function (*e.g.*, mental arithmetic) produced only minimal changes in cerebral blood flow; however, newer methods such as radioautography have shown bursts of metabolic activity and flow in very small, localized brain areas coincident with brain activity. For example, simple voluntary contraction of hand muscle is accompanied by a sizable increase in CBF in the localized contralateral hand area of the motor cortex; a light stimulus to the retina will increase blood flow to the superior colliculus and occipital cortex; and during speech, local metabolic activation of the motor speech area of the cortex has been observed.

Using radioactive xenon methods, Roland and his associates have reported that "pure" mental activity (*i.e.*, thinking), devoid of motor or sensory activity, also caused increases in regional cerebral oxidative metabolism and regional cerebral blood flow in several discrete areas of the cortex. Different subjects activated the same areas. Thus "function mapping" of the brain, using local flow and metabolism as indicators, has now become possible in animals and man and promises to add considerably to our understanding of neural function.

Characteristics and Control of Cerebral Circulation

Brain is the most vulnerable tissue of the body to ischemia; oxygen deprivation of only seconds may produce unconsciousness and, in a few minutes, irreversible damage. Fortunately, as many studies have shown, cerebral blood flow tends to remain remarkably constant under most physiological situations. This is due to a number of favorable factors that protect the cerebral circulation.

Hydrostatic Factors and CBF

The CNS vascular bed is, for example, better protected against changes in hydrostatic pressure than any other in the body. Enclosed within the rigid confines of the skull and spinal canal, CSF is in a continuous fluid-filled chamber whose hydrostatic pressure at any point will, in a manner similar to that of blood vessels, vary directly with body position (*i.e.*, with the height of the vertical fluid column). Thus the intravenous and extravascular (essentially CSF) pressures are balanced at all points in the spine and cranium. In the upright position, the CSF and venous pressures in the skull are both negative and in the lower spine are both positive. Thus venous collapse is prevented in the skull and venous distension in the lower spine, so the energy gradient is maintained across the CNS vascular bed regardless of position. This prevents the decrease in energy gradient that occurs, for example, in a hand lifted high over the head. In the latter situation there will be a hydrostatic fall in both arterial and venous pressures of 20 to 30 mm Hg, which in the veins will produce a negative pressure and collapse the walls, thereby effectively stopping blood flow. In spite of this protective feature, there is about a 20% reduction in CBF in the upright position.

General Regulation of Cerebral Circulation

In addition, the cerebral circulation has other safeguards. These include autoregulation, the baroreflexes, the CNS ischemic reflex, and specialized flow responses to Po_2 and Pco_2. Autoregulation, an important protective mechanism (Chapter 9), is also effective in hypertensive patients (Fig. 11.5). Because of its heavy dependence on aerobic metabolism, there is a tight coupling between metabolism and blood flow. It has been theorized that this strong control of metabolism over flow may be exercised through a metabolite or chemical agent such as oxygen, K^+ or adenosine (a breakdown product of the nucleoside adenosine, a potent cerebral vasodilator). However, the responsible agent is still uncertain.

While older studies reported the presence of autonomic fibers in the walls of cerebral vessels, it has been the consensus that they play only a minor role in normal cerebrovascular control. However, more recent studies have indicated wide species differences in this regard as well as the complicating effects of anesthesia. In monkeys and rabbits, for example, constrictor responses to nerve stimulation have been reported. There currently remains, therefore, a serious difference of opinion regarding the neural control of cerebral circulation in normal subjects. Recent reports have indicated that in hypertension,

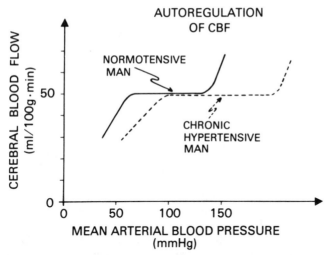

Figure 11.5. Autoregulation of cerebral blood flow in man in normotension and chronic hypertension. In hypertension the autoregulation persists, but the curve is shifted to the right. In this study, intracranial pressure, P_{CO_2} and P_{O_2} were maintained constant. (Reprinted with permission from N.A. Lassen, *Peripheral Circulation*, edited by P.C. Johnson. New York: John Wiley & Sons, 1978.)

vasoconstriction does occur and that it may play a role in attenuating the passive increase in CBF which would otherwise occur. Thus, it apparently acts to minimize the disruption of the blood-brain barrier and thereby may exert a protective effect in hypertension.

Recent studies have shown that during bicycle exercise in human subjects, there were (accompanying the usual increases in mean arterial pressure) increases of 31 to 58% in cerebral blood flow during submaximal and maximal exercise. P_{CO_2} however remained unchanged.

P_{CO_2} and Cerebral Blood Flow

The cerebral circulatory response to hypoxia is different than that of other beds. Resistance vessels in kidney and skeletal muscle, for example, reflexly constrict during systemic hypoxia—a sympathetic reflex response induced by activation of the arterial chemoreceptors. In contrast, the cerebral and coronary circulation dilate in response to hypoxia, a direct local tissue response due to dilation of distal intraparenchymal vessels. This protects the brain and myocardium, the tissues most dependent on aerobic metabolism. The CBF responds, however, only to rather severe hypoxia (*i.e.*, to P_{O_2} levels below 50 mm Hg). Arterial P_{CO_2} is an important regulator of cerebral flow and P_{CO_2} alterations exert a profound influence on CBF. Hypercapnia causes intense

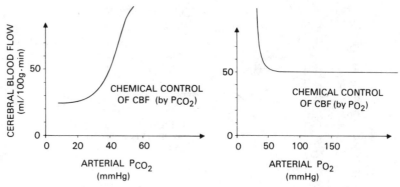

Figure 11.6. Effect of P_{CO_2} (*left*) and P_{O_2} (*right*) on cerebral blood flow. *Left*, note that the steepest part of the P_{CO_2} is near 40 mm Hg, indicating a high sensitivity of CBF to P_{CO_2} at physiological levels. *Right*, at the normal P_{O_2} levels of 80 to 120 mm Hg, the effect on CBF is practically nil. (Reprinted with permission from N.A. Lassen, *Peripheral Circulation*, edited by P.C. Johnson. New York: John Wiley & Sons, 1978.)

cerebral vasodilation, and hypocapnia is the cause of a marked vasoconstriction (Fig. 11.6A). The CO_2 effect is probably mediated by pH variations in cerebrospinal fluid and apparently serves primarily to maintain the pH of brain tissue. This objective is, in turn, probably associated with the fact that a decreased pH profoundly depresses neuronal activity. Arterial P_{O_2} changes within the physiological ranges have relatively little effect on CBF (Fig. 11.6B).

Pathophysiology of Cerebral Blood Flow

CBF is decreased in sleep, surgical anesthesia (as much as 50%), and in cerebral arteriosclerosis. The prevalence of the latter has important clinical implications since cerebral vascular disease is first in frequency among all neurological diseases and furthermore comprises 50% of all neurological hospital admissions to adult wards. The most serious consequence of cerebral arteriosclerosis is "cerebral vascular accident" (CVA or stroke). Whether the decrease in CBF is involved in the etiology of dementia or simply results from the decreased metabolic demand is debatable. Vascular stroke is the most common and devastating disease affecting the CNS, and in developing countries it is the third leading cause of death, ranking behind heart disease and cancer.

Vascular stroke may be due to a thrombus, embolus, or rupture of a cerebral artery, which can result in infarction of brain tissue or to a mass effect from a hematoma (tissue hemorrhage). The most common vascular distribution affected is that of the middle cerebral artery; the clinical results, depending on the branch affected and extent of the infarction, are varying degress of paralysis and fine sensory loss over the contralateral half of the body (hemiplegia and hemianesthesia) as well as speech (if the dominant hemisphere is involved) and visual problems. While flow to the infarcted area is diminished, that adjacent to the infarction may have increased flow, presumably due to the accumulation of metabolites at the periphery of the lesion.

In a recent investigation, Doppler ultrasound flowmeters were used to study cardiac output (CO) and common carotid blood flow in normal adults and cerebrovascular disease patients with more than a 50% reduction in diameter of their internal carotid arteries. In this study, the patients showed a 15% *increase* in common carotid flow (CCF) in the upright position and increases in their common carotid flow/cardiac output (CCF/CO) ratios in the upright position and in upright exercise. This was in contrast to normal adults, who showed the expected 20% decrease in CCF in the upright position and during upright exercise. It was concluded that patients with cerebrovascular disease have a diminished autoregulatory capacity, resulting in abnormal augmentation of cerebral blood flow with increases in CO. While the clinical significance of this flow aberration is not yet clear, it is anticipated that such studies will lead to a better understanding of the dynamics of CBF in stroke patients.

Coronary Circulation

Coronary circulation is critical not only because of the obvious central role of the heart but also because coronary artery disease (*i.e.*, ischemic heart disease) is the leading single cause of death in most of the "developed" countries of the world. There are special difficulties in the study of coronary circulation, for example, the marked anatomical vagaries of coronary arterial and venous vessels, the problem of high-fidelity recording on a constantly moving organ, and the significant species differences in the response of this bed. Moreover, the study of responses (*e.g.*, to a drug by the coronary circulation) is complicated by the indirect effect of the drug on the heart itself, whose altered activity will strongly affect the coronary circulation. In this chapter, the anatomy, characteristics, and control of the normal coronary circulation will be considered. Two of the most important manifestations of coronary pathophysiology, ischemic heart disease and congestive heart failure, are discussed in Chapter 14.

Anatomy

The adult human heart, which has a mass of 250 to 300 g, has three main arteries: the right coronary, supplying the right ventricle and a portion of the posterior left ventricle, and the left anterior descending and circumflex, which are the terminal branches of the left coronary and supply primarily the left ventricle (Fig. 11.7). A limited number of small arteries (arterioluminal) run from the main coronary arteries into the ventricles.

The "dominant" supply to the heart is usually determined by that artery that forms the posterior descending; the latter derives from the left circumflex in 85% of the cases in the dog (left dominance) but in man it is a continuance of the right coronary in about 90% of cases (right dominance). The conventional term "dominant" refers to the vessel that furnishes the major arterial supply to the inferior wall of the left ventricle and to the AV node; thus the term does not relate to the proportional mass of total myocardium supplied. From a functional standpoint, the anterior descending branch of the left coronary supplies the largest portion of the most important ventricle, *viz.*, the left, and in this sense is the predominant vessel.

The anterior cardiac vein from the right ventricle carries about 15 to 20% of the venous blood and drains into the right atrium. Most of the blood from the left ventricle empties into the great cardiac and other veins and finally into an expanded venous chamber, the coronary sinus. The coronary sinus, which carries 65 to 75% of coronary venous blood, drains into the right atrium. A few small thebesian veins, carrying about 3 to 5% of the total venous blood, drain directly into the cardiac chambers, mainly the right ventricle (Fig. 11.8).

Capillary and Collateral Circulation

As arteries pass across the surface of the heart, small branches come off at right angles to penetrate the myocardium and end in a rich network of arteries and capillaries. There are precapillary sphincters, which play an important role in opening up additional exchange beds during exercise (Fig. 11.8).

Since regional blood flow is highly important in the study of coronary disease, the development and validation of accurate methods assumes special significance. Recent studies have shown good agreement between the tritiated water and microsphere techniques, two of the most reliable of the regional flow methods.

Because coronary occlusion is a common clinical entity, the potential for development of collateral vessels becomes very important. Collaterals are anastomotic channels, usually small, preexisting arterial connections without intervening capillaries. These connections may be between main coronary arteries (intercoronary) or between branches of the same coronary artery (intracoronary) (Fig. 11.8).

The ability to develop collateral vessels varies with different species. In the dog, collateral vessels are located mainly near the epicardium and are relatively plentiful. In man, they are mainly subendocardial and less well developed; in man and in some animal species such as the pig (which has few collaterals), sudden occlusion of a large vessel usually results in a sig-

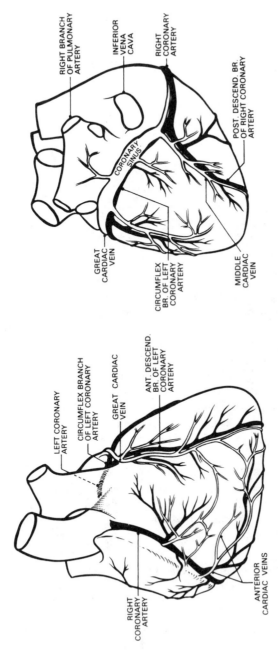

Figure 11.7.   Coronary vessels of the human heart. Anterior view (*left*) shows the right coronary artery and anterior descending artery; posterior view (*right*) shows the left circumflex artery and the posterior descending artery. The latter may be formed by the right coronary or left circumflex artery. The anterior cardiac veins from the right ventricle and the coronary sinus, draining primarily the left ventricle, empty into the right atrium.

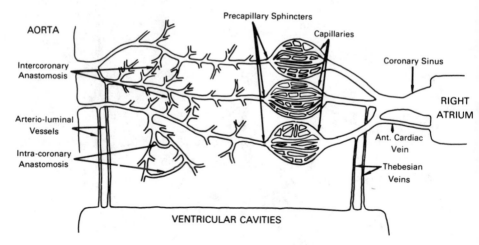

Figure 11.8. Diagrammatic sketch of the coronary vasculature showing arterioluminal vessels, thebesian veins, collateral arteries, and precapillary sphincters.

nificant infarction (necrosis) with possible cardiac arrest and death. However, with gradual occlusion of even 90% of the lumen of a large vessel (*e.g.*, in the dog), the collaterals open, there is proliferation of the vascular endothelium and smooth muscle cells, and within 4 to 8 weeks coronary flow may return almost to the preocclusion level.

A number of studies have suggested that after partial coronary artery occlusion, collateral vessels and myocardial capillary density will increase more rapidly in chronically exercised animals than in nonexercised animals. It is interesting that this enhanced capillarization seems to be related to the bradycardia of exercise since it will apparently occur also in nonexercised animals subjected to chronic bradycardic pacing. Whether this response is likely to occur in human coronary patients (many of whom are elderly) is not known. Collateral vessels apparently develop either because of (*a*) increased physical stress on the wall of the blood vessels due to heightened pressure gradients, or (*b*) the stimulating effect of hypoxia or other metabolites resulting from the ischemia.

Normal Values and General Characteristics

In man, coronary flow is usually measured either by the inert gas method (previously described) involving catheterization of the coronary sinus, or by a "washout" technique following injection of a radioactive agent such as ^{133}Xe or ^{85}Kr into the catheterized coronary artery. Direct measurement with

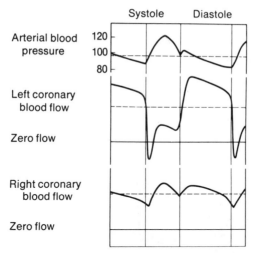

Figure 11.9. Right and left coronary arterial flow during systole and diastole. Note the greater effect of external compression on systolic flow to the left coronary as compared to the right. (Reprinted with permission from B. Folkow and E. Neil, *Circulation*. London: Oxford University Press, 1971.)

an electromagnetic or ultrasonic flowmeter in an experimental animal permits the recording of phasic flow as shown in Figure 11.9.

The smaller flow in the left coronary artery during systole (one-fifth of the total) is due to the external compression of the artery; the lesser pressures of the right ventricle produce less throttling and permit a proportionately greater systolic flow into the right coronary artery. The normal adult heart has a coronary blood flow of 70 to 80 ml/100 g/min and a total flow of about 250 ml/min (*i.e.*, 4 to 5% of the cardiac output).

How much reduction in coronary flow is required to impair myocardial contraction? While a full answer to this key question is not available, a recent study of experimental coronary stenosis in conscious dogs indicated that a 10 to 20% reduction in myocardial blood flow will cause significant impairment of regional myocardial contractility. Larger reductions in flow induce progressively greater decrements, but a 95% flow reduction was required to stop contractility entirely in the affected region. The investigators reported that this regional ischemia did not significantly affect general ventricular performance.

During these procedures, arterial blood pressure, heart rate, and LV systolic pressure were maintained, thus indicating that the nonischemic portions of the myocardium were able to compensate for the loss of regional contractility. In human patients, the clinical result of a coronary occlusion will depend on

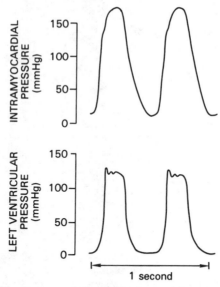

Figure 11.10. Simultaneous intraventricular and intramyocardial pressures from left ventricle of the dog. (Reprinted with permission from H. Kreuzer and W. Schoeppe, *Pfluegers Arch* 278:181, 1963.)

several factors including the rapidity of the occlusion, the area of the myocardium involved and the age and physical condition of the patient. The pathophysiological effects of human coronary occlusion are further discussed in Chapter 14 (Ischemic Heart Disease).

Control of Coronary Circulation

 The three main factors influencing flow are (*a*) *mechanical*, mainly external compression and perfusion pressure, (*b*) *metabolic*, and (*c*) *neural*.

Mechanical Factors and Coronary Flow

The compression effect is responsible for 25% of coronary flow resistance in the left ventricle at normal heart rates. For reasons that are not understood, resistance is significantly higher in the right ventricle. During tachycardia, when systole occupies an increasing percentage of the cycle, it can account for as much as 55% of vascular resistance. But external compression also affects intramyocardial flow distribution; as the left ventricle contracts, the pressure inside the muscle increases to a level comparable to and even higher than the intraventricular pressure (Fig. 11.10). Furthermore, the myocardial pressure is graded, being very low on the epicardial side and at its peak near the endocardium, so that subendocardial vessels are compressed the most.

As a result, subendocardial flow is primarily diastolic. In spite of this, injection of microspheres and other studies indicate that in the normal myocardium, subendocardial and subepicardial flow are about equal. However, when diastolic pressure is low, such as in shock, aortic stenosis, or coronary occlusion, subendocardial flow decreases disproportionately, so that this area is more vulnerable to ischemia. This seems to be borne out by the fact that after coronary occlusion, infarcts are more common in the subendocardial area.

Since at normal rates, about 80% of coronary flow occurs in diastole, it follows that aortic diastolic pressure becomes the primary determinant of coronary perfusion pressure. Theoretically, coronary flow would, therefore, fluctuate with the diastolic pressure; however (as discussed in Chapter 9) the coronary vessels show a high degree of "autoregulation," *i.e.*, between perfusion pressures of 60 to 180 mm Hg, flow remains relatively constant. Thus the increase in coronary flow which occurs in conditions in which diastolic pressure is elevated is due mainly to the increase in flow accompanying the increased afterload work and increased cardiac metabolism (as described below) rather than the elevated perfusion pressure.

Cardiac Metabolism and Coronary Flow

One of the most striking features of myocardial physiology is the close parallelism between metabolic rate and coronary flow; as previously discussed (Chapter 9) a general correlation exists in all tissues. Because of this close coupling, any increase of cardiac work as a result of exercise (Fig. 11.11), excitement, or administration of inotropic agents will induce a corresponding increase in coronary flow. The precise mechanism of this metabolic rate–blood flow coupling is not certain. Both increased PCO_2 and reduced pH will increase local flow, but unquestionably hypoxia (*i.e.*, decreased PO_2) is the most potent stimulus of all to coronary flow. The available evidence suggests that the chief metabolic mediator of the hypoxic vasodilation in the coronary bed is adenosine. Other factors, such as K^+, CO_2, pH, and prostaglandins, contribute to an unknown degree.

Neural Control of Coronary Flow

In order to study neural effects on myocardial blood flow, it is necessary to differentiate the direct effect on coronary vessels from an indirect effect that is secondary to stimulation of the myocardium. This is particularly important in the study of agents to counteract coronary vasospasm. Certain drugs as well as sympathetic stimulation, will, for example, increase the myocardial work and with it increase local accumulation of metabolites, which will in turn produce a secondary vasodilation of the coronary vascular bed. This will complicate any direct action the drug or neural stimulation may have on the coronary vessels themselves. This problem is usually circumvented by study-

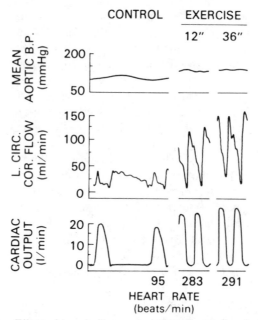

Figure 11.11. Effect of treadmill exercise on coronary flow in the dog. There is a large increase in coronary flow associated with the increased heart rate, blood pressure, and cardiac output. (Reprinted with permission from E.M. Khouri, D.E. Gregg, and C.R. Rayford, *Circ Res* 17:427, 1965.)

ing blood flow in the K$^+$ arrested, fibrillating heart or by using selective sympathetic and parasympathetic blocking agents (Chapter 9).

Studies using such procedures indicate that the main neural effects on coronary circulation are sympathetic. In the dog, cardiac sympathetic (stellate) stimulation usually results in increased myocardial blood flow. However, if the inotropic and chronotropic effects are blunted by β-blockade, a widespread adrenergic vasoconstriction, particularly to left stellate stimulations, is unmasked. It appears, therefore, that while the metabolic vasodilator effect is a dominant influence in controlling coronary flow, it is modulated by the α-adrenergic vasoconstrictors. β$_2$- and cholinergic receptors probably have only a secondary role in the normal regulation of coronary flow in the intact organism.

Renal Circulation

The kidneys have two major functions: (*a*) they excrete the primary end-products of bodily metabolism, and (*b*) they control the concentrations of most constituents of body fluids. Through these activities, they play a vital role in regulating the salt and water balance of the body. This section on renal circulation is mainly concerned with (*a*) the renal circulatory architecture and how it is adapted to kidney function, (*b*) some general characteristics of renal blood flow, and (*c*) the mechanisms affecting neurohormonal control of the kidney. The relationship of circulatory control mechanisms to plasma volume and to the genesis of hypertension are discussed in Chapters 10 and 15, respectively.

Functional Anatomy

The basic functional unit of the kidney, the nephron, is composed of (*a*) the glomerulus, which consists of a tuft of capillaries through which the plasma is filtered, and (*b*) long tubules adapted for reabsorption in which the filtered plasma is converted to urine. In man, about 85% of the nephrons are in the outer part, or cortex, of the kidney (cortical nephrons); the remaining fraction (15%), *i.e.*, the juxtamedullary nephrons, lie close to the inner portion, or medulla, of the kidney (Fig. 11.12). Huge quantities of plasma, about 180 L/day, are filtered through the porous walls of the glomerular capillaries; the main elements retained are the plasma proteins. In all, 98% to 99% of this plasma fluid is reabsorbed back into the blood through the renal tubules; the remaining 1.5 to 2.0 L/day passes through as urine.

From the renal artery, interlobar arteries ascend between the pyramids and divide into arcuate arteries that, in turn, subdivide into interlobular vessels and thence into afferent arterioles. The latter supply the glomerular capillaries (Fig. 11.12, *left*). The shorter, thin-walled, efferent arterioles subdivide to form the peritubular capillary plexuses that surround the cortical convoluted tubules. The efferent arterioles from the juxtamedullary nephrons form two branches, one of which divides into peritubular capillaries, while the other drains downward into vasa recta in the proximity of the loops of Henle before turning back upward to empty into the cortical veins.

Near the glomerulus, the afferent arteriolar wall is thickened asymmetrically and contains small specialized juxtaglomerular (JG) cells that are the site of renin formation. The portion of the distal tubule lying adjacent to the JG cells forms a small cellular plaque called the macula densa, which together with the JG cells is termed the juxtaglomerular apparatus, or JGA (Fig. 11.12, *right*), which constitutes an important humoral regulatory system.

Characteristics and Control of Renal Circulation

As described in Chapter 9, the kidneys are highly vascular organs. Although weighing only 300 g, they receive a blood flow of 1000 to 1200 ml/min, about 20% of the total cardiac output. Of this very large flow, only a modest portion is for metabolic needs, so the renal (A-V)O_2 difference is relatively small. The great part of the flow becomes glomerular filtrate and serves as the main regulator of the body's water and electrolyte balance. The renal

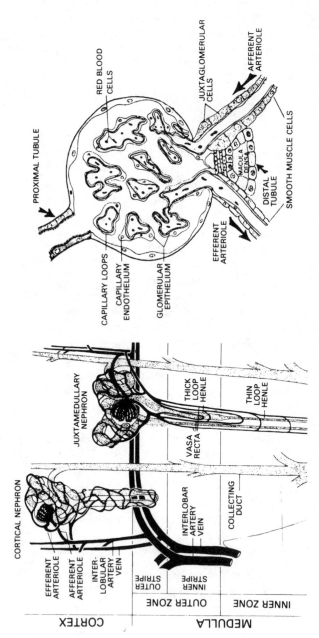

Figure 11.12. Renal circulation. *Left*, blood supply to cortical and juxtamedullary nephrons. *Right*, juxtaglomerular complex including JG cells and macula densa. (Reprinted with permission from R.F. Pitts, *Physiology of Kidney and Body Fluids*, 3rd ed. Chicago: Year Book Medical Publishers, 1974; A.M. Ham and T. Leeson, *Histology*, 4th ed. Philadelphia: J.B. Lippincott, 1961.)

circulation consists of two capillary beds arranged in series, the glomerular and the peritubular beds.

In passing through the afferent arterioles, the mean arterial pressure falls from 100 mm Hg to about 90 mm Hg in the glomerular capillaries. Passage through the efferent arterioles results in a large decrease of pressure to about 15 mm Hg in the peritubular capillaries. This pressure then further declines to about 8 mm Hg in the renal venules. The high-pressure glomerular capillary bed is adapted for filtration; the peritubular bed, with a relatively low hydrostatic pressure and high osmotic pressure, is well adapted for reabsorption.

Intrinsic (Local) Control of Renal Circulation

The glomerular filtration rate (GFR) of the kidney remains very constant. This ability to maintain a relatively constant GFR protects the body from large fluctuations in water and solute excretion that would otherwise occur with the fluctuations in arterial pressure. The evidence indicates that this GFR control takes place mainly in the efferent arterioles.

The mechanism responsible for this close relation between renal circulation and renal excretory function has been intensively studied. One of the primary controllers is tubuloglomerular feedback, which functions so that increased volume delivery to the distal tubule causes a direct decrease in GFR and a restoration of normal filtration. It has also been proposed that when arterial pressure, GFR, and distal delivery of electrolytes are reduced, activation of the renin-angiotensin system causes constriction of efferent arterioles, restoring glomerular perfusion pressure and GFR. Circulation and renal excretory function is complex and seems to depend on a balance between (a) capillary hydrostatic pressure, which can be altered by changing the relation between precapillary and post capillary resistance, and (b) capillary oncotic pressure, which can alter with changing blood flow and the filtration coefficient.

Renal blood flow shows a high degree of autoregulation, and changes in arterial pressure over a range of 80 to 200 mm Hg cause remarkably little change in renal blood flow. The mechanisms responsible for the autoregulation are not certain. The two most likely explanations appear to be a myogenic mechanism (Chapter 9) and the tubuloglomerular feedback responses of the juxtaglomerular apparatus.

Extrinsic Control of Renal Circulation

While the intrinsic control mechanisms provide considerable stability to the renal circulation, they do not prevent large variations in renal blood flow and GFR from occurring during activation of the sympathetic nervous system. Strong renal arterial vasoconstriction can result from emotional stress, the defense reaction (Chapter 10), exercise (Chapter 12), or as reflex responses to decreased central blood volume, hypotension (Chapter 10), hemorrhage

(Chapter 13) or shock (Chapter 15). Renal vasoconstriction lowers glomerular capillary hydrostatic pressure and filtration rate and thus tends to retain water and increase plasma volume. Renal vasoconstriction affects primarily the outer cortex, where most of the glomeruli are located. Vasodilators (*e.g.*, histamine, dopamine, and prostaglandins of the A and E series) generally induce greater fractional flow to the inner cortex and medulla. It is thought that PGE_2, a particularly potent renal vasodilator that is synthesized in the renal medulla, protects the renal parenchyma against the excessive salt and water-conserving action of the renin-angiotensin system. It has been suggested that PGE_2 deficiency may play a role in the genesis of essential hypertension, but the evidence thus far is only fragmentary.

Neurohormonal Control of Plasma Volume

There are three neurohormonal mechanisms that can significantly influence renal blood flow and plasma volume: (*a*) the renin-angiotensin-aldosterone (RAA) system concerned with the renal control of Na^+, (*b*) the antidiuretic hormone or ADH (vasopressin) system concerned with the renal control of free water, and (*c*) atrial natriuretic peptide, present in atrial tissue which dilates renal vessels and influences water and electrolyte balance.

In this section, these neurohormonal mechanisms are briefly described from the standpoint of the involvement of the circulatory system. Other important factors in fluid-volume control, such as thirst, other diuretic and saluretic hormonal mechanisms, and the interactions between the ADH and renin-aldosterone systems, have been omitted.

Renin-Angiotensin-Aldosterone System

The enzyme renin, produced by the modified smooth muscle cells (*i.e.*, the JGA cells), acts on the circulating α_2-globulin (renin substrate) and splits off a decapeptide, angiotensin I. Additional amino acids are subsequently split off (mainly in the lung) by a converting enzyme to yield the octapeptide angiotensin II. Although angiotensin II is a potent vasoconstrictor, its most important action is to stimulate aldosterone production and secretion by the cells of the zona glomerulosa of the adrenal cortex. An increased renin release by the kidney will therefore lead to greater release of aldosterone and to an increased reabsorption of Na^+ into the renal collecting tubule (and greater excretion of K^+). The reabsorbed Na^+ will carry water with it and thus increase plasma volume (Fig. 11.13). As with other self-correcting systems, when the volume deficit has been corrected, the RAA system is shut off.

The primary stimuli for renin secretion appear to be (*a*) increased sympathetic nerve activity, which may be produced reflexly by decreased central blood volume or arterial pressure or by other causes as described above, (*b*) decreased plasma Na^+ (sensed by the macula densa), or (*c*) decreased distension of renal arterioles. It should be noted that aldosterone is stimulated

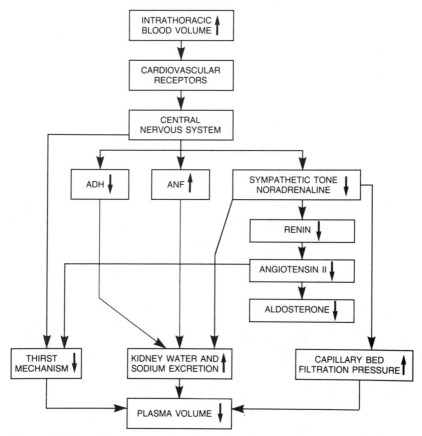

Figure 11.13.   Major pathways for the reflex control of plasma volume following expansion of intrathoracic blood volume (ADH = antidiuretic hormone; ANF = atrial natriuretic factor).

not only by angiotensin II but also by ACTH, plasma K^+ concentration, and other factors.

In the early hypovolemic stage of congestive heart failure, there is a suppression of the RAA mechanism, probably due to the continued elevation of central blood volume. However, in the later stages there appears to be an adaptation of the vagal endings with the resultant increase in the neurohormonal drive usually seen in chronic heart failure. This question is discussed further in Chapter 14 (Congestive Heart Failure).

ADH (Vasopressin) Mechanism

Antidiuretic hormone, or ADH (also called vasopressin), is an octapeptide synthesized in the hypothalamus and transported to and released from the posterior pituitary gland. As a messenger between the CNS and kidney, it plays a key role in maintaining the volume and osmolality of body fluids.

ADH is released from the posterior pituitary gland in response to a number of stimuli including: (a) activation of the sympathetic nervous system by emotion or decreased plasma volume as sensed by cardiopulmonary receptors, particularly of the left atrium; (b) increased osmolality of the interstitial fluid of brain (as sensed by osmoreceptors); and (c) increased plasma concentrations of angiotensin II. ADH acts on the collecting tubules of the kidney to increase reabsorption of free water, inhibit diuresis, and increase plasma volume (Fig. 11.13). As described in Chapter 10, increased distension of cardiopulmonary receptors will inhibit the secretion of ADH, and decreased distension will increase it. Diabetes insipidus, a rare disorder characterized by polyuria (excessive diuresis) and polydipsia (excessive thirst), is an ADH deficiency disease but usually has no primary blood-pressure abnormality.

In its second role, in which it is more commonly known as vasopressin, this hormone acts as an arterial vasoconstrictor, and its importance in circulatory physiology is becoming increasingly recognized. It is released in increasing quantities by the posterior pituitary gland during hemorrhage in which its constrictor action exerts a pressor effect adjunctive to that resulting from the arterial and cardiopulmonary baroceptor reflexes. It is now available as a highly purified synthetic arginine vasopressin (AVP) standard. A normal concentration in human plasma is about 4 to 6 picograms (pg) per ml of plasma. Its arteriolar vasoconstrictor action begins at a plasma concentration of about 30 pg/ml and is increased 50- to 100-fold after baroceptor denervation and 2000- to 8000-fold after ablation of the CNS. Cowley and his colleagues have presented increasing evidence that AVP may be importantly concerned with long-range regulation of arterial pressure.

Atrial Natriuretic Factor (ANF)

A 28 amino-acid peptide with potent diuretic and natriuretic properties has recently been reported. It is synthesized and released primarily from the cardiac atria. Distension of the atria causes renal vascular dilation, increased filtration, inhibition of Na^+ reabsorption, natriuresis, and a resultant reduction of extracellular fluid volume. The control of ANF and its ultimate role in Na^+ and H_2O balance have not yet been well defined. A simplified scheme of the relation of ANF to renal function is shown in Figure 11.13.

Splanchnic Circulation
Functional Anatomy

Splanchnic circulation is actually a collection of several grossly different circulations serving organs with very dissimilar functions. In the human adult,

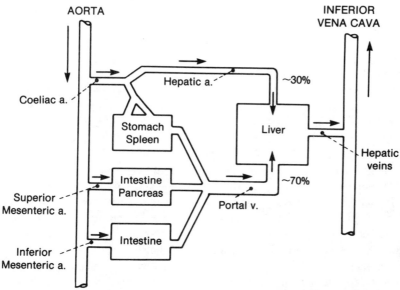

Figure 11.14. Simplified schema of splanchnic vascular bed showing the parallel arrangement of the circulation of the various gastrointestinal organs and their series arrangement with the portal circulation to the liver. Also shown is the dual blood supply to the liver and the common venous drainage of all these organs. (Reprinted with permission from L.B. Rowell, The splanchnic circulation. In: *The Peripheral Circulations*, edited by R. Zelis. New York: Grune & Stratton, 1975.)

the total splanchnic blood flow (SBF) is about 1500 ml/min (*i.e.*, approximately 25% of the cardiac output). The splanchnic vasculature has some unique characteristics, for example, the portal circulation is coupled with that of the gastrointestinal tract in series and with the hepatic artery in parallel. The arteries to the various splanchnic organs have many interconnecting branches. About 70% of the liver blood flow is from the portal vein, and about 30% travels *via* the hepatic artery. All SBF ultimately drains *via* the hepatic veins. Thus, in spite of providing blood flow to a great diversity of organs, the splanchnic circulation has an anatomical commonality of final flow and, in this sense, can be considered as a single hypothetical flow tract (Fig. 11.14).

Characteristics and Control

Most arterial beds in the splanchnic circulation have approximately normal arteriovenous pressure relations. The portal bed, however, is a low-pressure, low-resistance system with a portal pressure of about 8 to 10 mm Hg and a hepatic venous pressure of about 0 to 2 mm Hg. Pressure-flow studies of the portal circuit indicate that it is a relatively "passive" bed (*i.e.*, it generally imposes little active resistance to flow). There is a partial reciprocity between hepatic artery and portal vein that tends to maintain a constant total liver blood flow. The hepatic sinuses are lined with a very porous, "discontinuous" type of endothelium that offers little resistance to either proteins or fluid. As a consequence, the volume flow of hepatic lymph is great, and its protein content is almost as high as that of plasma. The normal O_2 extraction of splanchnic blood is low (only about 15 to 20%) so there is a considerable oxygen reserve available in low-flow states.

All splanchnic organs are richly innervated with sympathetic α-receptors that receive innervation primarily from the splanchnic nerves. Sympathetic stimulation, whether as a response to exercise or increased temperature or through baroceptor stimulation (as a result of hemorrhage, upright posture, or lower body negative pressure), will invoke strong splanchnic vasoconstriction. This serves to redistribute the splanchnic flow and is a key factor in maintaining arterial pressure during low cardiac output states. Splanchnic venous constriction in response to sympathetic stimulation is also a very effective aid in hypotensive states, since about 20 to 25% of the total blood volume is contained in the splanchnic region.

There is no evidence of neural vasodilators in the splanchnic bed and very little indication of autoregulation in the intact, innervated organism. During gastric and intestinal digestion, there is hyperemia, which indicates a close coupling of blood flow and functional state. The mechanism of this effect is not known but has been ascribed to neural influences, to the action of gastrointestinal hormones such as secretin or gastrin, or to other agents such as serotonin or bradykinin.

Pathophysiology

During *hemorrhage*, the splanchnic circulation plays an important role. A strong splanchnic vasoconstriction is initiated by the low-pressure cardiopulmonary baroceptors and, as arterial pressure falls, is strengthened by the arterial baroceptors. In severe shock this response is further reinforced by the reflex effect of the chemoreceptors. Venous constriction is an important part of this response, and it has been estimated that as much as 50% of additional blood volume mobilized from "blood reservoirs" in shock may come from the splanchnic region. Some venoconstriction is "active," but a significant portion is "passive," *i.e.*, it is due to the recoil of veins onto the smaller venous volume, which is, in turn, a result of constriction of the precapillary resistance vessels. Vasoconstriction can persist unabated for prolonged periods.

In *physical exercise* there is a constriction of both arteries and veins in the splanchnic area. The venous constriction is primarily responsible for the 35% decrease in splanchnic blood volume that occurs during mild supine exercise. SBF decreases in proportion to the intensity of the exercise. Rowell has made the interesting observation that in normal subjects, trained athletes, and mitral stenosis patients the rate of decrease of SBF with increasing intensity of exercise ($\dot{V}O_2/\dot{V}O_2$max) was similar, (*i.e.*, had the same slope and similar intercepts). Although the patients, normal subjects, and athletes had, in that order, progressively larger $\dot{V}O_2$max values, (that is, maximum rate of O_2 consumption) they all reduced their SBF by about 80% at their $\dot{V}O_2$max. The $\dot{V}O_2$max, in effect, diverts this flow (about 250 to 300 ml O_2/min) into the general circulation. However, this O_2 transport capacity represents a much higher fraction of $\dot{V}O_2$max in the patients with a limited cardiac output than in normal subjects or athletes. As a consequence, this capacity provides to these patients a substantial boost to their O_2 transport.

The importance of the sympathetic vasoconstrictor mechanism, particularly in cardiac patients, is demonstrated by Rowell's estimate that constriction of the combined splanchnic, renal, cutaneous and nonworking muscle bed provides 42% of the total capacity for O_2 delivery in mitral stenosis patients at their $\dot{V}O_2$max. The vasoconstrictor response obviously has its greatest significance in patients with low cardiac output.

Heat stress with increase in body temperature also causes a splanchnic vasoconstriction and diminished SBF. With combined heat and exercise stress the tendency toward splanchnic vasoconstriction in the two stresses is additive, so that there is a tendency toward an even greater shunting of splanchnic blood into the general circulation. However, additional skin blood flow is now needed to dissipate the added heat. Cardiac patients with a limited myocardial reserve are often unable to increase cardiac output to supply this additional need and so must try to divert flow from other sources. When they become unable to do this they reach the point of decompensation.

This vasoconstrictor capacity of the splanchnic, renal, and nonworking muscle bed provides a most important reserve. However, additive stresses (*e.g*, exercise and heat) may rapidly deplete these reserves in patients whose cardiac output is compromised.

One of the most serious of liver diseases is cirrhosis, an irreversible alteration of liver architecture consisting of diffuse fibrosis with wide-spread necrosis of liver parenchyma and areas of nodular regeneration. It is usually the aftermath of chronic chemical (usually alcoholic), bacterial, or other toxic damage to the liver. Portal venous hypertension (up to 20 or 25 mm Hg) may occur with ascites (accumulation of intraperitoneal fluid). In an effort to bypass the hepatic circulatory obstruction, many portal-systemic collaterals develop, among them, large vessels in the esophageal mucosa called esophageal varices. Hemorrhage from an esophageal varix with hemoptysis (spitting up of blood) and massive bleeding into the stomach is a major complication of portal hypertension, with a mortality rate as high as 50 to 60% for each bleeding episode.

Cutaneous Circulation

The main function of skin circulation is to maintain temperature balance by providing (a) insulation against cold and (b) efficient heat transfer between the body core and the periphery. This heat-regulating mechanism, aided by sweat production and evaporative cooling, is much better adapted to protect against overheating than against excessive cold.

Anatomy of Skin Vasculature

Skin has a variable thickness, generally 1 to 3 mm, a surface area in the 70-kg adult of 1.7 to 1.8 m² and an aggregate mass of 2 to 2.5 kg, about 4% of the total body weight. From a functional standpoint, the vasculature is of two general types. The first is an extensive, superficial arteriolar-capillary-venular network of the usual architecture with an extensive, slow-flowing subcutaneous venous plexus. This general structure prevails over most of the body, with particularly rich networks in the forearm, legs, and thighs.

The second vascular arrangement, which is found in palms of the hands, soles of the feet, and in the face (especially the ears, nose, and lips), is similar to the above but has, in addition, a large number of unique arteriovenous anastomoses (AVAs). Skin in these areas is studded with numerous such capillary bypasses which consist of coiled arterial vessels about 50 μm in diameter with thick muscular walls, well supplied with sympathetic nerve fibers. These vessels do not have capillary exchange surfaces and by virtue of their unusual vascularity are capable of large heat exchanges (Fig. 11.15).

Normal Values and Response Range

Skin blood flow is commonly determined in man with the venous occlusion plethysmograph (Chapter 6). Such studies have shown that this tissue is capable of extreme flow ranges; under maximum heat stimulation, hand skin flow can increase about 30-fold from the normal values of 3 to 5 ml/100 g tissue/min and with cold application of 15°C, 10-fold decreases to 0.3 to 0.5 ml/100 g/min. With further cooling (e.g., to 10°C) there follows, however, a cold-induced vasodilation, a protective, local, nonneurogenic reaction, sometimes called the "hunting response." Its mechanism is unknown.

Control of Skin Blood Vessels

While there are direct blood flow effects of heat and cold on skin (as described above), by far the main mechanism is an "indirect" sympathetic reflex re-

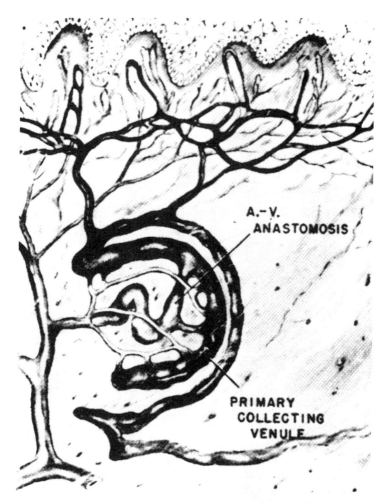

Figure 11.15. Schematic drawing of blood vessels of the finger showing superficial plexus and an AV anastomosis that connects directly to a venule of the subcutaneous plexus. When dilated, the AVAs are capable of huge increases in flow. (Reprinted with permission from A.C. Hseih. In: *The Peripheral Circulations*, edited by R. Zelis. New York: Grune & Stratton, 1975).

sponse. This is due to a stimulation of heat-sensitive thermoreceptors in the skin and in the hypothalamus (*via* warmed blood), which markedly vasodilate resistance vessels (arterioles and AVAs) as well as capacitance vessels. The result is a large increase in both arterial flow and in the slow-velocity, subcutaneous venous flow, the latter being especially well adapted to transfer

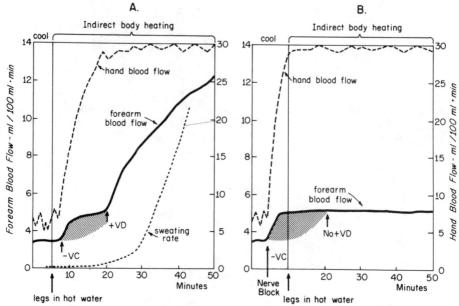

Figure 11.16. Reflex effects of indirect heating on skin blood flow in normal hand and forearm, *i.e.*, changes in finger and forearm blood flow when legs were put in hot H_2O. A, Vasodilation in the hand is mediated only by release of tonic sympathetic vasoconstrictor tone ($-VC$); this "passive" vasodilation accounts, however, for only a small part of the blood flow in the forearm ($-VC$ to $+VD$). The remainder, as well as the sweating, is due to active sympathetic vasodilation and can be prevented by sympathetic blockade, B; note in B the abrupt increase in hand (skin) blood flow after nerve block illustrating the neurogenic control of skin blood flow. However, (in B) the nerve block prevented the increase in forearm blood flow. (Reprinted with permission from J.T. Shepherd, *Physiology of Circulation in Human Limbs in Health and Disease*. Philadelphia: W.B. Saunders, 1963.)

heat to the environment. Vasodilation in the hands, feet, and face is "passive" (*i.e.*, due to reduction in sympathetic tone) but in other areas is mainly "active" (Fig. 11.16).

This active vasodilation is carried out by arterioles, but not by AVAs. Some investigators have proposed that this dilation mechanism is similar to that prevailing in certain glandular tissues and sweat glands and that it involves the local release of an enzyme that acts on a globulin substrate to liberate bradykinin, a potent vasodilator.

The reflex response to cold, while less marked, is significant and includes not only reduction of arterial flow but also venoconstriction, with a resultant decrease in subcutaneous venous volume and an increase in velocity of venous blood flow (a distinct advantage in minimizing heat loss). During severe and prolonged cold, the direct effects, added to the indirect reflex effects, may so reduce skin flow that it is almost immeasurable, with the distinct risk of frostbite and severe tissue damage. Frostbite was previously discussed in Chapter 2 under blood viscosity.

Pathophysiological Responses

Inflammation of the skin or pressure on the skin surface induces a vascular reaction depending on the intensity of the stimulus. After light stroking there is pallor and after a heavier stroking, a red line due to venular dilation. Upon repeated or heavier pressure, the reddening or "flare" will occur and spread because of arteriolar involvement. With still greater trauma, wheals will result. This sequence has been called the "triple response" and is ascribed to the local production and spread of histamine; it involves a local vascular mechanism and is thought to be an axon reflex.

Blood vessels of skin are unusually sensitive to central nervous and hormonal influences. Fear may be marked by vasoconstriction and pallor, cold sweats may occur due to nervous tension, and blushing will follow certain emotional stimuli (although the latter response is reportedly becoming extinct in Western civilization).

The unusual sensitivity of skin vessels to nervous and hormonal influences makes this tissue vulnerable to certain vasospastic disorders of the extremities. *Raynaud's disease*, a chronic condition of this type, affects the hands and occurs particularly in women in colder climates. It is characterized by frequent vasospasms and blanching of the fingers of both hands followed by vasodilation, ischemic pain, and in some cases eventual tissue necrosis. The condition is thought to be an exaggerated vasoconstrictor response to continued sympathoadrenal stimulation associated with nervous tension. Bilateral upper thoracic sympathectomy is sometimes helpful but usually does not afford lasting relief.

Circulation in Skeletal Muscle

The primary function of these vessels is to serve the metabolic needs of skeletal muscle, needs that can increase as much as 100-fold over the resting level. Because of the great muscle mass, a secondary role is to provide a reserve of vascular resistance for certain emergencies such as circulatory shock. Muscle circulation has two quite different mechanisms to discharge these two different functions: a local metabolic and a central neural control system.

General Flow Characteristics and Normal Values

As mentioned in Chapter 9, at rest, 20 to 25% of the cardiac output supplies the skeletal muscles with about 4 to 6 ml of flow per 100 g/min. However,

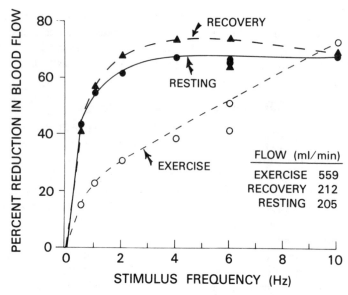

Figure 11.17. Effect of frequency of electrical stimulation of the lumbar sympathetic chain on limb flow in the dog. At rest there was marked flow reduction with increase in frequency. During exercise the stimulation was less effective because the bed was under metabolic control. (Reprinted with permission from D.E. Donald, D.J. Rowlands, and D.A. Ferguson, *Circ Res* 26:185, 1970.)

at maximal exercise almost 90% of the cardiac output may be diverted to the working muscles (Chapter 12, Exercise). Rapid, phasic (white) fiber units, which comprise 80 to 85% of the muscle mass, may upon contraction increase their flow 10-fold from a resting level of 2 to 4 ml/100 g/min while the slow, tonic (red) fibers, may experience a 4-fold increase from somewhat higher resting values of 20 to 30 ml/100 g/min. In experimental animals such flow determinations are usually made by direct flowmetering of the arteries and in man by means of venous occlusion plethysmography (Chapter 6).

Muscle arterioles have a high resting tone, most of which is inherent in the vascular muscle itself (myogenic tone) and the remainder due to a tonic sympathetic vasoconstrictor outflow with a frequency of about 1 impulse/sec. An increase in the stimulation frequency to 4 to 5 impulse/sec produces about a 70% reduction in flow but has a lesser effect on exercising muscle (Fig. 11.17). An important advance in flow dynamics has been the development of methods to study regional circulation and the degrees of nonuniformity of flow (*e.g.*, perfusion heterogeneity using tritiated water).

Local (Metabolic) Control of Muscle Circulation during Exercise

At rest the neural factors are primary, but during muscle contraction the local metabolism becomes practically the exclusive regulator of the muscle flow.

Skeletal muscle has well-developed autoregulatory and reactive hyperemic properties, a further manifestation of the link between metabolism and flow in this bed. During physical exercise the skeletal muscles achieve their tremendous increase in oxygen exchange through (a) an extreme metabolic dilation of the microcirculation, (b) an increase in the number of perfused capillaries (recruitment), and (c) an increased oxygen extraction in the capillary bed.

During rhythmic exercise, flow is intermittent because of the mechanical compression effect on the vasculature. Flow interference begins at about 30% of maximum tension with complete stoppage at about the 70% level. This deprives the fiber of oxygen at its time of greatest need, although the myoglobin of red muscles provides some assistance through its oxygen "accumulator" and release action. On the venous side, this intermittent compression of veins, in conjunction with venous valves, produces a strong phasic milking action (Chapter 6, Venous Return). The resultant lowering of net venous pressure is thought to play an important role in increasing perfusion through lower extremity muscles during exercise such as running.

As with other vascular beds, considerable effort has been directed to the study of the possible mechanism of the hyperemia during increased metabolism. A number of vasodilator agents have been proposed, most prominently Po_2, H^+, K^+ and adenosine; as yet there is no agreement.

Some investigators believe that local hyperosmolality may be a factor, at least in initiating the hyperemic response. With exercise there is known to be a metabolic breakdown within the muscle cell of many large molecules into smaller ones, which increases osmolality and causes transfer of water into the cell. This is probably responsible for the 10 to 15% decrease in plasma volume which is usual after exercise.

Central (Neural) Control of Muscle Circulation

Sympathetic vasoconstriction is the primary circulatory control mechanism of skeletal muscle in nonexercise situations. Vasodilation can be brought about either passively by decreased stimulation of vasoconstrictors (the most common mechanism) or actively via sympathetic cholinergic or β-adrenergic vasodilators. Cholinergic vasodilation mainly results from cerebral activity such as mental effort or emotion. It is thought that these descending impulses from the higher centers may bypass the medullary cardiovascular centers.

Skeletal muscle vessels are also important participants in reflex response. Increased stimulation of arterial baroceptors and certain cardiopulmonary receptors will result in decreased sympathetic tone and passive vasodilation of skeletal muscle resistance vessels. It is thought that some active vasodilation also occurs, at least initially. Conversely, decreased stimulation of arterial and cardiopulmonary receptors will result in reflex sympathetic vasoconstriction in skeletal muscle (Fig. 11.18).

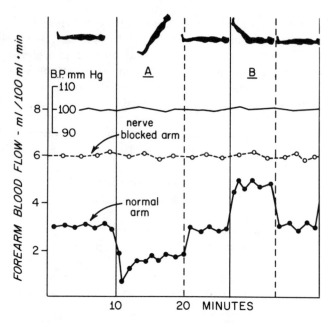

Figure 11.18. Response of forearm skeletal muscle blood flow to decreased (A) and increased (B) cardiopulmonary receptor stimulation due to intrathoracic blood volume changes. These changes were produced by head-up tilt and leg raising, respectively. Sympathetic blockade in the control arm prevented the flow changes. Arterial baroreceptors were not involved, since arterial pressure did not change. (Reprinted with permission from J.T. Shepherd, *Physiology of the Circulation in Human Limbs in Health and Disease.* Philadelphia: W.B. Saunders, 1963.)

Stimulation of aortic and carotid body chemoreceptors (*e.g.*, during hypoxia or shock) will also induce reflex vasoconstriction in skeletal muscle. If, however, a vasodilation stimulus is imposed on a bed previously vasoconstricted (*e.g.*, by hemorrhage or hypoxia), such sudden inhibition—accompanied as it sometimes is by vagal bradycardia—can lower peripheral resistance sharply and result in fainting (Chapter 13).

It should also be mentioned that muscle veins, in sharp contrast to splanchnic and cutaneous veins, are practically devoid of adrenergic nerve endings in their walls, and as a consequence these veins react little if at all to sympathetic vasomotor constriction and so do not serve a significant reservoir function.

Neurohormonal Effects

Under certain circumstances, catecholamines may influence muscle vasculature. As described in Chapter 9 (Neural Control of Flow) the arterioles of skeletal muscle contain sympathetic α-, β- and cholinergic receptors, so that the result of sympathetic stimulation is usually a balance between two or more effects. Norepinephrine (NE) injection has a small β-dilator but a much stronger α-constrictor action. A moderate intravenous dose of NE in the intact organism will, therefore, raise the blood pressure and thereby activate the arterial baroceptors, producing a subsequent reflex vasodilation and corrective fall in pressure. Epinephrine usually induces a marked but transitory β-dilator action that is enhanced if its secondary effect, an α-constrictor action, is blocked (Chapter 9).

Pulmonary Circulation

Anatomy

The pulmonary and systemic circuits are in series, and in the normal resting adult, each ventricle has an output of about 70 ml/kg/min or 5 L/min. The pulmonary circulation, with only one-tenth the capacity of the systemic, must, in the same time period, accommodate the same ejected volume. The pulmonary vessels, which are much shorter, accommodate this volume without excessive pressure fluctuations because of their thinner walls and greater compliance. The pulmonary capillaries form a very thin, rich, vascular network around the alveoli, which facilitates blood-gas exchange.

The blood supply to the lung itself, the bronchial circulation, constitutes only 1 to 2% of the left ventricular output. Venous drainage is mainly *via* the azygous system. Bronchial veins form a latticework in the adventitia and submucosa of the bronchial tree. In the presence of post–pulmonary capillary hypertension (*e.g.*, in mitral stenosis), the bronchial veins become congested and frequently form varicosities. With sudden, strong respiratory movements, damage to these venous walls may result in hemoptysis (spitting up of blood).

Pressure and Flow in the Pulmonary Vessels

The mean pressures in the right ventricle and pulmonary artery are about one-sixth as great as those in the left ventricle and aorta (Fig. 11.19). Since the total flows are equal, the pulmonary vascular resistance is only one-sixth that of the systemic. However, the pressure waves, flow patterns, and cardiac valvular movements of these two circuits are quite similar. The normal mean pressure in the pulmonary artery is about 15 mm Hg, in the capillaries about 10 mm Hg, and in the pulmonary veins and left atrium about 5 mm Hg. Thus the pulmonary arterial-capillary gradient is about equal to the pulmonary capillary-venous gradient (about 5 mm Hg) indicating that these two segments contribute about equally to pulmonary vascular resistance, a very different situation than in the systemic circuit. The mean pulse pressures in the left atrium are somewhat higher than those of the right (Fig. 11.19) because of the more forceful contractions of the left atrium and ventricle.

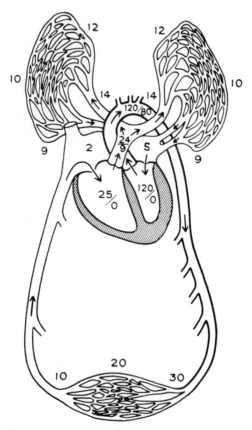

Figure 11.19.   Representative pressures (mm Hg) in normal adult pulmonary and systemic circulation. (Reprinted with permission from J.H. Comroe, *Physiology of Respiration*, 2nd ed. Chicago: Year Book Medical Publishers, 1974.)

The total thoracic blood volume (TBV), which in the normal 70-kg adult is about 1200 ml, includes the pulmonary blood volume (*i.e.*, that within the lung), which is about 500 ml. In the discussion on vascular volumes and pressures (Chapter 1), it was mentioned that the TBV (also called central blood volume) represents about a quarter of the total blood volume and provides an important reserve filling pressure for the ventricles. The volume contained in the vena cavae and right heart, (about 350 ml) constitutes right heart reserve, and that in the pulmonary artery, lungs, and pulmonary veins (about 900 ml) serves as left heart reserve.

As a low-pressure system, about one-half of the TBV (about 500 ml) is readily dislocated into the lower extremities upon assumption of the upright position. A substantial fraction of the TBV is also displaced into the general venous circulation during hemorrhage, dehydration, or other vascular stress in which there is a fall in systemic venous pressure. Conversely, thoracic blood volume and pressure rise in the supine position, in exercise, during generalized systemic vasoconstriction, water immersion in the upright position, or left heart failure (*i.e.*, any condition in which extrathoracic venous volume and pressure rise). It should also be noted that TBV fluctuates during each breathing cycle because of rhythmic alterations of intra- and extrathoracic pressure. During inspiration there is a net increase of about 250 ml of blood in the chest and during expiration, a similar decrease (Venous Return, Chapter 6).

Distribution of Blood Flow in the Lung

In order to carry out its primary mission of blood-gas exchange, it is necessary that the oxygen-poor blood delivered *via* the pulmonary arteries be maximally exposed to oxygen-rich air of the alveoli (*i.e.*, that perfusion and ventilation be kept in balance). An imbalance between these two is, however, a common occurrence and is responsible for most gas-exchange problems in pulmonary disease. One factor contributing to the ventilation-perfusion imbalance is the effect of posture on flow distribution: in the upright position, there is minimal flow to the lung apex and a progressively increasing rate of flow toward the base. What is the reason for this inequality?

As described in Chapter 6 (Respiratory Pump), respiratory excursions induce fluctuating negative intrathoracic pressures. These pressures are exerted, however, mainly on the pulmonary arterial and pulmonary venous vessels. Pulmonary capillaries on the other hand are more strongly influenced by alveolar pressures. Because the alveolocapillary membrane is thin and pliant, the effective extravascular capillary pressure normally approximates the alveolar pressure (P_A) rather than the more negative intrathoracic pressure. But in the upright position there may be a hydrostatic pressure difference of 30 cm H_2O (23 mm Hg) between the apex and base of the lung. Since the normal pulmonary artery pressure is only about 20 cm H_2O, this hydrostatic pressure difference has important pulmonary hemodynamic consequences.

Since at the lung apex (*i.e.*, above the heart) the pulmonary intracapillary pressure may be lower than alveolar pressure, some of the capillaries may collapse, and flow at the apex will be less than at the base (Fig. 11.20, *zone 1*). However, at the base (Fig. 11.20, *zone 3*), the added hydrostatic pressure increases the capillary transmural pressure well beyond the alveolar pressure, so the vessels will not only remain patent but are distended and flow will be increased. In this situation it is seen that flow depends not only on the usual longitudinal driving pressure gradient but also on the transmural pressure gradient, which must be positive in order to prevent collapse.

In the upright subject the ventilation-perfusion ratio is greater than one at the apex and decreases to values below one at the base. In the normal individual this is not a serious handicap to gas exchange. However, if there is a

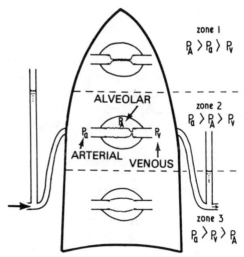

Figure 11.20.   Illustration of hydrostatic effect of body position on pulmonary capillary flow. In *zone 1* above the heart level, the extramural pulmonary alveolar pressure (P_A) may be greater than the pulmonary capillary pressure and some capillaries may collapse. In *zone 2*, flow may be intermittent; in *zone 3* below the heart, with increased hydrostatic pressure, the capillaries distend, and flow is increased. (Reprinted with permission from J.B. West, C.T. Dollery, and A. Naimark, *J Appl Physiol* 19:713, 1964.)

pathological deficiency of either ventilation or perfusion, this potential handicap can be exaggerated and present a serious threat to possible gas exchange.

Control of Pulmonary Vessels

The pulmonary circulation acts mainly as a passive, compliant, vascular bed, adapting to the demands of the circulation at large. Most studies indicate that although the vessels are well supplied with vagal and sympathetic fibers, these apparently have little functional role. Pulmonary vessels will, however, constrict strongly under the influence of hypoxia. This is a regional phenomenon that occurs in the area of the hypoxia, and it may be due to local release of a vasoconstrictor substance. It should be noted that this pulmonary vasoconstrictor response is directly opposite to the usual vasodilator effect of hypoxia in all other circulatory beds. The hypoxic vasoconstriction is reinforced by similar vasoconstrictor action of decreased pH, which often coexists. Hypoxic vasoconstriction serves a useful purpose in diverting the flow from poorly ventilated regions to other lung areas with more abundant oxygen, thus improving the overall gas exchange. Hypoxic vasoconstriction, which may occur at altitude or in patients with chronic obstructive pulmonary disease, can— if prolonged—lead to pulmonary hypertension.

Drugs that constrict pulmonary vessels include norepinephrine, serotonin, histamine, and a number of the prostaglandins. Isoproterenol and acetylcholine are vasodilators.

Pulmonary Capillary Dynamics and Edema

The combination of a plasma osmotic pressure of about 28 mm Hg and a low pulmonary capillary hydrostatic pressure of 10 mm Hg results in a rather unusual net inward force of about 18 mm Hg. This factor, coupled with a rather "tight" capillary endothelium, helps to maintain narrow interstitial spaces between the capillary and alveolar surfaces, which in turn expedite gaseous diffusion. This negative pressure gradient represents a safety factor, reducing the chances of interstitial fluid accumulation. Pulmonary edema will, for example, usually not occur in experimental animals until left atrial pressure exceeds 20 mm hg.

However, in the case of severe left ventricular failure or mitral stenosis, left atrial pressure and volume will steadily increase with an eventual damming effect and an increase in pulmonary venous and capillary pressures. Interstitial edema will then develop, and if the process continues, fluid will also accumulate in the alveoli, resulting in progressive interference with oxygenation, shortness of breath, and difficulty in breathing, *i.e.*, dyspnea (see Congestive Failure, Chapter 14).

Pulmonary edema may also develop in certain cases of elevated cerebrospinal fluid pressure (P_{CSF}), for example, following head injury. When P_{CSF} reaches levels sufficient to induce large increases in systemic arterial pressure, pulmonary capillary pressure rises, along with left atrial pressure and cardiac output. Recent studies by Maron and Dawson have shown that the pulmonary hypertension in this condition is probably the result of a strong pulmonary venous constriction due to adrenal catecholamines liberated during the elevation of P_{CSF}.

Suggested Readings

General

Abboud FM, Fozzard HA, Gilmore JF, and Reis DJ. *Disturbances in Neurogenic Control of the Circulation*. Bethesda, Md: American Physiological Society, 1981.

Donald DE and Shepherd JT. Autonomic regulation of the peripheral circulation. *Annu Rev Physiol* 42:429–439, 1980.

Johnson PC. *Peripheral Circulation*. New York: John Wiley & Sons, 1978.

Korner PI. Control of blood flow to special vascular areas: brain, kidney, muscle, skin, liver and intestine. In: *Cardiovascular Physiology, MTP International Review of Science*, edited by AC Guyton and CE Jones. Baltimore: University Park Press, 1974.

Mellander S and Johansson B. Control of resistance, exchange and capacitance functions in peripheral circulation. *Pharmacol Rev* 20:117–196, 1968.

Olsson RA. Local factors regulating cardiac and skeletal muscle blood flow. *Annu Rev Physiol* 43:385–395, 1981.

Rowell LB. *Human Circulation-Regulation During Physical Stress*. New York: Oxford University Press, 1986.

Shepherd JJ and Mancia G. Reflex control of the human cardiovascular system. *Rev Physiol Biochem Pharm* 105:1–99, 1986.

Shepherd JT. *Physiology of the Circulation in Human Limbs in Health and Disease*. Philadelphia: W.B. Saunders, 1963.

Zelis R. *The Peripheral Circulations*. New York: Grune & Stratton, 1975.

Cerebral Circulation

Cagle G, Greene ER, Miranda JP, and Reilly PA. Non-invasive ultrasound measurements of cardiac output and common carotid blood flow in cerebrovascular disease patients as a function of posture and exercise. *Physiologist* 25:3233, 1982.

Heistad DD and Kontos HA. Cerebral Circulation. *Handbook of Physiology*, Sec 2, Vol. 3, pp 137–182, 1983.

Kety SS and Schmidt CF. The nitrous oxide method for the determination of cerebral blood flow in man: theory, procedure and normal values. *J Clin Invest* 27:476, 1948.

Lassen NA. Brain. In: *Peripheral Circulation*, edited by PC Johnson. New York: John Wiley & Sons, 1978.

Patton HD, Sundsten JW, Crill WE, and Swanson PD. *Introduction to Basic Neurology*. Philadelphia: W.B. Saunders, 1976.

Roland PE. Changes in brain blood flow and oxidative metabolism during mental activity. *NIPS* 2:120–124, 1987.

Sokoloff L. *Brain Imaging and Brain Function*. New York: Raven Press, 1985.

Symposium on Cerebral Circulation: Chairmen—FM Abboud and DD Heistad. *Fed Proc* 40:2296–2334, 1981.

Thomas SN, Schroeder T, Secher NH, and Mitchell JW. Cerebral blood flow during dynamic exercise in humans. *J Appl Physiol* 67:744–748, 1989.

Coronary Circulation

Berne RM and Rubio R. Coronary circulation. In: *Handbook of Physiology, Section 2: The Cardiovascular System*, edited by RM Berne, N Sperelakis, and SR Geiger. Bethesda, Md: American Physiological Society, 1979, Vol. I, pp 873–952.

Braunwald E, Ross J, and Sonnenblick EH. Regulation of coronary blood flow. In: *Mechanisms of Contraction of the Normal and Failing Heart*. Boston: Little, Brown, 1976.

Cohen MV, Yipinotosi T, and Scheuer J. Coronary collateral stimulation by exercise in dogs with stenotic coronary arteries. *J Appl Physiol* 52:664–671, 1982.

Feigl EO. Coronary physiology. *Physiol Rev* 63:1–205, 1983.

James TN. *Anatomy of the Coronary Arteries*. New York: Hoeber Medical Division, Harper & Row, 1961.

Rinkema LE, Thomas J, and Randall WC. Regional coronary vasoconstriction in response to stimulation of stellate ganglia. *Am J Physiol* 243:H410–415, 1982.

Rubio R and Berne RM. Myocardium. In: *Peripheral Circulation*, edited by PC Johnson. New York: John Wiley & Sons, 1978, pp 231–253.

Santamore WP and Bove AA. *Coronary Artery Disease*. Baltimore: Urban and Schwarzenberg, 1982.

Sarnoff SJ, Braunwald E, Welch GH, Case RB, Stainsby WN, and Macruz R. Hemodynamic determinants of oxygen consumption of the heart with special reference to the tension-time index. *Am J Physiol* 192:148–156, 1958.

Tripp MR, Meyer MW, Einzig S, Leonard JJ, Swayze CR, and Fox IJ. Simultaneous regional myocardial blood flow by tritiated water and microspheres. *Am J Physiol* 232:H173–190, 1979.

Wright AJA and Hudlicka O. Capillary growth and changes in heart performance induced by chronic bradycardial pacing in the rabbit. *Circ Res* 49:469–477, 1981.

Vatner SF. Correlation between acute reductions in myocardial blood flow and function in conscious dogs. *Circ Res* 47:201–207, 1980.

Young MA and Vatner SF. Regulation of large coronary arteries. *Circ Res* 59:579–596, 1986.

Renal Circulation

Brenner BM, *et al*. *Glomerular Ultrafiltration*. In: *The Kidney*, Vol. 1, 3rd Ed., edited by BM Brenner and FC Bector. Philadelphia: W.B. Saunders & Co., 1986.

Cowley AW Jr. Vasopressin and cardiovascular regulation. In: *Cardiovascular Physiology IV, International Review of Physiology*, Vol. 26. Baltimore: University Park Press, 1982, pp 189–242.

Cuneo RC, Espiner EA, Nicholls MG, *et al*. Hemodynamic, renal and hormonal responses to ANP infusion in man. *J Clin Endo Metab* 63:946, 1986.

Echtenkamp SF, Zucker IH, and Gilmore JP. Characterization of high and low pressure baroceptor influences on renal nerve activity in the primate *Macaca fascicularis*. *Circ Res* 46:726–730, 1980.

Groban L, Ebert TJ, Kreis DU, *et al*. Hemodynamic, renal and hormonal responses to incremental ANF infusion in the human. *Am J Physiol* 256:780–786, 1989.

Gauer OH and Henry JP. Neurohormonal control of plasma volume. In: *Cardiovascular Physiology II, International Review of Physiology*, Vol. 9, edited by AC Guyton and AW Cowley. Baltimore: University Park Press, 1976, pp 145–190.

Hall JE. Regulation of renal hemodynamics. In: *Cardiovascular Physiology IV, International Review of Physiology*, Vol. 2, edited by AC Guyton and JE Hall. Baltimore: University Park Press, 1982, pp 243–321.

Wiedmann P, Hasser L, Gnadiger MP, *et al*. Blood levels and renal effects of atrial natriuretic in normal man. *J Clin Invest* 77:734–742, 1986.

Splanchnic Circulation

Granger DN and Kvietys PR. The splanchnic circulation: intrinsic regulation. *Annu Rev Physiol* 43:409–418, 1981.

Jacobson ED and Tepperman BL. (eds.). Splanchnic circulation (Symposium). *Fed Proc* 41:2079–2116, 1982.

Rowell LB. The splanchnic circulation. In: *The Peripheral Circulations*, edited by R. Zelis. New York: Grune & Stratton, 1975, pp 163–192.

Cutaneous and Skeletal Muscle Circulation

Greenfield ADM. The circulation through the skin. In: *Handbook of Physiology*, Section 2: *Circulation*, Vol. II, edited by WF Hamilton and P Dow. Washington, D.C.: American Physiological Society, 1963, pp 1325–1351.

Heistad DD and Abboud FM. Factors that influence blood flow in skeletal muscle and skin. *Anesthesiology* 41:139–156, 1974.

Hseih ACL. The cutaneous circulation. In: *The Peripheral Circulations*, edited by R. Zelis. New York: Grune & Stratton, 1975, pp 79–94.

Paradise NF, Swayze CR, Shin DH, and Fox IJ. Perfusion heterogeneity in skeletal muscle using tritiated water. *Am J Physiol* 220:1107–1115, 1971.

Rowell LB. The cutaneous circulation and circulation to skeletal muscle. In: *Physiology and Biophysics*, 20th ed., edited by TC Ruch, HD Patton and AM Scher. Philadelphia: W.B. Saunders, 1974, pp 185–214.

Rowell LB. Human cardiovascular responses to exercise and thermal stress. *Physiol Rev* 54:75–159, 1974.

Shepherd JT. *Physiology of the Circulation in Human Limbs in Health and Disease.* Philadelphia: W.B. Saunders, 1963.

Sparks HV. Skin and muscle. In: *Peripheral Circulation*, edited by PC Johnson. New York: John Wiley & Sons, 1978, pp 193–230.

Pulmonary Circulation

Cumming G. The pulmonary circulation. In: *Cardiovascular Physiology, MTP International Review of Science*, edited by AC Guyton and CE Jones. Baltimore: University Park Press, 1974.

Green JF. The pulmonary circulation. In: *The Peripheral Circulations*, edited by R Zelis. New York: Grune & Stratton, 1975, pp 193–210.

Maron MB and Dawson CA. Pulmonary venoconstriction caused by elevated cerebrospinal fluid pressure in the dog. *J Appl Physiol* 49:73–78, 1980.

Schreiner BF Jr and Yu PN. Pulmonary circulation, congestion and edema: anatomic and physiologic conditions. In: *Clinical Cardiovascular Physiology*, edited by HJ Levine. New York: Grune & Stratton, 1976, pp 635–706.

Slonim NB and Hamilton LH. *Respiratory Physiology*, 4th ed. St. Louis: C.V. Mosby, 1981.

West JB. *Respiratory Physiology*, 2nd ed. Baltimore: Williams & Wilkins, 1979.

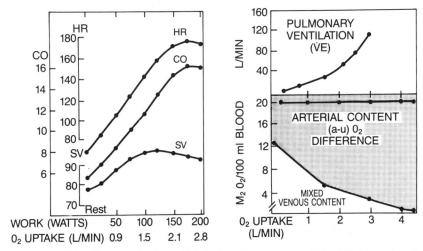

Figure 12.1. Progressive exercise in healthy, young adults: Effect on heart rate (HR), cardiac output (CO) (L/min), and stroke volume (ml), (*left*) and on pulmonary ventilation and blood O_2 content (*right*). (Adapted from Astrand P and Rodahl K, *Textbook of Work Physiology*, 2nd ed. New York: McGraw-Hill 1977.)

(Figure 12.1). This increased O_2 extraction is an important means of increasing O_2 uptake during exercise.

The increased cardiac output is accomplished through increases in both heart rate and stroke volume (SV). Cardioacceleration at low levels of exercise is due to vagal release, but at high levels it is due to combined vagal release and sympathetic activation. The maximal heart rate (HR_{max}), which is usually achieved at $\dot{V}O_{2max}$, is an important limiting factor in cardiovascular performance. HR_{max} decreases progressively with age. Although there is considerable individual variability, it can be approximated by the formula $HR_{max} = 220 - age$ (in years).

The increase in SV is due to increased filling of the ventricles (Frank-Starling mechanism) and heightened myocardial contractility induced by sympathetic stimulation. Some of the past controversy regarding SV response to exercise is now known to have been due to postural effects. In supine exercise, because of increased filling pressure, SV is greater (than in the upright position) and with increasing exercise it is maintained nearly constant, so that the CO increase in the supine position is achieved mainly through increase in HR.

In the sitting or standing position, SV is about one-third less than in the supine position. Thus, in upright exercise SV is initially smaller but increases progressively at increasing work levels until about 40% of $\dot{V}O_{2max}$, at which point it reaches its maximal value (for the upright position) and plateaus.

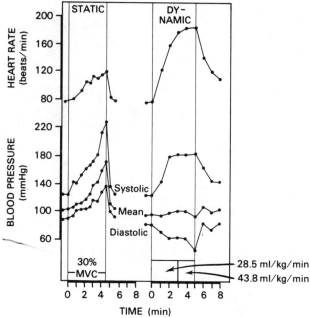

Figure 12.2. Hemodynamic response to static and dynamic exercise in healthy young adults. Note the much greater rise in heart rate and pulse pressure in dynamic exercise. (Reprinted with permission from A.R. Lind and G.W. McNicol, *Can Med Assoc J* 96:706, 1967.)

However, the SV at $\dot{V}O_{2max}$ is still lower in upright than in supine exercise. Final CO levels are very similar at equivalent work loads in the two positions.

Thus, at submaximal workloads the increase in CO is due to increases in both HR and SV. But at high work levels—because of earlier leveling off of the SV—the increase in CO is achieved mainly by the increase in HR (Fig. 12.1, *left*).

During exercise, there is a pronounced rise in systolic pressures (SP), which reach levels of 170 to 200 Hg at $\dot{V}O_{2max}$. In spite of a 4- to 5-fold increase in CO, diastolic pressure is changed little and may decrease, mainly because of the decreased vascular resistance in exercising muscle. Thus, in dynamic exercise, the result is an increase in pulse pressure that roughly parallels the rise in systolic pressure, and a moderate increase or no change in mean arterial blood pressure (Fig. 12.2). It has been suggested by Mitchell *et al.* that an important mechanism involved in these circulatory changes is the "exercise pressor response." They postulate that physical exercise (either dynamic or static) stimulates small myelinated (group III) and unmyelinated (group IV) fibers in skeletal muscle, which invoke a sympathetic response of

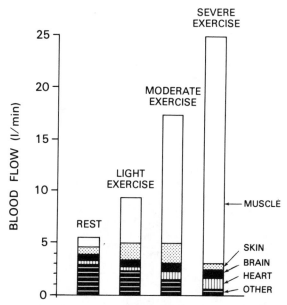

Figure 12.3. Distribution of blood flow with increasing levels of exercise in man. In severe exercise there is about a 20-fold increase in skeletal muscle flow and a 4-fold increase in coronary flow, with little change in brain blood flow and a marked decrease in flow to almost all remaining tissues. (Reprinted with permission from E.H. Starling and L. Evans, *Principles of Human Physiology.* Philadelphia: Lea & Febiger, 1968).

peripheral vasoconstriction, tachycardia, increased myocardial contractility, and hypertension. The degree of response is approximately proportional (in both dynamic and static exercise) to the muscle mass involved and the intensity of the exercise. Similar responses can be induced in experimental animals by electrical stimulation of skeletal muscles (particularly fast-twitch fibers) or of the group III or group IV afferent fibers from these muscles. The central pathways of the exercise pressor reflex are not yet known.

Distribution of Blood Flow in Exercise

A rise in blood flow to the exercising muscles is brought about through both an increase and a redistribution of CO. At rest, only about 15 to 20% of CO is distributed to skeletal muscle, in contrast to 85 or 90% during maximal exercise. This represents a 15- to 20-fold increase in flow to the skeletal muscles and a 3- to 4-fold increase to the myocardium (Fig. 12.3); muscle is the only tissue in the body that can markedly increase its own blood flow.

In skeletal muscle, the increased flow is initiated by anticipatory sympathetic cholinergic vasodilation and is reinforced by the metabolic hyperemia.

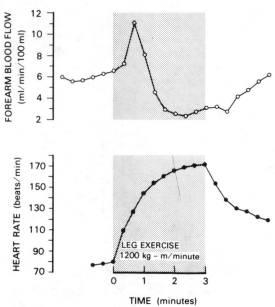

Figure 12.4. Changes in forearm blood flow during severe leg exercise in human subjects. After a temporary increase in forearm (muscle) flow during leg exercise, there was a constriction and flow reduction to about 50% of control. (Reprinted with permission from B.S. Bevegard and J.T. Shepherd, *J Appl Physiol* 21:123, 1966.)

As the exercise continues, the general tendency to sympathetic vasoconstriction is, in skeletal muscle, overwhelmed by metabolic vasodilation, thereby resulting in a massive increase in blood flow to this tissue. The vasodilation in the capillary bed of working muscle is probably due to increases in P_{CO_2}, K^+ and H^+.

The redistribution of flow, which is highly important in the shunting of oxygenated blood to active muscle, results not only from a decreased vascular resistance in skeletal muscle but also from strong sympathetic vasoconstriction in other tissues such as kidney, splanchnic area, and nonexercising muscle. Blood flow to the vasculature of the brain and myocardium (which have few α-receptors) is unchanged or increased (Fig. 12.3).

Thus, as might be expected, during leg exercise, blood flow to the nonexercising forearm muscles is decreased (Fig. 12.4). However, this normal forearm response to leg exercise may be reversed in certain disorders. Mark *et al.* reported that during leg exercise, vasodilation (instead of vasoconstriction) occurs in the forearm (and perhaps in other muscle tissue as well) in aortic stenosis patients. They suggested that this altered response may be due to reflexes from left ventricular baroceptors stimulated by the dilated ventricle and theorized that this reaction may be responsible for the exertional dyspnea and syncope that may occur in aortic stenosis and pulmonary hypertension patients. This vasodilator reaction of the forearm to exercise will usually revert to the normal vasoconstrictor response after surgical implantation of an efficient valve.

Although there is wide vasodilation of skeletal muscle arterioles, the veins of both exercising and nonexercising tissues are constricted, particularly those of the splanchnic venous bed. This is a sympathetic effect that assists in shunting blood into the central circulation, thereby aiding cardiac output.

During running there is a remarkable decrease in venous pressure at the ankle because of muscle pump action (Chapter 6, Skeletal Muscle Pump). However, pressure in the common femoral veins and inferior vena cavae increases to levels of 20 to 25 mm Hg, probably due to the high abdominal pressure that is mechanically necessary to fix and hold the pelvis, a condition that is essential to the running motion. This heightened intraabdominal venous pressure is a significant energy barrier for the heart.

Thermoregulatory adjustments are essential in any exercise that lasts more than a few minutes, since 80% of the total energy produced is thermal and must be carried to the skin surface to be dissipated. In moderate exercise, skin blood flow usually increases 3- to 4-fold. In severe exercise a constrictor tendency manifests itself, and flow returns toward baseline levels, apparently in an effort toward maximum conservation of venous return and cardial output. A conflict therefore develops, which is resolved in favor of maintaining cardiac output. This represents a problem in certain cardiac patients. The limited exercise capability of congestive heart failure patients is due partly to their diminished skin blood flow and consequent inability to dissipate heat and reduce their body core temperature. The hypothalamus is the essential integrator for both the vasomotor and the thermoregulatory changes (Chapter 10, Role of Hypothalamus).

Arm vs. Leg Exercise

At submaximal work intensities, the $\dot{V}O_2$ for arm and leg work is not significantly different. However, the achievable $\dot{V}O_{2max}$ is dependent on the mass and type of muscle involved. The $\dot{V}O_{2max}$ in arm ergometry is only 60 to 80% of that of leg ergometry or of combined arm and leg ergometry. The reason for the $\dot{V}O_{2max}$ limitation when smaller muscle masses such as the arm are involved has been attributed to (a) a lesser mechanical efficiency (i.e., a smaller ratio of work output to caloric expenditure) or (b) a lesser degree of conditioning (which usually prevails in arm vs. leg muscles).

But regardless of the cause, there is almost invariably a greater HR and pressor response to arm work compared to a similar level of leg work (Fig. 12.5). This phenomenon is usually held responsible for the oft-repeated history

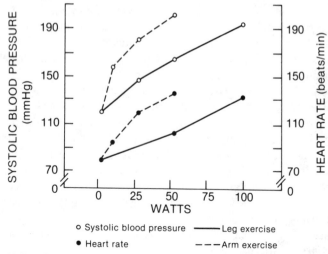

○ Systolic blood pressure ──── Leg exercise
● Heart rate ─ ─ ─Arm exercise

Figure 12.5. Systolic blood pressure and heart rate response at rest and at various levels of arm and leg ergometer exercise in patients with ischemic heart disease. At every work level the SBP and HR responses were greater during arm exercise. (Reprinted with permission from H.K. Hellerstein and B.A. Franklin. In: *Rehabilitation of the Coronary Patient*, edited by N.K. Wenger and H.K. Hellerstein. New York: John Wiley and Sons, 1978.)

of the keen sensitivity of angina pectoris patients to arm exercise. Aside from the lesser mechanical efficiency of small muscle groups, there is also a lesser "myocardial efficiency." For an equivalent degree of work, arm exercise induces a greater systolic pressure–HR increment than leg work. Since the pressure-rate product is a close correlate of myocardial oxygen consumption, arm work is more likely to produce myocardial ischemia in angina patients.

Systemic Response to Exercise

With the onset of exercise, respiratory changes occur rapidly, so there is increased gas exchange by the first or second breath. In the normal individual, the arterial Po_2 is unchanged even in severe exercise, which suggests that the factor limiting the exercise is not pulmonary ventilation. There is, however, a progressive decrease in venous O_2 saturation (Fig. 12.1) and, therefore, an increasing $(A-V)O_2$ difference, indicating a heightened extraction of O_2 by the tissues (Fig. 12.1). The O_2 extraction, which is greater in congestive failure patients at similar work loads, is sometimes used as a rough index of decreased cardiac output in cardiac decompensation.

  Important changes occur in blood chemistry. Because of the intense metabolic activity in the active muscles, the Pco_2, H^+ ion concentration, and blood temperature are all considerably increased in the tissues. This results in a shift of the HbO_2 dissociation curve to the right, which facilitates the release of O_2 to the tissues (Fig. 1.8). The accumulation in muscle of certain metabolites (*e.g.*, K^+, lactic acid and H^+ ions) during exhausting exercise is thought to be the main factor responsible for local discomfort, muscle pain, and fatigue. The increase in blood lactate reflects the anaerobic glucose breakdown necessary to maintain the exercise; the capacity to develop an O_2 debt is important in achieving maximal work.

Both aerobic (oxidative) and anaerobic (nonoxidative) metabolism contribute to the production of ATP necessary for muscle contraction. Muscle work that requires an energy expenditure greater than that which can be supplied by the ongoing oxidative processes is termed anaerobic. This situation prevails at the onset and during the intensive stages of exercise (*i.e.*, those which exceed 50 to 60% $\dot{V}O_{2max}$). This level is referred to as the "anaerobic" or "ventilatory" threshold. The lactic acid and other metabolites that accumulate during anaerobic exercise represent an oxygen debt that must be repaid during recovery in order to restore the metabolic system. Within the muscle there is, with exercise, increased glycogenolysis with increased production and release of pyruvate and lactate, increased lipolysis of muscle triglycerides, and increased free fatty acid (FFA) oxidation.

At high work rates, lactate increases disproportionately to pyruvate; the increased rate of lactate accumulation and greater lactate/pyruvate ratio usually occur at the threshold O_2 consumption for a given individual. For sustained exercise, the muscles are supplied with increased glucose and FFA by the liver and adipose tissue. The sympathetic nervous system and various hormones (particularly insulin and glucagon) are importantly concerned with metabolic regulation.

Plasma catecholamines increase markedly, depending on the intensity of the exercise and the active muscle mass involved. This reflects the sympathetic hyperactivity that is characteristic of the exercise response. Plasma levels of epinephrine may increase 3- to 4-fold and norepinephrine levels 5- to 7-fold in intensive exercise. The plasma catecholamines increase only slowly during submaximal exercise, but when approaching $\dot{V}O_{2max}$, rise steeply. The plasma levels of renin activity, vasopressin, and prolactin also increase with exercise. Farrell *et al.* reported that plasma levels of β-endorphin are elevated during exercise and suggested that endogenous opioids moderate the increases of epinephrine and other glucogenic hormones during exercise, thus serving to create a more appropriate milieu for handling the imposed stress.

The limitation to maximal dynamic exercise performance does not lie in the respiratory system but in the transport of O_2 to the tissues and removal of CO_2 and waste products. The specific limitation is either in the limited CO or in the enzymatic capabilities of the muscle tissue to extract the oxygen.

Static (Isometric) Exercise

As noted above, dynamic or isotonic exercise involves rhythmic movement of large muscle groups and requires increased O_2 uptake and heightened activity of the circulatory system. On the other hand, static or isometric exercise involves the development of muscular tension and strength, usually against resistance. Static exercise, because it induces a diastolic pressure increase, results in an afterload on the heart—a pressure load—rather than a flow-load.

In static (isometric) exercise, the energy expenditure is small compared to dynamic (isotonic) work, but the hemodynamic changes are equally pronounced. Experimentally, static exercise is often induced through maintenance of a sustained handgrip contraction at 30% of maximum voluntary tension to fatigue, which for most subjects is about 4 to 7 minutes. The sustained contraction calls forth a powerful cardiovascular reflex that results in a marked increase in both systolic and diastolic pressure.

If the responses to dynamic and static exercises are contrasted, it will be seen that in both cases there are large increases in systolic pressure; however, in dynamic exercise the increase in HR is much greater and the response of diastolic pressure much less (Fig. 12.2). Pushing, lifting, or carrying weights can elicit a hemodynamic reflex similar to the standard isometric test; for example, carrying or holding a 20-kg suitcase for 2½ minutes can induce a systolic blood pressure increase of about 45 mm Hg, a diastolic rise of about 30 mm Hg, and an HR increase of about 24 beats/min. Because of the pronounced increase in diastolic pressure and therefore of afterload, static exercise greatly increases myocardial O_2 demand. However recent studies by Hanson and Nagle have shown that patients with uncomplicated myocardial infarction can carry weights of 30 to 50 lbs without difficulty and with graduated isometric training can be returned to occupational tasks requiring isometric exercise.

Isometric exercise has been used as a myocardial stress test during cardiac catheterization. Patients with cardiac disease but with normal ventricular function at rest often develop ventricular pressure and wall motion abnormalities during static exercise, which help to uncover latent myocardial disease.

At lower muscle tensions (30 to 40% of maximum), the blood flow to the contracting muscles is increased, but at higher tensions (70% or more) the blood flow is stopped by the muscle compression. Blood flow in the exercising muscle is a compromise between the metabolically induced vasodilation and the compression of the blood vessels by the contracting muscles.

In a healthy subject the arterial pressure increase during static exercise is due mainly to the increase in CO, which in turn is due primarily to the increase in HR. This is particularly true during strenuous static exercise when the intrathoracic pressure increase—associated with the exercise effort—impedes

Table 12.1.
Oxygen Requirements at Different Stages of the Bruce Treadmill and Bicycle Ergometer Exercise Tests[a]

Functional Class	Clinical Status	O_2 Requirement (ml O_2/kg/min)	Bruce Treadmill Test 3 min stages		Bicycle Ergometer Test kg-m/min
			mph	% grade	
I normal	Healthy active	46	4.2	16	1500
I normal	Healthy sedentary	35	3.4	14	1050
I borderline	Borderline	28	3.0	13	850
II	Symptomatic patients	17	1.7	10	450
III	Symptomatic patients	10	1.5	8	200

[a]The maximum work level achieved defines the $\dot{V}O_{2max}$, and the left hand columns give approximations of the clinical status associated with such work performance.

venous return and therefore stroke volume (Chapter 13, Valsalva Maneuver). The degree of blood pressure response depends on several factors but mainly on the intensity of exercise and the amount of muscle mass involved.

The circulatory response to static exercise involves both central and peripheral mechanisms. The cerebral or "central command" factor is a direct effect of the motor cortex on medullary CV centers. The blood pressure increase is partially related to the intensity of the "command" (*i.e.*, the subjective effort exerted), which probably affects the number of motor units recruited. One peripheral mechanism involves the somatic afferent fibers, which activate the exercise pressor response in a manner similar to that in dynamic exercise. In static exercise there may be additional peripheral reflex factors initiated by metabolic or chemical agents (*e.g.*, K^+ ions) liberated in the muscle tissues.

In static exercise—as in dynamic exercise—plasma catecholamines and blood lactate levels are elevated.

Exercise Tests

The use of exercise as a screening test in cardiac disease has grown enormously in the last 20 years to become common procedure in cardiovascular medicine. The primary purposes are (*a*) to reveal latent ischemic heart disease and (*b*) to determine the functional capacity of the circulatory system.

While there are numerous test procedures, the most common in the United States is a prescribed treadmill test with progressive levels of physical work, designed to bring the subject to his limit of work capacity. Within narrow limits, each work level requires a specific O_2 uptake per kg body weight per min; thus, $\dot{V}O_{2max}$ may be estimated from the stage of the test at which the subject reaches his highest work level (Table 12.1). For example, if the subject is forced to stop at the end of the third stage of the Bruce test (*i.e.*, at 3.4 mph at a 14% grade) his $\dot{V}O_{2max}$ will be about 30 to 35 ml O_2/kg/min, which is approximately average for middle-aged, sedentary American men and would place him in a functional Class 1. On the other hand, a maximal work capacity of about 17 ml O_2/kg/min is considered below normal and would indicate a reduced tolerance for daily activities.

An alternate method of expressing physical fitness is the work level at which the subject attains his peak HR. Each individual has a definable HR_{max}, which declines progressively with age. The average HR_{max}, which is about 190 to 200/min at age 20, will decrease to about 165/min at age 60. By setting the mean age-predicted HR_{max} (or 90% of HR_{max}) as a reasonable goal, a better assessment can be made of the individual's work tolerance.

The presence of cardiac disease is not always easy to distinguish from poor physical condition. Coronary disease is suggested by inability to achieve maximum HR, by abnormal increase in arterial pressure during exercise, by high values of the (A-V)O_2 difference, but particularly by an ischemic S-T segment change in the ECG or angina.

The most definitive evidence of ischemic heart disease is the characteristic anginal pain (described in Chapter 14) or a 1-mm (*i.e.*, 0.1 mV) horizontal or downsloping S-T segment depression on the ECG during the exercise test. Even these signs, while highly suggestive, are not absolute, since in both cases false positives or false negatives may occur. As shown in Figure 12.6, S-T displacement of 1 mm or more occurs in a high percentage of patients with angina but also in a significant percentage of the normal population.

One difficulty in the diagnosis of coronary disease (particularly milder disease) is that a degree of coronary sclerosis as well as some decrease in cardiac functional ability is inherent with normal aging. In this regard, Bruce and coworkers have suggested that the response alterations in maximal exercise caused by cardiovascular disease and those attributable to aging can be separated by comparison with age-predicted values for healthy subjects. Deviations from the predicted norm in HR_{max} would suggest deficiencies in $\dot{V}O_{2max}$ (*i.e.*, work capacity); deviations in systolic pressure–HR (double) product values would suggest myocardial $\dot{V}O_2$ or left ventricular deficiencies (Chapter 11). Residual differences between these two values would represent peripheral circulatory impairment. These investigators have found this approach useful in separating a deficiency in circulatory delivery of oxygen into left ventricular and peripheral components.

Because of the variability of response of coronary heart disease (CHD) patients, the use of exercise tests has in recent years become somewhat controversial. The ability of a 1 mm S-T depression to correctly prognosticate CHD (*i.e.*, the "sensitivity" of the test) is only 66%, varying from 40% in mild (one vessel) disease to 90% in disease of two vessels or more. Thus it predicts severe disease more accurately than mild disease. On the

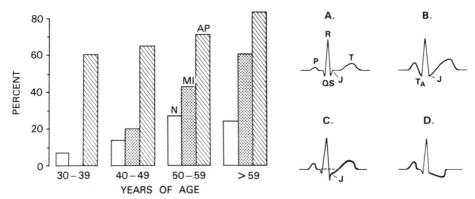

Figure 12.6. S-T segment displacement in myocardial ischemia. *Left*, prevalence of S-T segment depression after maximal exercise in normal subjects (*N*), patients with healed myocardial infarcts (*MI*), and patients with angina pectoris (*AP*). Note the relative independence of age in angina patients but age dependence in other groups. *Right*, types of S-T changes in exercise: *A*, normal ECG; *B*, false junctional J depression due to atrial T wave; *C*, true junctional S-T depression; *D*, S-T downslope segment depression. (Reprinted with permission from E. Simonson, *Physiology of Work Capacity and Fatigue*. Springfield, Ill.: Charles C Thomas, 1971.)

other hand, its "selectivity" (*i.e.*, its ability to properly exclude those without disease) is 84%, also not ideal. This means that in about 16% of cases, there is a "false" negative result (*i.e.*, the test is positive in 16% of individuals who on later coronary angiography apparently have normal coronary arteries). For reasons that are not clear, false positives are 6 to 8 times more common in females than males. Thus, while it is evident that ischemia of the myocardium due to narrowing of the coronary arteries is a primary cause of ECG disturbances such as S-T depression, there are also other causes, whose nature is presently unknown. It should be pointed out, however, that exercise testing has additional important uses: to follow the progress of post–myocardial infarct patients, to evaluate the degree of disability or recovery for occupational purposes, to assist in fashioning a personal exercise prescription for a recuperating patient, and for testing of various therapeutic regimens.

Ellestad and others have pointed out that there is a group of patients who have a decreased ability to achieve the usual heart rate levels during exercise. Those whose maximum HRs fall outside the 90% confidence limits for HR_{max} are termed "chronotropic incompetents." These subjects have a rate-pressure product (HR × systolic BP) lower than other patients (*i.e.*, a deficient myocardial O_2 supply) and have a 4-fold greater incidence of future coronary events. The cause of "chronotropic incompetence" is unknown.

Exercise Training

General

Repeated physical exercise will induce significant training effects that markedly increase the body's ability to perform work. A minimum regimen necessary to achieve such effects would involve large muscle masses continuously for at least 20 to 30 minutes, in two to three exercise sessions per week, at 60% $\dot{V}O_{2max}$ for a minimum period of 8 to 10 weeks. In addition to frequency, the type of exercise and intensity of effort are also important determinants of the degree of training achieved. Many studies on normal people, trained athletes, and animals trained to exercise, have indicated that during such "conditioning," important metabolic and circulatory adaptations are made. The changes are most marked in young adults who start training at a low fitness level. There is currently widespread interest in exercise-training effects with particular reference to their possible preventive and therapeutic role in certain cardiovascular disorders, especially ischemic heart disease.

Certainly exercise physiology has emerged as one of the most important fields of study of our time. It is obvious that the human body was never meant to be sedentary, and coping with the results of sedentary living poses some of the greatest health problems of our day.

Type of Exercise

As mentioned above, there are two types of exercise: (*a*) dynamic or isotonic, which refers to rhythmic contraction and relaxation of muscle groups, and (*b*) static or isometric exercise in which the muscles are kept at continued tension or contraction with little or no movement. Repetition of dynamic exercise is usually called endurance or aerobic training, and of isometric exercise, strength or power training. There are significant differences in cardiac effects depending on the type of physical training. In endurance training (*e.g.*, running, cycling, or rowing), there is an increase in heart volume due mainly to an increase in size of the cardiac cavities and to a lesser extent to an increase in muscle mass. There is an increase in SV/heart volume ratio and an increase in ejection fraction (EF). With strength or power training (weight lifting, shot putting, etc.), there is an increase in LV wall thickness (*i.e.*, a concentric hypertrophy similar to that seen in early hypertension). The increase in wall thickness is at the expense of volume, so that end-diastolic volume is either decreased or unchanged in relation to body weight. In power athletes, there is a decrease in SV/heart volume ratio and in EF. Reports indicate no myocardial damage in either type of training.

There are few, if any, cardiovascular benefits from strength training. While physical activity usually involves some elements of both types of exercise, the following discussion refers only to exercise training of the endurance type.

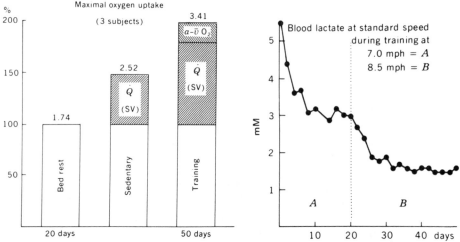

Figure 12.7. Effect of physical training on $\dot{V}o_{2max}$ (L/min) and blood lactate (mM/L) during exercise. *Left,* comparison of $\dot{V}o_{2max}$ of normal subjects after 20 days of bed rest, while sedentary, and after 50 days of physical training. *Right,* progressive decrease of blood lactate for a standard exercise: *A,* during first 20 days of training, and *B,* during next 30 days of training. (Reprinted with permission from P. Astrand and K. Rodahl, *Textbook of Work Physiology.* New York: McGraw-Hill, 1977.)

Cardiovascular Changes

The enhanced ability to perform physical work is particularly evidenced by substantial increases in $\dot{V}o_{2max}$ as well as lesser accumulation of blood lactate (Figure 12.7). The rise in $\dot{V}o_{2max}$ is due mainly to the elevation in CO (usually about 20 to 25%) and only to a limited extent to an increase in the (A-V)O_2 difference. The increased CO is facilitated by the decreased vascular resistance that is an important facet of the training response. There is an inverse relationship between $\dot{V}o_{2max}$ and systemic peripheral resistance. At the same work load, the "conditioned" individual will have a lower HR and a more rapid postexercise HR recovery; however, his HR_{max} is usually unaffected. With training, stroke volume (SV) will be increased at rest and at both submaximal and maximal exercise. Paulsen *et al.* found that, compared with sedentary controls, trained runners also had lower rate-pressure (HR × systolic pressure) products at rest and during submaximal exercise.

Endurance athletes usually have a lower systolic pressure at rest and at various levels of exercise. The fit subject often has a lower diastolic pressure during exercise, probably as a manifestation of his greater ability to decrease the peripheral vascular resistance of the arterioles in his exercising muscles.

There is increasing evidence that prolonged physical training will produce small but definite decreases in arterial blood pressure in hypertensive patients. Animal studies have indicated that prolonged physical conditioning will result in increased myocardial fiber mass, increased capillary/fiber ratio, improved myocardial contractility, and increased coronary artery size. The cardiac hypertrophy of the human endurance athlete also occurs in the physically trained animal, and with it there is improved hemodynamic performance. The evidence on the formation of new collateral vessels in the myocardium is conflicting. However, one definitive study indicates that the effect of ischemia on opening new capillaries is enhanced in the physically trained heart, suggesting that training plays at least an adjunctive role in promoting new capillary formation. It is, however, very significant that almost all of the above training effects occurred mainly in young animals and only to a very limited extent in older ones, suggesting that physical training, if it is to have lasting myocardial effects, might have to be started at an early age. Di Carlo *et al.* found that endurance training in dogs significantly reduced adrenergic coronary vasoconstrictor tone, thus apparently permitting a greater role for the coronary β-adrenergic vasodilators during exercise.

Systemic Responses to Training

With exercise training, adaptive changes occur in many other bodily systems. There is usually a decrease in blood viscosity and hematocrit. Sustained intensive physical training has been shown to induce a mild, transient "sports anemia," which usually subsides in several days. Endurance conditioning also enhances the fibrinolytic response to exercise and results in a decrease in plasma triglycerides and an increase in plasma high-density lipoprotein levels, changes associated with a lesser risk for ischemic heart disease. In addition, physical training, especially in the obese subject, reduces body weight and body fat percentage, increases lean body mass, and causes a general reduction in the "fat envelope." The influence of exercise training on some typical physiologic and metabolic parameters is shown in Table 12.2.

A recent report indicates that aerobic fitness (endurance training) enabled middle-aged men to maintain their ability to cope with heat stress; more profuse sweating enabled trained men to maintain lower core and skin temperature. In an analysis of physiological adaptation to aerobic training, Nadel expressed the belief that the increase in absolute blood volume is probably the most important benefit of all, since it increases both central blood volume and stroke volume. These changes enhance O_2 and heat transport and thus greatly increase the ability of the body to maintain skin blood flow and a lower core temperature during exercise.

Table 12.2.
Representative Physiological and Metabolic Values Before and After Aerobic Exercise Training[a]

Variable	Untrained	Trained	Difference (%)
Max stroke volume (ml/beat)	120	180	50
Max cardiac output (1/min)	20	30–40	75
Resting heart rate (beats/min)	70	40	−43
Max heart rate (beats/min)	190	180	−5
Max (A-V)O$_2$ diff. (ml/100 ml)	14.5	16.0	10
Max $\dot{V}$O$_2$ (ml/kg-1/min)	30–40	65–80	107
Blood volume (1)	4.7	6.0	28
Hemoglobin (g/kg)	11.6	13.7	18
$\dot{V}_E$ max (1/min)	110	190	73
Percent body fat	15	11	−27
Glycogen (mmol/g wet muscle)	85.0	120	41
Resting ATP (mmol/g wet muscle)	3.0	6.0	100
Resting CP (mmol/g wet muscle)	11.0	18.0	64
Aerobic enzymes			
Succinate dehydrogenase (mmol/kg wet muscle)	5–10	15–20	133

[a]Values are approximate; trained values are from endurance athletes but the differences may be partly due to genetic factors. (From McArdle WD, Katch FI, and Katch VL. *Exercise Physiology* 2nd ed. Philadelphia: Lea & Febiger, 1986).

The levels of plasma norepinephrine (NE) at rest and at the same relative work loads (*i.e.*, at the same percentage of $\dot{V}$O$_{2max}$) are unchanged with endurance training. However, the increase in plasma NE at the same absolute work load is much less after training, which indicates a lesser sympathetic response for the same exercise level.

It has been reported that physical training also has psychological manifestations. Some studies have shown that physical fitness can attenuate emotional stress, reduce anxiety, and improve social adjustment. However, only limited data are available on this question. In some endurance athletes, a euphoria-like state, sometimes called a "runner's high," occurs after distance runs. Other reports indicate a diminished sensitivity to pain after endurance events and on occasion have termed distance running as a "near addiction." It has been theorized that such subjective sensations may be due to the liberation of endorphins, which are amino acid complexes released by the CNS or pituitary gland and transported to specific CNS or peripheral sites. It is believed that endorphins react with opiate receptors located within the brain and play an important role in pain modulation, sleep, and stress reactions. Farrell *et al.* have recently reported a 2- to 5-fold increase in plasma β-endorphins after a strenuous 30-minute treadmill run in endurance athletes.

However, mood state and perceptual data showed no significant relationship to the β-endorphin levels, so that the role of endorphins in these psychological alterations remains speculative.

Cross Adaptation and Detraining

As indicated above, there is abundant evidence that repeated, vigorous, endurance-type exercise will greatly increase cardiac output, lower resting heart rate and blood pressure, decrease body fat, and improve musculoskeletal function. Some studies have indicated that physical training will lessen the risk of ischemic heart disease (IHD). But does physical fitness improve general resistance to the physical inroads of stress and disease (e.g., IHD) when they occur? The answer to this interesting question is not known and investigations of this type are still in their early phases.

A few preliminary studies have indicated some degree of cross adaptation to physical training. During generalized hypoxia, for example, physically trained rats maintained significantly greater cardiac output and cardiac work performance than untrained rats even though O_2 delivery and lactate production were similar. The trained animals were capable of more efficient energy utilization for external cardiac work.

Physical training also improves heat tolerance. Rats that were treadmill-trained in a cool environment performed better on a work-heat tolerance test and suffered less tissue damage than untrained animals. Physically trained human subjects also have better circulatory adaptation to heat.

German investigators, on the other hand, have reported postural intolerance in some endurance athletes, for example, a lower resistance to gravity stresses such as head-up tilt after similar exposure to prolonged water immersion. The mechanism of this effect is not certain but may be due to a lower baroceptor sensitivity, or to a sluggish cardioaccelerator response in the athletes, or both.

The mechanisms for the above-described "training effects," particularly the increase in $\dot{V}O_{2max}$, are not certain but are probably due to a combination of an increased oxygen delivery to the muscles (mainly an increase in CO) and an increase in the size and number of muscle mitochondria (i.e., increased oxidative capacity of the muscle cell). It is interesting, however, that one training effect, bradycardia, if achieved with repetitive exercise of certain large muscle groups, is operative only when the same trained muscles are used and does not occur with exercise involving the untrained muscles. These findings would suggest that peripheral mechanisms are involved and that cross adaptation is minimal.

Detraining or deconditioning of the trained endurance athlete is rapid, occurring within about 12 to 20 weeks after cessation of exercise training.

Bed rest, which will induce even more rapid deconditioning, will cause a substantial decrease in $\dot{V}o_{2max}$ (Fig. 12.7), shortening of exercise endurance time, and decreases in plasma volume within 2 to 3 weeks. Bed rest or exposure to zero gravity eliminates the usual relocation of venous blood to the dependent veins, which would ordinarily occur in the sitting or standing position; plasma volume then tends to accumulate in the thoracic veins. A hypovolemia of 15 to 25% will result from the diuresis induced by the continued effect of this increased central blood volume on the cardiopulmonary "volume" receptors (Chapter 10). The detraining effect in these situations is also due to decreased muscle activity with a consequent diminution of muscle mass (*i.e.*, a "disuse atrophy"). The importance of the blood-volume changes in detraining is underscored by the fact that infusions of 6% dextran in saline can largely reverse the circulatory effects.

Clinical Application of Physical Training

As discussed in Chapter 14, there are both controllable and uncontrollable risk factors for ischemic heart disease. To date, the primary controllable factors have been considered to be hypertension, high blood cholesterol, and smoking. However, recent findings have strongly suggested that physical inactivity should be added to this list of "majors."

British investigators in the 1950s were among the first to suggest a link between exercise and heart disease, when they reported fewer heart attacks in those who walked rather than remained seated on the job (*e.g.*, bus conductors *vs.* bus drivers, and postmen *vs.* sedentary postal workers). Subsequent studies of large populations have shown that activity that burns about 300 calories/day—the equivalent of an hour's brisk walk—results in a markedly lowered chance of an initial heart attack (*i.e.*, such activity is effective in primary prevention).

Given the methodological problems of biological—particularly human—research, these findings do not constitute "proof" that habitual exercise will reduce the risk of heart disease. It may be that certain occupations or physical activities attract people with less disease or lower vulnerability to heart disease. It has been suggested that physical activity may not be directly related to the atherosclerotic process but may enable the heart to better tolerate the ischemia and lessen the manifestations of coronary disease. The issue of whether it is physical fitness or the physical activity which is beneficial has also been raised. Recent studies have indicated that physical fitness rather than activity is an independent protective factor against ischemic heart disease. It appears likely that two separate processes are at work. Aside from the diminished likelihood of ischemic heart disease, other effects, perhaps not directly related to cardiovascular function, such as increased physical mobility, improved carbohydrate metabolism, better heat tolerance, and lessened psychological tension may, particularly in older individuals, greatly improve the "quality" of life and considerably expedite successful aging.

Most patients who have undergone physical training after their myocardial infarct (MI) can achieve performance levels at least equivalent to those of normal, sedentary subjects. However, the response to training is sometimes restricted in patients with more extensive infarcts, presumably because of reduced myocardial function. After physical training, MI patients will have decreased body fat and plasma triglycerides compared with nontrained control patients. In other studies performed after 8 weeks of training, MI patients performed subanginal work loads at lower rate-pressure product levels (*i.e.*, with a lesser increase in myocardial O_2 consumption). One group of IHD patients who exercised intensively for more than one year developed a capacity for endurance exercise equal to that of trained normal subjects. These patients equaled the normal subjects in running endurance, in spite of a lower $\dot{V}O_{2max}$, by developing a higher lactate threshold. Thus some post-MI patients with limited $\dot{V}O_{2max}$ can undergo training adaptations enabling them to approximate a metabolic steady state during exercise that elicits $\dot{V}O_{2max}$.

The obvious beneficial effects of supervised physical exercise for coronary patients has prompted increased efforts to provide much-needed physical rehabilitation programs for such patients. The ability of many coronary patients to achieve a well-adjusted and productive future life depends largely on a well-planned and well-executed physical-training rehabilitation program (Chapter 14, Cardiac Rehabilitation).

Effects of Aging
Aging and the Circulation—General

It is well known that the combination of a low fertility rate in the post–baby boom years and a low mortality has made ours an aging population. Pifer and Bronte have projected that by 2050 the over-65 population in this country—presently about 12%—will increase to 22%, or about 67.4 million. The over-85 population—presently 1.1%—will increase about 4½ times, to about 5.2%. This massive demographic shift will have profound social, economic, and medical implications. Not only does the incidence of cardiovascular disease increase steeply with age but there is also (as mentioned previously) a striking similarity between the effects of age *per se* and early coronary heart disease. This sometimes poses a serious problem in differential diagnosis and makes it particularly important to establish norms for cardiovascular function in the aged before reaching conclusions regarding cardiovascular pathology.

At rest there are only minor changes in cardiac function with age. However, with exercise, older individuals show significant differences in their circulatory responsiveness. In adults, $\dot{V}O_{2max}$ tends to be highest at about age 27

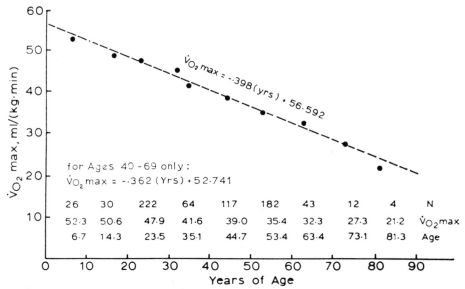

Figure 12.8.   Regression of mean $\dot{V}_{O_{2}max}$ per decade of age in 700 boys and men (corrected for body weight) showing a steady decline of oxygen uptake during maximal exercise with advancing age. (Reprinted with permission from M.M. Dehn and R.A. Bruce, *J Appl Physiol* 33:805, 1972.)

and, thereafter, steadily decreases by about 1% per year, so that at age 65 it is about 60% of the former value (Fig. 12.8).

A recent study has shown that sedentary young men have about a 30% greater $\dot{V}_{O_{2}max}$ than sedentary young women, but the rate of decline with age was significantly greater in the men than in the women. The sedentary young men also had higher HR_{max}, cardiac index$_{max}$ and stroke index$_{max}$ values than the young women, but again (except in the case of the SI) the rate of decrease was greater in the sedentary men. The decline of $\dot{V}_{O_{2}max}$ is also more rapid in the obese and in smokers.

A number of physiological and psychological studies have separated the elderly population into the young-old (65-75 years), the old-old (75-85 yrs) and the very old (over 85 yrs) on the basis of the degree and rate of the changes. Geriatrics, the systematic study of aging, is a relatively new specialty. The following outline of the physiological alterations with age is based on a brief survey of the relatively limited data available.

Circulatory System—Structural Changes

During aging there are a number of cardiopulmonary structural changes that have far-reaching physiological consequences. The decreased arterial distensibility and venous compliance with age (Chapter 1) occurs in both man and animals and is related to a progressive increase in the collagen/elastin ratio of the vessel wall. There is increasing stiffness of the aorta and large arteries in both a radial and longitudinal direction as determined by pressure-volume curves (Fig. 1.7).

This arterial rigidity is the result of a diffuse process involving the replacement of elastin with connective tissue. The result is due to an alteration of the viscoelastic properties of the wall at large and not to atherosclerosis, which is generally a patchy and irregular process. While (as mentioned in Chapter 1) the increase in aortic volume, especially after age 60, provides some hemodynamic buffering, this is quite inadequate to offset the marked compliance changes. The aortic volume change required to induce a pressure change of 100 mm Hg is, at age 70, only about ½ that at age 20 (Fig. 1.7). With increasing age, there is, in peripheral arteries, a rise in the systolic and a drop in the diastolic pressure wave due to this alteration in arterial distensibility.

The decreased aortic distensibility along with the increase peripheral resistence of the arterial bed also serves to increase the mechanical impedance of the aortic bed and imposes a heavier afterload on the aging left ventricle. This increased impedance to ejection is very likely an important factor in limiting the increase in left ventricular stroke volume (LVSV) during exercise in the older subject. Associated with the increased aortic impedance there is also an increase in left ventricular chamber size. The limited data available indicate a decreased LV compliance, which could be a significant factor in limiting both LV end-diastolic volume and the Starling response. In older subjects, increased stiffness of the heart valves and pericardium may also exert a functional handicap.

As Kenney has pointed out, aside from the alterations in the cardiovascular system, each step in the path that O_2 takes from the outer air to the metabolizing cell is vulnerable to aging. The pulmonary alveoli become smaller and more shallow, so there is a steady decline in vital capacity and about a 20% decrease in alveolar surface area by age 70. There is a decrease in pulmonary elastic recoil and lung compliance, and because of the stiffened rib cage there is increasing reliance on diaphragmatic breathing. Since skeletal muscle typically shows prolonged contraction and relaxation periods, all the timed, ventilatory functions are slower.

The alveolar-arterial O_2 difference increases with age. Although Hb concentration is maintained in the healthy older person, there is a small alteration in RBC metabolism and a resultant decreased concentration of 2,3-diphosphoglycerate. As a consequence, there is a shift of the HbO_2 dissociation curve to the left, thereby making the tissue unloading of O_2 more difficult (Figure 1.8).

Age Effect on Circulation at Rest

A number of studies have shown that in addition to the decline in $\dot{V}O_{2max}$ there is, in older individuals, a gradual decline in the resting values of cardiac index (CI), stroke index (SI) and (A-V)O_2 difference.

The decrease in cardiac output (described above) is a very significant circulatory handicap; it means a decline of about 1/3 from age 20 to age 80. The fundamental cause is the steady decline in metabolic rate, which, in turn, is probably due to the decreased efficiency of the tissue oxidative enzymes (as manifested by the continuing decline in (A-V)O_2 difference). It is most likely that the heart, if healthy, plays mainly a permissive role in the circulatory system and is not a primary cause of the declining cardiac output. Cross-sectional studies have generally shown a progressive rise in systolic and diastolic pressure (Fig. 6.5) and peripheral vascular resistance with age. However, physiological age does not always parallel chronological age, and there are wide individual differences, depending primarily on physical condition and hereditary, dietary, and socioeconomic factors. Some recent reports have indicated that in some individuals, arterial pressures do not rise with age and that many of these subjects do not have increased systemic vascular resistance (Lakatta, 1986).

Age Effect on Stress Response

While the above structural changes impose relatively little handicap on the normal, older individual at rest, circulatory stresses such as exercise will uncover the depth of the physiological reserve and will reveal significant functional deficiencies with increasing age. As mentioned above, beginning at about age 25, dynamic work capacity (*i.e.*, $\dot{V}O_{2max}$ per unit body weight) decreases steadily with age. Older men and women respond to exercise with progressively lower increases in HR, SI, CI, and (A-V)O_2 differences and greater increases in systolic pressure.

It has been consistently observed that in man, peripheral resistance at rest and at comparable work loads is increased with age and that in exercise there is a decreased dilator capability in vascular smooth muscle. It is also significant that during exercise the elderly have elevated pulmonary arterial wedge pressures and increased right ventricular end-diastolic pressures, suggesting a diminished reserve capacity in older hearts. While younger individuals usually respond to exercise with an increased ejection fraction (EF), there is a progressive decline in the LVEF response to exercise with age, and an increasing frequency of myocardial wall motion abnormalities in subjects 50 years and older. Generally, the attainment of steady-state levels of HR, blood pressure, and ventilatory responses is slower and the rate of recovery more prolonged with increasing age. Translated into practical terms, this means that the quantity of work that can be performed during a given work period is reduced in the aged, and more frequent or prolonged rest periods may be needed.

The reason for the decreased myocardial response to exercise in the elderly is not certain. It may be associated with (*a*) increased aortic impedance and the afterload limitations it imposes on LV ejection, (*b*) decreased responsiveness of the Frank-Starling mechanism (*i.e.*, a preload deficiency), or (*c*) decreased myocardial contractility, perhaps due to a diminished sympathetic response of cardiac muscle (which has been shown to occur in animals). Recent studies suggest that, in the absence of overt disease, the overall decline in functional cardiovascular capacity with age is due mainly to a progressive decrease in skeletal muscle mass (or more specifically to a decline in skeletal muscle protein), a decrease in the capillary to muscle fiber ratio, and a decrease in the arterial vascular cross-sectional area and mass. It is widely believed that an active life-style with habitual exercise will enable the individual to retain cardiovascular function for a longer period and delay these changes.

Autonomic Responsiveness and Aging

As described above, the older individual generally has an impaired response to physical exercise, which is associated with a heightened aortic impedance, a decreased myocardial performance, and an inadequate peripheral circulatory response. It is not certain, however, to what extent these pathophysiological manifestations are due to anatomical deficiencies, defective autonomic reflexes, or insufficient neurohumoral stimulation.

Autonomic stress tests in normal subjects of different ages have shown decreased resting cardiac vagal tone, a lesser rise in heart rate and diastolic pressure in the older subjects during head-up tilt, and lesser heart rate increments in the standard Valsalva test. Whether the defect lies in the afferent or efferent limb of the autonomic reflex or in a higher, integrating CNS center is not certain. Studies in animals and man indicate that the arterial baroceptors may become less sensitive with advancing age (Fig. 12.9). It has been suggested that this decreased baroceptor sensitivity may be due to an increased rigidity of the aorta and carotid arteries, which would result in less deformation of the receptors and less stimulation for equivalent pressure changes.

Animal and human studies have shown a decreased responsiveness of the myocardium and a decreased heart rate response to β-adrenergic binding sites in the tissue with age. It seems likely therefore that the diminished performance of the circulatory system is due to both a decrease in autonomic responsiveness and anatomical and functional defects within the cardiovascular system itself.

Increased plasma NE levels are found consistently in older individuals, both at rest and in response to standard stresses such as exercise or upright posture. However, age apparently does not affect the plasma epinephrine response, which might suggest a selective age effect on certain neurohormonal pathways.

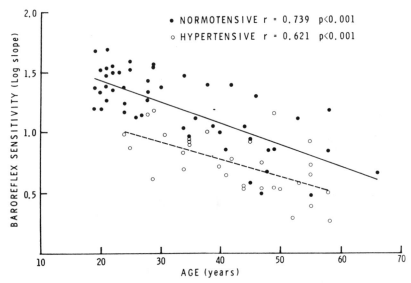

Figure 12.9. Effect of age on baroreflex sensitivity, indicating a progressive fall in the sensitivity index (pulse interval/Δ systolic pressure) with increasing age in both normotensives and hypertensives. (Reprinted with permission from B. Gribbin, T.G. Pickering, P. Sleight, and R. Peto, *Circ Res* 39:424, 1971.)

As mentioned above, the elderly are more vulnerable, not only to exercise but also to general stresses such as sodium depletion and orthostasis. Studies have shown, for example, that temporary Na^+ depletion in older subjects (65 to 80 yrs) lessened their response to orthostasis, while younger subjects were not affected by this relatively mild stress (Fig. 12.10); aside from inadequate systolic pressure reactions, these older subjects also had diminished increases in heart rate and had tendencies toward fainting.

Orthostatic Tolerance in the Elderly

The normal circulatory response to the upright posture (discussed in Chapter 13) is quite well maintained until about 65 to 70 years of age. However, at about age 75 or more, there is a progressive tendency in many subjects toward postural hypotension (*i.e.*, a decrease of ≥20 mm Hg in systolic or diastolic pressure upon standing). The specific cause of this disorder is not known. There are, however, five main hemodynamic deficiencies that might theoretically predispose to orthostatic hypotension in the elderly: inadequacy of cardioacceleration, left ventricular ejection, thoracic blood volume, the skeletal muscle pump (Chapters 6 and 13), and the vascular resistance response. As mentioned above, there is clear evidence of a diminished capacity for cardio-acceleration and ventricular contractility during stress in the elderly.

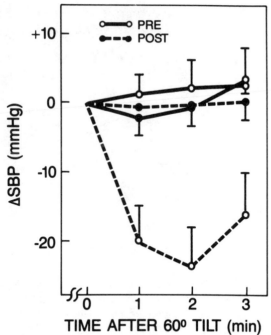

TIME AFTER 60º TILT (min)

Figure 12.10. Changes in systolic blood pressure (SBP) responses to the 3 min, 60° upright tilt in healthy young (25–35 years) and old (65–80 years) subjects before and after a moderate two-day diuretic-induced Na$^+$ depletion. Three of the six older subjects had symptoms of postural intolerance. Black dots represent young healthy subjects; white dots represent old healthy subjects. Solid lines represent systolic pressures before Na$^+$ depletion; dotted lines represent systolic pressure after Na$^+$ depletion. (From R.P. Shannon *et al. Hypertension* 8:438, 1986.)

Previous studies have suggested a particular deficiency in heart-rate response in the critical first 15 to 30 sec of standing which may lead to cerebral ischemia and contribute to postural instability.

Orthostatic hypotension of the elderly is a serious clinical problem that is amplified because of its increasingly progressive incidence with age. It is important partly because of its role in the causation of falls in the elderly—a considerable medical problem—and partly because it is a major deterrent to ambulation in the aged. Decreased ambulation in turn has a crippling effect on the social autonomy and quality of life of the older citizen.

Aging and the Circulation—Summary

It appears that in aging, the normal function of the heart and blood vessels is highly dependent on the physical properties of distensibility, contractility, and elasticity, all of which involve connective tissue as well as muscle. With increasing age there is an increasing ratio of collagen to muscle. Significantly, the collagen itself changes and becomes cross-linked with calcium deposits and thus less compliant. The anatomical and physiological changes result in (a) a heightened aortic impedance with an increased work load on the left ventricle, (b) a less distensible myocardium that has longer contraction and relaxation periods, and (c) a lowered autonomic responsiveness with age, resulting in a diminished heart-rate rise during standing and the Valsalva maneuver.

Functionally these changes are associated with a steadily decreasing work capacity ($\dot{V}O_{2max}$), the rate of decrease being heavily dependent on individual factors such as physical training and obesity. The decreasing work capacity is, in turn, associated with an altered hemodynamic response to exercise. In particular, there is a decrease in HR_{max}, SV_{max}, and CO_{max} with increasing end-diastolic and arterial blood pressure.

The structural changes that occur with normal aging produce little or no functional handicap at rest and only a minor handicap at moderate work levels in normal, physically fit elderly persons.

However, these changes do lead to a reduction of hemodynamic reserve and a lowered ability to cope with environmental stress. In individuals over age 75, these hemodynamic deficiencies may lead to orthostatic intolerance and, in some cases, to orthostatic hypotension, an important clinical problem in the elderly.

Suggested Readings

Exercise and Physical Training

Astrand P and Rodahl K. *Textbook of Work Physiology*, 2nd ed. New York: McGraw-Hill, 1977.

Blomqvist CG. Cardiovascular adaptions to physical training. *Annu Rev Physiol* 45:169–189, 1983.

Bruce RA, DeRouen TA, and Hossack KF. Value of maximal exercise tests in risk assessment of primary coronary heart disease events in healthy man. *Am J Cardiol* 46:371–378, 1980.

Bruce RA, Fisher LD, Cooper MN, and Gey GO. Separation of effects of cardiovascular disease and age on ventricular function with maximal exercise. *Am J Cardiol* 34:757–763, 1974.

Di Carlo SE, Blair RW, Bishop VS, *et al*. Role of β-adrenergic receptors on coronary resistance during exercise. *J Appl Physiol* 64:2287–2293, 1988.

Ellestad MH. *Stress Testing: Principles and Practice*. 3rd ed. NYC Davis FA. 1986.

Farrell PA, Gates WK, Maksud MG, and Morgan WP. Increases in plasma β-endorphin/β-lipotropin immunoreactivity after treadmill running in humans. *J Appl Physiol* 52(5):1245–1249, 1982.

Farrell PA, Gustafson AB, Garthwaite TA, *et al*. Influence of endogenous opioids on the response of selected hormones to exercise in humans. *J Appl Physiol* 61:1051–1057, 1986.

Froelicher VF. *Exercise and the Heart*. Chicago: Yearbook Publishers, 1987.

Hanson P and Nagle FJ. Isometric exercise: Cardiovascular responses in normal and cardiac populations. *Cardiology Clinics* 5(2):157–170, 1987.

Lind AR and McNicol GW. Local and central responses to sustained muscle contractions and the effect of restricted arterial inflow. *J Physiol* 192:575–593, 1967.

McArdle WD, Katch FI, and Katch VL. *Exercise Physiology: Energy, Nutrition and Human Performance*, 2nd ed. Philadelphia: Lea & Febiger, 1986.

Mitchell JH, Kaufman MP, and Iwamoto GA. The exercise pressor reflex: its cardiovascular effects, afferent mechanisms and central pathways. *Annu Rev Physiol* 45:229–242, 1983.

Montoye HJ, Christian JL, Nagle FJ, and Levin SM. *Living Fit.* Menlo Park, Ca: Benjamin/Cummings Pub. Co., 1988.

Nadel ER. Physiological adaptations to aerobic training. *American Scientist* 73:334–343, 1985.

Paulsen W, Boughner DR, Ko P, Cunningham DA, and Persaud JA. Left ventricular function in marathon runners: echocardiographic assessment. *J Appl Physiol* 51(4):881–886, 1981.

Peronnet P, Cleroux J, Perrault H, Cousineau D, deChamplain J, and Nadeau R. Plasma norepinephrine response to exercise before and after training in humans. *J Appl Physiol* 51(4):812–815, 1981.

Radomski MW, Sabiston BH, and Isoard P. Development of "sports anemia" in physically fit men after daily sustained submaximal exercise. *Aviat Space Environ Med* 51(1):41–45, 1980.

Sandler H and Vernikos-Danellis J. *Inactivity: Physiological Effects.* New York: Academic Press, 1986.

Seals DR, Washburn RA, Hanson PG, Painter PL, and Nagle FJ. Increased cardiovascular response to static contraction of larger muscle groups. *J Appl Physiol* 54:434–437, 1983.

Shepherd J. Behavior of resistance and capacity vessels in human limbs during exercise. *Circ Res* 20 and 21 (Supl. I):70–82, 1967.

Stegemann J, Busert A, and Brock D. Influence of fitness on the blood pressure control system in man. *Aerosp Med* 45:45–48, 1974.

Wasserman K, Hansen JE, Sue DY, and Whipp BJ. *Principles of Exercise Testing and Interpretation.* Philadelphia: Lea & Febiger, 1987.

Wenger NK and Hellerstein HK (eds.). *Rehabilitation of the Coronary Patient.* New York: John Wiley & Sons, 1978.

Aging

Collins KJ, Exton-Smith AN, James MH, and Oliver DJ. Functional changes in autonomic nervous responses with aging. *Age & Ageing* 9:17, 1980.

Dambrink JHA and Wieling W. Circulatory response to postural change in healthy male subjects in relation to age. *Clin Sci* 72:335, 1987.

Ebert TJ, Hughes CV, Tristani FE, Barney JA, and Smith JJ. The effect of age and coronary heart disease on the circulatory responses to graded lower body negative pressure. *Cardiovasc Res* 16:663–669, 1982.

Guyton AC. *Cardiac Output and Its Regulation.* Philadelphia: W.B. Saunders, 1963.

Hodgson JL and Buskirk ER. Physical fitness and age with emphasis on cardiovascular function in the elderly. *J Am Geriatrics Soc* 25:385–392, 1977.

Hossack KF and Bruce RA. Maximal cardiac function in sedentary normal men and women: comparison of age-related changes. *J Appl Physiol* 53(4):799–804, 1982.

Kenney RA. *Physiology of Aging: A Synopsis.* Chicago: Year Book Medical Publishers, 1982.

Lakatta EG. Hemodynamic Adaptation to Stress with Advancing Age. *Acta Med Scand* Supp 711:39, 1986.

Lakatta EG. Cardiac muscle changes in senescences. *Ann Rev Physiol* 49:519–521, 1987.

McDermott DJ, Tristani FE, Ebert TJ, Porth CJ, and Smith JJ. Age-related changes in cardiovascular response to diverse circulatory stresses. In: *Arterial Baroceptors and Hypertension*, edited by P Sleight. Oxford: Oxford University Press, 1980, pp 361–364.

Masoro EJ. *CRC Handbook of Physiology in Aging.* Boca Raton, Fla: CRC Press, 1981.

Pifer A and Bronte DL. *Our Aging Society: Paradox and Promise.* New York: W.W. Norton, 1986.

Rowe JW and Kahn RL. Human aging: usual and successful. *Science* 237:143–149, 1987.

Shephard RJ. *Physical Activity and Aging.* Chicago: Year Book Medical Publishers, 1978.

Shock NW. *Normal Human Aging: The Baltimore Longitudinal Study of Aging*. NIH Pub. No 84–2450. Washington, D.C.: Supt. of Documents, U.S. Govt. Printing Office, 1984.

Smith JJ, Hughes CV, Ptacin MJ, Barney JA, Tristani FE, and Ebert TJ. Homodynamic response to graded postural stress in normal males: the effect of age. *J Gerontology* 42:406–411, 1987.

Smith JJ and Porth CJ. Age and the response to orthostatic stress. In: *Circulatory Response to Upright Posture*, edited by JJ Smith. Boca Raton, Fla: CRC Press, 1990.

Strandell T. Circulatory studies on healthy old men. *Acta Med Scand* 175(Suppl. 414):1–44, 1964.

Weisfeldt ML (ed.). *The Aging Heart: Its Function and Response to Stress*. New York: Raven Press, 1980.

chapter 13

Circulatory Response to Nonexercise Stress

Stress is the result of a real or imagined threat to the well-being of the individual. It usually involves the autonomic nervous system and if sufficiently serious, there is activation of the defense center of the hypothalamus with a powerful sympathoadrenal release (Chapter 10). Individuals vary widely in their responses to stress depending upon their age, physical and emotional state, and the nature and severity of the stress. The effects of physical exercise, both dynamic and static, as well as the principles of exercise stress testing were discussed in Chapter 12.

In this chapter are included brief descriptions of a few comm(
physical stresses and the clinical tests that are sometimes us
them. Because inadequate reactions to such tests are often th
impending disease, compensatory stress responses and their mechanism
be analyzed.

Postural and Gravity Effects on the Circulation

Normal Postural Responses

The effect of gravity on the circulatory system and the important factors influencing venous return, such as the skeletal muscle pump, have been discussed in detail in Chapter 6. A review of those elements is essential to an understanding of the circulatory response to postural changes.

Displacement of Thoracic Blood Volume

For normal man, standing erect presents no problem, but an inadequate orthostatic response may be an indication of a serious clinical disturbance. The upright posture requires proper functioning and coordination of the musculoskeletal system, the nervous system, and the circulatory system. From a circulatory standpoint the two main elements concerned in postural abnormalities are the skeletal muscle pump and the baroceptor reflexes.

Postural changes are often simulated through use of a tilt table or by "lower body negative pressure"; in the latter procedure, air is evacuated and pressure reduced in a box enclosing the lower body below the iliac crests. These devices produce hemodynamic changes similar to but not identical with standing erect and have the advantage of facilitating physiological measurements.

In recumbent, resting man, the total blood volume is about 70 to 75 ml/kg. About 25 ml/kg (*i.e.*, about one third of the total blood volume) is thoracic or "central" blood volume. Upon assumption of the upright posture, 7 to 10 ml/kg of thoracic blood volume (a total of about 500 to 700 ml in the average-sized adult) migrates quickly to the lower body, to buttocks, pelvis, and mainly to lower extremities. The migration is in two phases—fast and slow. The first, or fast, phase begins immediately, is about 90% complete in 2 to 3 minutes, and constitutes about 90% of the total thoracic blood migration. The second, or slow, phase of blood migration involves transcapillary diffusion of cell-free and protein-free fluid into the interstitial tissues of the lower extremities. This plasma filtrate comes, therefore, from the blood and not the thorax. The plasma diffusion rate is slow, comprising a total of only about 1.5 ml/kg during the first 10 min of standing.

The fast and slow phases of blood migration are shown in Figure 13.1A & B. Figure 13.1A shows the rate of decrease of thoracic blood volume in normal adult males during the first 20 min of 70° headup tilt (which is

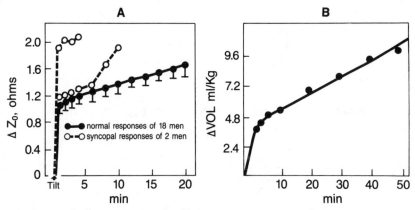

Figure 13.1.   Fast and slow phases of blood volume migration in upright position. *A,* Decrease in thoracic blood volume (increase in transthoracic Z_0) during 20 min 70° headup tilt in healthy young men. The unusual thoracic blood volume changes in two subjects who fainted are discussed further in the section on Abnormal Postural Responses. *B,* Increase in volume of both lower extremities (legs and thighs) during headup tilt in normal human subject. (Adapted from T.S. Ebert, J.J. Smith, J.A. Barney, *et al. Aviat Space Environ Med* 57:49, 1986 and Asmussen, E. *et al., Surgery* 8:604, 1940.)

comparable to a free stand). The decrease in thoracic blood volume is illustrated by an increase in transthoracic electrical impedance (which varies inversely with the amount of thoracic blood). In Figure 13.1*A,* the alteration in thoracic blood volume was determined with the impedance cardiographic method described in Chapter 7 (Figure 7.8). Figure 13.1*B* shows the accumulation of blood in the lower extremities in a normal adult male during the first 50 min of headup tilt. These two bimodal curves show that the great bulk of the thoracic blood migrates quickly to the lower extremities in the first 2 to 3 minutes. The syncopal (fainting) responses of the two subjects in Figure 13.1*A* are discussed later in this chapter. Studies of "graded" postural stress, for example the tilting of subjects to different angles, showed that the sine of the tilt angle—which constitutes the gravity force vector—is closely correlated with the degree of migration of thoracic blood. These studies also showed that the percentage of thoracic blood volume loss is the best index of the degree of postural stress.

Thus, free standing, headup tilt (to an angle of 70° more), or lower body negative pressure will reduce thoracic blood volume by about one-third and reduce central venous pressure levels of 4 to 6 mm Hg to about 0 to 2 mm Hg. Although the blood remains within the circulatory system, it is sequestered in the lower body and so long as the subject is upright, the blood is not available to the heart and circulation. As discussed in Chapter 7, these reductions in thoracic blood volume and central venous pressure will result in substantial decreases in venous return, cardiac filling pressure, and cardiac output.

In healthy, younger adults there is rapid circulatory compensation for these deficiencies and frequent postural changes are effortless and entirely asymptomatic. However, in many subjects who are elderly or on autonomic blocking medication, and in certain patients with cardiovascular or autonomic disturbances, postural intolerance may develop, as discussed later in this chapter.

Compensatory Responses to Postural Changes

Among the circulatory adaptations to postural change, the most important are those of the autonomic reflexes and the skeletal muscle pump. As the central blood volume and cardiac output decrease and the arterial pressure begins to fall, there is a strong vasoconstriction, particularly of the splanchnic, renal, and skeletal muscle beds, with a consequent net rise in total peripheral resistance. The increases in resistance (about 40%) and in heart rate (about 20%) not only maintain but increase the diastolic and mean arterial pressure (about 10%). Systolic pressure shows little or no change.

Representative circulatory responses of healthy young adults to the upright posture are shown in Figure 13.2. Although the blood pressure and heart rate changes are fairly consistent among normal individuals of similar age, other parameters show variations. For example, in some cases blood pressure is maintained with only a small decrease in cardiac output and a modest increase in peripheral resistance. In other subjects there is a greater fall in stroke volume and cardiac output and a larger rise in peripheral resistance. The significance of such variations is not known at present.

With prolonged standing, renal vasoconstriction leads to a progressive decrease in renal blood flow. In the upright posture there is also a 20% decrease in cerebral blood flow and, for reasons that are not clear, a hyperventilation, with a tendency toward hypocapnia. This combination of factors undoubtedly contributes to the 5 to 10% fainting rate usually encountered during prolonged postural tests. Cerebrospinal fluid protects the brain from excessive postural variations in blood flow as discussed in the section on hydrostatic factors and cerebral blood flow (Chapter 11).

Several neurohormonal systems are activated in the upright posture or during lower body negative pressure (LBNP). There are rapid and significant increases in plasma catecholamine levels with a 60 to 80% increase in norepinephrine and a 20 to 30% increase in epinephrine. In addition there is activation of the renin-angiotensin system and arginine vasopressin (AVP) (especially during presyncope or syncope) and decreased activation of atrial natriuretic factor (ANF). In general, neurohormones seem to play only a minor role in the rapid hemodynamic adjustment to the upright posture.

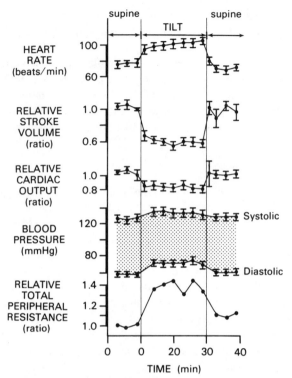

Figure 13.2. Response of normal young men to a 20-minute head-up tilt, showing means and standard error of means. Note the prompt increase in heart rate, vascular resistance, and diastolic pressure and the decrease in stroke volume, cardiac output, and pulse pressure. (Reprinted with permission from J.J. Smith, J.E. Bush, V.T. Wiedmeier, and F.E. Tristani, *J Appl Physiol* 29:133, 1970.)

However, AVP, ANF, and other hormones are undoubtedly important in the long-term effort to maintain plasma volume.

Mechanism of Circulatory Response to Upright Posture

The cardiac and peripheral resistance changes are due to the autonomic reflex responses of the arterial and cardiopulmonary baroceptors. Curiously enough, venoconstriction is transient and limited. Recent evidence suggests that the human arterial baroceptor reflexes play the major role in the cardiac responses, while the cardiopulmonary reflexes are more important in controlling peripheral resistance.

There is strong evidence that in the upright posture, the skeletal muscle pump (SMP) is a vital factor in assisting venous return. During walking and running the importance of the SMP is unquestionable (Fig. 6.7). As discussed at some length in Chapter 6, it is becoming increasingly evident that the SMP also plays a major role in maintaining venous return during quiet standing. The continuous swaying movements of the body, which are characteristic of quiet standing in the human, involve trains of somatic, proprioceptive reflexes that begin at the plantar surfaces of the feet and extend upward to cause alternate waves of contraction and relaxation of the entire antigravity muscle system. These reflexes not only maintain the mechanical stability of the upright body but also are essential as a circulatory muscle pump in maintaining venous return in the upright posture. It is evident that the importance of the SMP in counteracting the orthostatic caudal sequestration of thoracic blood has, in the past, been considerably underestimated.

Reports indicate that in normal young adults, a change from the recumbent to the sitting position will result in diastolic pressure increases of about 90% and heart rate increases of about 55% of those occurring during the change from the recumbent to the upright position. The systolic pressure does not alter significantly in either case.

Abnormal Postural Responses

A number of investigators have reported a 5 to 10% rate of presyncopal symptoms or syncope in normal adults subjected to 20 min or longer of quiet free stand or headup tilt. This fainting rate will be greater upon exposure to high temperature and humidity and in subjects more prone to psychologic stress, as discussed in the fainting section later in this chapter. As shown in Figure 13.1, two subjects who developed presyncopal symptoms during headup tilt showed sharp decreases in thoracic blood volume (increases in transthoracic electrical impedance) coincident with the development of fainting symptoms. The reason for this sudden additional decrease in thoracic blood volume is not known; it has been theorized that it may be due to a sudden fall in systemic venous pressure resulting either from a collapse of arterial pressure (vasovagal syncope) or from abrupt withdrawal of skeletal muscle pump activity.

Postural intolerance develops even in healthy elderly people with increasing frequency after 75 yrs of age, presumably due to diminished skeletal muscle pump action (from deconditioning) or to decreased autonomic responses, or both.

Decreased tolerance to the upright posture will occur if the skeletal muscle pump effect on venous return is inadequate (Chapter 6) or if the baroceptor reflexes (Chapter 10) are interrupted. As described in the section on fainting (in this chapter), loss or diminution of the muscle pump action may result in severe postural intolerance. Partial or complete loss of sympathetic vasoconstrictor responses may occur (*a*) in certain systemic diseases such as diabetes

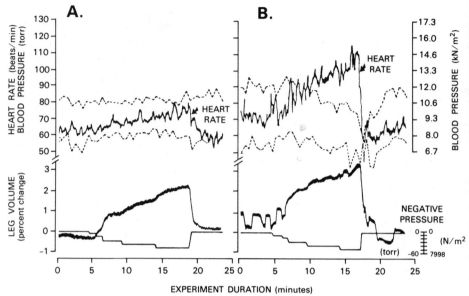

Figure 13.3.   Response of Skylab commander to lower body negative pressure test before (A) and on 20th day (B) of zero gravity. in B there is a greater rise in heart rate and a decrease in blood pressure during LBNP; with the sudden fall in heart rate, fainting was imminent and the test was discontinued. (Reprinted with permission from R.L. Johnson, G.W. Hoffler, A.E. Nicogossian, S.A. Bergman, and M.M. Jackson, *Third Manned Skylab Mission*, NASA Tech Memo TMX 58154, November, 1974.)

or syphilis, (*b*) in primary idiopathic hypotension, or (*c*) after administration of α-adrenergic blocking agents. Such patients, upon standing or being tilted, experience a rapid fall in blood pressure and often faint abruptly without the usual premonitory symptoms of pallor, sweating, and nausea.

Transient postural hypotension will also occur after prolonged bed rest, water immersion of 6 hours or longer, or exposure to the weightless or zero gravity state (Fig. 13.3). The hypotension in these situations has been attributed to the decreased plasma volume (common in these conditions) and to the lessened gravity effect on the arterial baroceptors. The latter explanation seems less likely since gravity changes affect all parts of the body equally, and theoretically should not influence the arterial stretch induced by internal pressure changes.

Cardiac patients with congestive failure may show increased tolerance to postural stress, and head-up tilt often results in an increased stroke volume and cardiac output associated with relief of dyspnea (Fig. 13.4). It has been suggested that this paradoxical effect may be associated with (*a*) a leftward

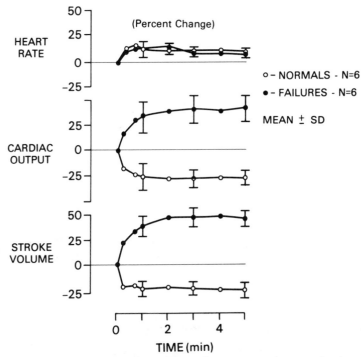

Figure 13.4. Comparison of hemodynamic response of congestive heart failure patients and normal subjects to head-up tilt. In contrast to the normal subjects, note the increased stroke volume and cardiac output in the patients. (Courtesy of Dr. W.V. Judy, University of Indiana.)

shift of the failing heart on the "Starling curve" to relative compensation, permitting an increased stroke volume at lesser filling pressure or (b) increased lung capacity due to caudal migration of thoracic blood. Hypertensive patients may show hemodynamic alterations to head-up tilt depending on the stage of their disease. Early hypertensives tend toward orthostatic hypertension while severe hypertensives may have orthostatic hypotension (Fig. 15.1).

Upon assumption of the upright posture or rapid headup tilt, normal subjects experience an immediate increase in heart rate—a sequence termed the "initial heart rate complex." It is characterized by a sharp 30 to 35% increase in heart rate, which peaks at 13 to 16 sec, then falls rapidly. Since these heart-rate changes are due to autonomic reflexes, this complex is considerably blunted in certain cases of neurological disease. Some clinical investigators have developed postural tests for autonomic neuropathy based on these changes, and (as shown in Fig. 13.5) the initial heart-rate increase is much diminished in diabetic patients with autonomic neuropathy.

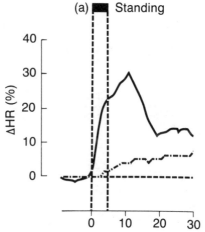

Figure 13.5. "Initial heart rate complex" induced in the first 30 sec of standing. Average changes in five healthy adults (average age 45 years) (−) and five age-matched diabetic patients with cardiac vagal neuropathy (-··-). (After Wieling *et al.*, *Clin Science* 64, 581, 1983.)

Increased Intrathoracic Pressure (the Valsalva Test)

Normal Valsalva Responses

In 1707 the Italian anatomist, Valsalva, described a maneuver in which the subject closes the mouth and nose, expires forcibly, and thereby increases the pressure inside the pharynx and lung passages. The original purpose was to inflate the middle ear *via* the eustachian tubes; today the test is more commonly used as a means of assessing autonomic responsiveness to circulatory changes. By increasing intrathoracic pressure and thereby impeding venous return, cardiac output and arterial pressure are reduced. The resulting hemodynamic strain tests the circulatory system and particularly the integrity of the autonomic circulatory reflexes.

As commonly performed, the subject blows into a mouthpiece (attached to a manometer) against a 40 mm Hg resistance for 15 seconds. There is a sudden rise in intrathoracic, intraabdominal, and cerebrospinal fluid pressure. The peripheral venous valves shut, and the blood, prevented from flowing into the vena cavae, accumulates in the peripheral veins, and venous pressure increases sharply. Central venous pressure rises about 7 mm Hg for each 10 mm Hg increase in mouth pressure. This induces a sharp reduction in venous return, and as a result, aortic flow decreases to about 40 to 50% of control with rapid and profound changes in blood pressure.

The Valvalsa response is classically divided into four phases as illustrated in Figure 13.6. At the start of the strain (phase I) there is a sudden rise in

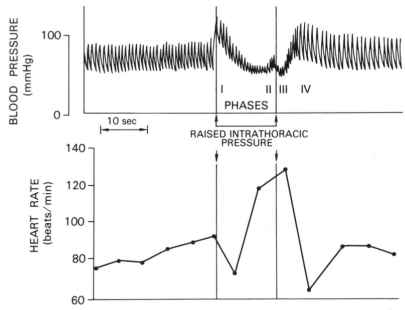

Figure 13.6. Blood pressure and heart rate response to Valsalva test in a normal young adult. Intrathoracic pressure, 40 mm Hg. Note (*top*) the falling arterial pressure and tachycardia in phase II. The highest (phases II and III) and lowest (phases I and IV) heart rates for the respective phases are shown in the bottom figure. The pressure overshoot and bradycardia in phase IV (*top*) and the large heart rate decrement from phases III to IV (*bottom*) indicate functional baroceptor reflexes.

arterial pressure as the heightened intrathoracic pressure is transmitted directly through the aorta to the arterial tree; the heart rate usually shows a small decrease. In phase II there is diminished venous return to the right heart; cardiac filling becomes inadequate, and the mean arterial and pulse pressures begin to fall; then follow a reflex tachycardia and peripheral vasoconstriction, which limit the pressure drop. Mean arterial pressure may actually rise above control at the end of phase II. In phase III, immediately after release, blood pressure drops quickly because of the sudden fall in intrathoracic pressure, and the heart rate increases further. In phase IV, the blood pressure rebounds as a result of the rapid surge of venous return and the ejection of the increased stroke volume into the constricted arterial system. About 5 to 6 seconds after release, the blood pressure overshoots, reflexly inducing a marked bradycardia (Fig. 13.6).

Since heart rate, a noninvasive measurement, is reportedly as valid an autonomic indicator as blood pressure, it may also be used to assess the Valsalva response. In the normal individual, the heart-rate changes, as might

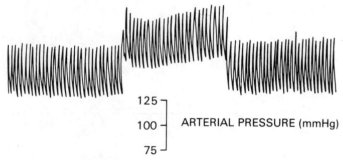

125 ⎤
100 ⎦ ARTERIAL PRESSURE (mmHg)
75 ⎦

Figure 13.7. "Square wave" blood pressure response to the Valsalva test in hypertensive heart failure. There is no change in pulse pressure, no pressure overshoot, and very little change in heart rate. (Reprinted with permission from E.P. Sharpey-Schafer, *Handbook of Physiology*, Section 2: *Circulation*, edited by W.F. Hamilton and P. Dow. Washington, D.C.: American Physiological Society, 1965, Vol III).

be predicted, are roughly opposite to those of the blood pressure as shown in Figure 13.6.

The Valsalva test simulates the type of stress often associated with lifting, pushing, blowing a musical instrument, straining at stool, coughing, etc. The maneuver tests the ability of the circulatory system to cope with a decreasing venous return and a falling arterial pressure and thus is a measure of the integrity of the baroceptor and cardiopulmonary reflexes. In addition to the pronounced arterial constrictor reaction, peripheral venoconstriction is a prompt response, not only to a Valsalva maneuver, but also to a deep breath or to hyperventilation. It has been suggested that the venoconstriction is mediated *via* sympathetic adrenergic fibers; the afferent source is probably in the chest wall, the diaphragm, or in cardiopulmonary mechanoreceptors.

Abnormal Valsalva Responses

Most clinical abnormalities of the Valsalva are due either to (*a*) an increased intrathoracic blood volume, (*b*) interruption of the baroceptor reflex arc, or (*c*) a combination of these two.

Increase in intrathoracic blood volume occurs in congestive heart failure and results in a "square wave" Valsalva response in which there is little or no change in pulse pressure in phases II and III and very little or no overshoot in phase IV (Fig. 13.7). Since the blood pressure changes are diminished, the heart rate alterations are less marked.

The arterial pressure is maintained because (*a*) the increased central blood volume and atrial filling pressure provide a reservoir of venous return which

A.   **B.**

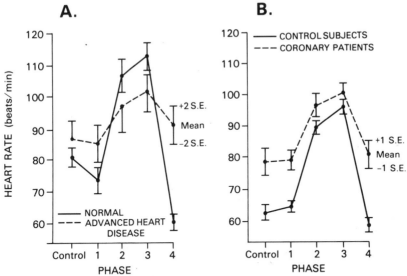

Figure 13.8.   Heart-rate response to Valsalva test (40 mm Hg for 15 sec); A, in congestive heart failure patients (reprinted with permission from E.I. Elisberg, *JAMA* 186:200, 1963); and B, coronary patients not in congestive failure. Note in both cases the "flattened" response compared to control subjects. (Reprinted with permission from F.E. Tristani, D.G. Kamper, D.J. McDermott, B.J. Peters, and J.J. Smith, *Am J Physiol* 233:H694, 1977.)

maintains the cardiac output, and (*b*) the heightened peripheral venous pressure that usually accompanies the increased central blood volume, reduces venous distensibility and helps maintain a higher venous pressure gradient toward the right atrium. As the congestion lessens, the Valsalva response becomes more normal because of the abatement of these factors. In congestive heart failure, because the blood pressure changes are greatly diminished, the heart rate response is also flatter than normal (Fig. 13.8A).

Recent reports have indicated that ambulatory coronary heart disease patients not in congestive failure also have decreased heart-rate responses to the Valsalva test (Fig. 13.8B). This lessened heart-rate response may be due either to a subclinical intrathoracic congestion or to decreased baroreflex responsiveness.

Interruption of the baroreflex arc may occur in other neurological disorders involving the autonomic nervous system, such as primary idiopathic hypotension. In such cases, the Valsalva test will show a continued pressure fall in phase II and no arterial pressure rebound or bradycardia in phase IV because of the failure of vasoconstriction and cardioacceleration (Fig. 13.9). These individuals, as previously mentioned, are also prone to postural hypotension.

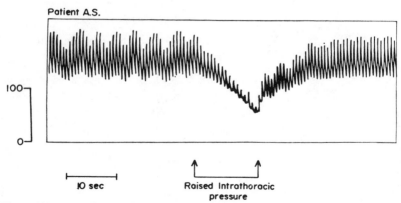

Figure 13.9. Valsalva response in a patient with idiopathic orthostatic hypotension. There is an excessive fall in blood pressure in phase II and an absence of overshoot and bradycardia in phase IV. (Reprinted with permission from R.H. Johnson and J.M.K. Spalding, *Disorders of the Autonomic Nervous System.* London: Blackwell Scientific Publications, 1974.)

Diving (Face Immersion) Response

This unique reflex represents the ultimate defense of the submerged vertebrate against asphyxia, namely, a gross redistribution of the circulation in order to concentrate oxygen in the brain and heart. This remarkable response enables the domestic duck to remain submerged for 15 minutes, the sea lion for 30 minutes, and the whale for 2 hours. Its residual counterpart in man can be activated by diving or by immersion of the face in cold water.

Hemodynamic Changes

The three key elements of the diving response are apnea, an intense vagal bradycardia, and a powerful, extensive peripheral vasoconstriction, most marked in vessels of the muscle, kidneys, skin, and splanchnic areas.

In the duck, hemodynamic changes involve a sudden decrease in cardiac output and heart rate to about 6% of the control values. Except for the coronary and cranial vessels, there is a massive vasoconstriction of the entire arterial tree so that the circulation becomes in effect a heart-brain circuit. The stroke volume and arterial pressure are relatively unchanged. When the animal surfaces, these changes are reversed within seconds, with a large overshoot in cardiac output and heart rate (Fig. 13.10A). The face immersion reflex in man will induce a comparable but less intense response characterized by a quick reduction in heart rate (about 25%), skin blood flow (75%), and muscle flow (50%). Arterial blood pressure increases by about 20% (Fig. 13.10B).

Breath holding alone will cause similar but less marked effects. The brad-

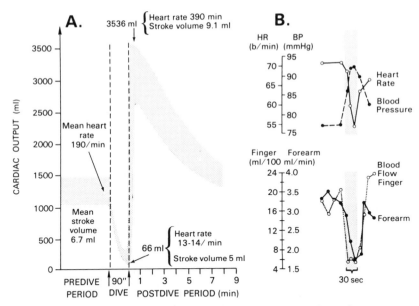

Figure 13.10. Diving and face immersion reflex: *A*, hemodynamic responses to 90-second head submersion in a duck (reprinted with permission from B. Folkow, N.J. Nilsson, and L.R. Younce, *Acta Physiol Scand* 70:347, 1967); *B*, responses to 30-second face immersion in normal male subjects. (Reprinted with permission from D.D. Heistad, F.M. Abboud, and J.W. Eckstein, *J Appl Physiol* 25:542, 1968.) In man the decrease in heart rate and blood flow are of lesser degree.

ycardic effect is greater with cold (rather than cool) water, and an attenuated response can be elicited by dry cold. An unusual feature is that the bradycardic effect of face immersion is increased during physical exercise so that paradoxically, the combination of a tachycardic stimulus (dynamic exercise) and a bradycardic stimulus (diving reflex) may yield a stronger bradycardic tendency than diving alone.

Blix has recently pointed out that when assessing the diving responses of animals, a distinction should be made between "forced submersion" where the animal is threatened, and natural dives, since in the latter case the bradycardia and vasoconstriction are less.

In contrast to the face immersion response, which is activated by cold receptors in the trigeminal area, cold water to other parts of the body causes reflex increases in heart rate and blood pressure. The cold pressor test (Chapter 10), involving immersion of the hand in ice water (0°C), will stimulate pain fibers as well as cold receptors and produce a greater rise in blood pressure and heart rate than cold water (10°C).

Mechanism of Diving Response

In a series of interesting studies, Daly and his colleagues have demonstrated the role of the arterial chemoreceptors in the central modulation of this response. Stimulation of receptors of the face or upper airway initiates the reflex, inhibits the respiratory center (producing the apnea), and elicits vagal bradycardia and generalized vasoconstriction. The apnea leads to hypoxemia and hypercapnia; both of these would ordinarily induce a reflex hyperventilation, sympathetic vasoconstriction (mainly in skeletal muscle), and vagal bradycardia through the action of the arterial chemoreceptors (Chapter 10). It is theorized that during the apnea and the absence of activity of the pulmonary stretch receptors and central inspiratory neurons, the hyperventilation stimulus is suppressed; the cardiovascular limbs of the chemoreceptor reflex are retained and are responsible for the continuation and reinforcement of the existing vasoconstriction and bradycardia.

Due to the massive, generalized increase in peripheral resistance, the arterial pressure is maintained, and in the absence of coronary and cerebral vasoconstriction, the blood is made available to the heart and brain. The importance of the chemoreceptors in maintaining the response is underscored by the fact that experimental withdrawal of chemoreceptor drive by perfusion of the carotid bifurcation region of the seal with normoxic blood during the later stages of the dive results in a reversal of the bradycardia. The integrating center for the diving reflex is not known. A cerebral connection is likely since threatening motions toward a seal will induce the reflex even before immersion.

Clinical Implications

Because of the powerful vagal action, pathological arrhythmias, such as ventricular premature contraction and idioventricular rhythm, as well as T wave inversion, commonly occur after only 30 seconds of diving in man. On the other hand, immersion of the face in a basin of cold water has been used to invoke the vagal effect to advantage in order to terminate supraventricular paroxysmal tachycardia. In certain situations the reflex apnea may be protective against the inhalation of liquids or noxious fumes. Since the response is potent in the newborn, it may serve to protect the fetus at birth.

In clinical cardiovascular studies, the face immersion response is sometimes used as a test for relatively ''pure'' vagal bradycardia. While sympathetic vasoconstriction is simultaneously activated, the bradycardiac effect is relatively immune to other reflex restraints (e.g., by baroceptors or physical exercise). The bradycardiac response decreases linearly with age and reportedly is diminished in coronary patients after myocardial infarction, while sympathetic pressor responses remain intact.

Table 13.1.
Arterial Blood Pressure and Clinical Result of Hemorrhage

Loss of Blood Volume	Mean Arterial Pressure— Immediate Response	Likely Result
5–10%	Little change	Spontaneous recovery
15–20%	80–90 mm Hg	Moderate hypotension, spontaneous recovery
20–30%	60–80 mm Hg	Early shock—usually reversible
30–40%	50–70 mm Hg	Serious shock— irreversible in some cases

Hemorrhage

Circulatory Changes in Hemorrhage

The clinical results of blood loss depend on many factors, but particularly on the rate and degree of bleeding, the age and health of the patient, and the availability of treatment. The blood pressure and general response in an uncomplicated, untreated hemorrhage in a normal adult occurring within a relatively brief period (15 to 30 min) might be roughly estimated as shown in Table 13.1.

The brief description in this section refers mainly to short-term responses to moderate bleeding (less than 30% of blood volume). Protracted hemorrhagic hypotension generally leads to circulatory shock, a quite different pathophysiological entity, which will be discussed in Chapter 15.

The immediate consequences of hemorrhage are (*a*) a decrease in blood volume, (*b*) a fall in venous return and cardiac output, and (*c*) a resultant decline in arterial and venous pressure.

Compensatory Response to Hemorrhage

Within seconds after bleeding begins, the fall in central blood volume and arterial pressure will activate cardiopulmonary and baroceptor reflexes (particularly from the carotid sinuses) and as a result, the sympathoadrenal defense system is fully mobilized. In the case of a relatively small hemorrhage (*e.g.*, a standard phlebotomy of 500 ml), there is a modest rise in peripheral resistance and a small decrease in pulse pressure (Fig. 13.11).

With a greater blood loss and more marked hypotension, the responses will be correspondingly greater. There are two main compensatory changes.

1. *Increase in heart rate and contractility.* Tachycardia does not usually occur, however, in uncomplicated hemorrhage until the blood loss exceeds 700 to 800 ml.

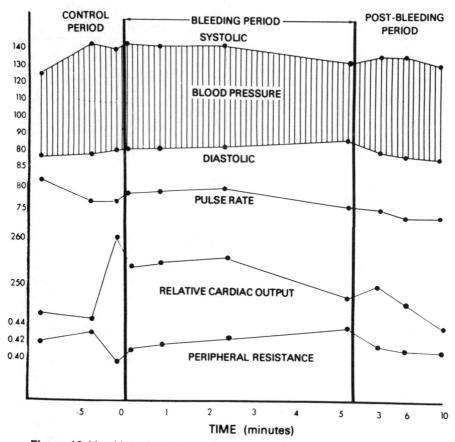

Figure 13.11. Mean hemodynamic response of normal male donors to 540 ml phlebotomy (*n* = 25). Uncomplicated hemorrhage of about 10% of blood volume. Note the preliminary fall in peripheral resistance and rise in cardiac output just after insertion of the needle and before bleeding was begun. Note also the immediate widening of the pulse pressure as the bleeding is stopped. (Reprinted with permission from J.R. Logic, S.A. Johnson, and J.J. Smith, *Transfusion* 3:83, 1963.)

2. *Strong generalized constriction of both resistance and capacitance vessels.* In particular, vessels of skin (producing a marked pallor), splanchnic area (with resulting ischemia of gut and liver), skeletal muscle and kidney are affected. Cerebral and coronary beds are unaffected.

The renal vasoconstriction reduces glomerular filtration leading to oliguria and sometimes to anuria. Venoconstriction is a prominent aspect of the compensatory reaction. For example, in the splanchnic bed, which contains about

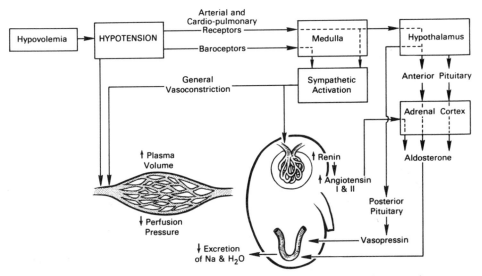

Figure 13.12. Schema of factors tending to restore plasma volume and extracellular fluid during and after hemorrhage. Reduced general capillary pressure and renal vasoconstriction are key elements in maintaining plasma volume; increased vasopressin and aldosterone levels are helpful adjuncts.

20% of the total blood volume, a translocation of even half of this amount to the central veins can provide a significant autotransfusion.

Maintenance of Plasma Volume

Vasoconstriction assists the circulation in two ways: (*a*) by decreasing the circulatory capacity so the remaining blood volume will create a greater venous filling pressure, and (*b*) by lowering the general capillary hydrostatic pressure and thus promoting fluid transfer from tissues to the plasma. Certain hormonal mechanisms are also activated during hemorrhage to help maintain the plasma volume (Fig. 13.12). Renal vasoconstriction reduces glomerular filtration and urine formation; renin and angiotensin production is increased *via* renal ischemia. The decreased atrial stretch causes reflex release of vasopressin (ADH) and (along with other factors) is responsible for the release of aldosterone from the adrenal cortex. These two hormones maximize H_2O and Na^+ reabsorption from renal tubules and help conserve plasma volume.

Other Responses to Hemorrhage

There is a pronounced increase in plasma catecholamines; epinephrine is responsible for the hyperglycemia in hemorrhage, but it is unlikely that any of the circulatory hormones (catecholamines, angiotensin, or vasopressin) contribute significantly to the general vasoconstriction. There is a decrease in RBCs, hematocrit, and plasma protein concentration in blood because of the dilution by the absorbed tissue fluid. After the hemorrhage, the plasma proteins are usually replaced in about 3 to 6 days and the RBCs in about 4 to 6 weeks. Therapy is logically directed at fluid replacement, whole blood if the hematocrit is low, but if not available, plasma or plasma substitutes.

Fainting (Syncope)

Fainting is the loss of consciousness due to cerebral ischemia. Clinically a differentiation is usually made between "organic" and "functional" causes. Among the more common "organic" causes (*i.e.*, those in which an apparent known disease process is involved) are cerebrovascular syncope (usually associated with cerebral arteriosclerosis), orthostatic hypotension (often associated with central or peripheral disorders of the sympathetic nervous system), and cardiac syncope.

The most common causes of cardiac syncope include supraventricular tachycardia, disorders of the His-Purkinje system, Stokes-Adams syndrome (complete heart block, see Chapter 4), carotid sinus hypersensitivity, and intrinsic sinus node dysfunction. Fainting tendencies are also a frequent accompaniment of α-adrenergic blockade, the latter occurring, for example, as a side effect of antihypertensive therapy. As previously mentioned, these patients usually faint abruptly upon standing, without showing the usual preliminary symptoms.

Functional syncope or ordinary fainting (also called vasodepressor or vasovagal syncope) has multiple causes. It may occur in unusually sensitive individuals after a purely psychic stimulation such as emotional shock or the sight of blood. On the other hand, practically everyone will faint during extreme somatic stress such as a 1500-ml phlebotomy or a 30- to 40-minute passive, suspended tilt. However, clinical fainting in the healthy individual is usually due to a combination of stresses; the most common predisposing factor is decreased circulating blood volume induced, for example, by a previous blood withdrawal, excessive physical exercise, diarrhea, protracted bed rest, or prolonged standing in the heat.

Circulatory Responses during Fainting

The usual preliminary symptoms of extreme pallor, nausea, sweating, and abdominal discomfort are sometimes attributed to sympathoadrenal activation but are more likely due to the liberation of vasopressin. These symptoms are usually accompanied by a decreasing systolic and pulse pressure, a rapid heart rate, and decreasing right atrial pressure. At the moment of vascular failure, there is a sudden sharp decrease in mean arterial and pulse pressure, a marked

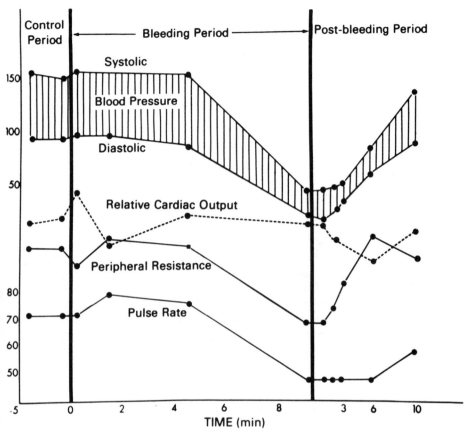

Figure 13.13. Hemodynamic response of blood donor (53-year-old healthy male) to a 580-ml phlebotomy. Toward the end of the bleeding, subject developed pallor, nausea, and abdominal discomfort. Blood pressure just before end of bleeding was 46/25. Note the sharp fall in mean and pulse pressure, peripheral resistance, and heart rate. Cardiac output was maintained. (Reprinted with permission from J.R. Logic, S.A. Johnson, and J.J. Smith, *Transfusion* 3:83, 1963.)

bradycardia, cerebral ischemia, and loss of consciousness—all occurring very rapidly, sometimes within seconds (Fig. 13.13).

The right atrial pressure usually falls further, but cardiac output remains relatively unchanged. The key defect is a powerful vagal stimulation accompanied by a sudden loss of peripheral vascular resistance, primarily in skeletal muscle. The mechanism is probably a massive sympathetic inhibition from the hypothalamic cardioinhibitory center (Chapter 10). Cholinergic vasodilators do not seem to be involved.

Mechanism of Vasodepressor Syncope

While it is generally agreed that the immediate prelude to fainting is cerebral ischemia, there are few data and no agreement on the final common pathway through which the circulatory collapse is brought about. Because of the unusual autoregulatory ability of cerebral vessels, signs of cerebral ischemia usually do not occur until arterial pressures reach very low levels, (*i.e.*, about 40 mm Hg). However, a heightened cerebral arterial tone decreases autoregulatory ability so that cerebral ischemia develops at higher arterial pressures than is usually the case. Two conditions that increase cerebral vascular tone are hypocapnia and hypertension.

Hyperventilation and its resultant hypocapnia commonly occur not only in emotional strain but also during hemorrhage and postural stress. The hypocapnia will, in turn, induce tachycardia and increased cardiac output. However, the most striking effect of hypocapnia is the cerebral vasoconstriction, which can reduce cerebral flow by 40% after only 1 or 2 minutes of active hyperventilation. Although uncomplicated hyperventilation rarely causes syncope in normal subjects, it can be an important contributing factor. Similarly, certain hypertensive patients develop cerebral ischemia at higher than normal levels of arterial pressure and have fainting tendencies in spite of increased arterial perfusion pressures. The cause is not certain, but it is probably due to cerebral arteriosclerosis or decreased autoregulatory capability of cerebral vessels.

For fainting to occur consistently, both hypotension and an adjunct factor are necessary. For example, a moderate hemorrhage (10% of blood volume), a Valsalva maneuver, or prolonged standing will all cause a decrease in cardiac output and a modest hypotension, but none will by itself ordinarily produce fainting. However, in all of them, a fainting tendency may be precipitated by an unnoticed hyperventilation.

While practically all individuals have one or two fainting episodes in their lifetime, there is a small but consistent fraction of the adult population, without apparent organic disease, which is prone to repeated fainting episodes. About 5% of blood donors, for example, have such fainting tendencies. Reports indicate that such "fainters," compared to control subjects, experience a greater fall in arterial pressure and a greater decrease in alveolar P_{CO_2} to a standard 500-ml phlebotomy. Psychological tests further showed that the fainters also had a greater tendency toward hypochondriasis and depression than did control subjects. Such studies suggest an interrelationship between psychic factors and hemodynamic response to stress which might account for the tendency toward circulatory collapse in these individuals. As described in Chapter 10, such psychogenic fainting may involve the depressor area of the hypothalamus.

Suggested Readings

Angell-James JE and Daly M deB. The diving response: some possible clinical implications. In: *Advances in Psychological Sciences*, Vol. 20: *Advances in Animal and Comparative Physiology*, edited by G Pethes and VL Frenyo. Oxford: Pergamon Press, 1981, pp 277–284.

Blix AS. Diving responses: fact or fiction. *NIPS* 2:64, 1987.

Blomqvist CG and Stone HL. Cardiovascular adjustments to gravitational stress. In *Handbook of Physiology*, Section 2, *The Cardiovascular System*, edited by JT Shepherd, FM Abboud, and SR Geiger. Bethesda, Md: *American Physiological Society*, 1025, 1982.

Fox IJ, Crowley WP, Grace JB, and Wood EH. Effects of the Valsalva maneuver on blood flow in the thoracic aorta in man. *J Appl Physiol* 21:1553–1560, 1966.

Frey MAB and Kenney RA. Changes in left ventricular activity during apnea and face immersion. *Undersea Biomed Res* 4:27, 1977.

Gauer ON and Thron HL. Postural change in the circulation. In: *Handbook of Physiology*, Section 2: *Circulation*, edited by WF Hamiton and P Dow. Washington, D.C.: American Physiological Society, 1965, Vol. III, pp 2409–2440.

Heistad DD, Abboud FM, and Eckstein JW. Vasoconstrictor response to simulated diving in man. *J Appl Physiol* 25:542–549, 1968.

Klein LJ, Saltzman HS, Heyman A, and Sicker HO. Syncope induced by the Valsalva maneuver. *Am J Med* 37:263–268, 1964.

Korner PI, Tonkin AM, and Uther JB. Reflex and mechanical circulatory effects of graded Valsalva maneuvers in normal man. *J Appl Physiol* 40:434–440, 1976.

Logic JR, Johnson SA, and Smith JJ. Cardiovascular and hematologic responses to phlebotomy in blood donors. *Transfusion* 3:83–93, 1963.

McHenry LC, Fazekas JF, and Sullivan JF. Cerebral hemodynamics of snycope. *Am J Med Sci* 241:173, 1961.

Porth CJ, Bamrah VS, Tristani FE, and Smith JJ. The Valsalva maneuver: mechanisms and clinical implications. *Heart Lung* 13:507–518, 1984.

Rowell LD. *Human Circulation during Physical Stress*. London: Oxford University Press, 1986.

Ruetz PD, Johnson SA, Callahan R, Meade RE, and Smith JJ. Fainting: a review of the mechanisms and a study in blood donors. *Medicine* 46:363–384, 1967.

Ryan C, Hollenberg M, Harvey DB, and Gwynn R. Impaired parasympathetic responses in patients after myocardial infarction. *Am J Cardiol* 37:1013–1018, 1976.

Sharpey-Schafer EP. Effect of respiratory acts on the circulation. In: *Handbook of Physiology*, Section 2: *Circulation*, edited by WF Hamilton and P Dow. Washington, D.C.: American Physiological Society, 1965, Vol. III, pp. 1875–1886.

Shepherd JT and Mancia G. Reflex control of the human cardiovascular system. *Rev Physiol Biochem Pharm* 105:1, 1986.

Smith JJ, Bonin ML, Wiedmeier VT, Kalbfleisch JH, and McDermott DJ. Cardiovascular response of young men to diverse stresses. *Aerospace Med* 45:583–590, 1974.

Smith JJ, Bush JE, Wiedmeier VT, Tristani FE. Application of impedance cardiography to the study of postural stress in the human. *J Appl Physiol* 29:133–137, 1970.

Smith JJ and Ebert TJ. General response to orthostatic stress. In, *Circulatory Response to the Upright Posture*, edited by JJ Smith. Boca Raton, Fla: CRC Press, (In Press).

Smith JJ and Porth CJM. Age and response to orthostatic stress. In, *Circulatory Response to the Upright Posture*, edited by JJ Smith. Boca Raton, Fla: CRC Press, (In Press).

Tristani FE, Kamper DG, McDermott DJ, Peters BJ, and Smith JJ. Alteration of postural and Valsalva responses in coronary heart disease. *Am J Physiol* 233:H694–699, 1977.

chapter 14

Pathophysiology: Ischemic Heart Disease and Congestive Heart Failure

Circulatory Pathophysiology—General

The next two chapters are intended to show in a limited sense how disease may alter physiology and how the disordered state often helps us to better understand the normal. An understanding of pathophysiology often requires basic investigation as well as observation of the patient. Dr. Carl J. Wiggers, one of our truly great cardiovascular physiologists, was fond of saying that the mistakes of nature (*i.e.*, disease) can best be solved by shuttling the problems back and forth between the clinic and the experimental laboratory. In these chapters, in which we present capsule descriptions of four of the more common cardiovascular diseases, we have, therefore, also included accounts of basic studies and animal experiments insofar as they relate to the disease process.

In the following discussions of pathophysiology, the term *anoxia* refers to a complete absence of an oxygen supply, local or general. *Hypoxia* denotes a state of reduced oxygen supply. *Ischemia* is a condition of reduced perfusion of blood, local or general. Hypoxia (or anoxia) is classically subdivided into four types: hypoxic, anemic, stagnant, and histotoxic.

Hypoxic hypoxia is a condition in which there is a reduction of the P_{O_2} of arterial blood. This may be caused by an inadequate partial pressure of oxygen in inspired air (*e.g.*, by ascent to altitude), by hypoventilation, or by lung disease in which there is an inadequate transfer of oxygen from the alveoli to the pulmonary capillary blood. *Anemic hypoxia* is the result of an inadequate amount of hemoglobin to carry the oxygen (*i.e.*, a reduced oxygen carrying capacity), such as may occur in anemia or carbon monoxide poisoning. *Stagnant hypoxia* is a condition in which blood flow is so diminished that insufficient oxygen is delivered to the tissues despite a normal blood P_{O_2} and normal hemoglobin concentration. This commonly occurs in low-flow states such as circulatory shock or congestive heart failure.

In *histotoxic hypoxia*, both the oxygen carrying capacity of blood and tissue perfusion are adequate, but the oxygen is denied to the cells because of a toxic agent. This may occur as a result of cyanide poisoning in which cellular hypoxia is produced through paralysis of the electron transfer function of cytochrome oxidase. *Cyanosis* is a bluish discoloration of the tissues due to reduced hemoglobin. The discoloration becomes evident particularly in the nail beds of the fingers, in the lips, and in the mucous membranes when the blood concentration of reduced hemoglobin exceeds 5 g/dl. It commonly accompanies states of severe heart failure and advanced lung disease.

Asphyxia is a simultaneous decrease in P_{O_2} (hypoxic hypoxia) with an increase in P_{CO_2} (hypercapnia) of the blood produced by a restriction or cessation of respiratory ventilation. With acute, complete asphyxia, there follows in sequence and within a matter of minutes unconsciousness, failure of the respiratory center with respiratory arrest, failure of the vasomotor center with a consequent fall in arterial pressure, and finally, ventricular ischemia and fibrillation. While pure hypoxia is usually painless and may even induce euphoria (*e.g.*, in high altitude flying), asphyxia, because of the associated hypercapnia, usually evokes extreme discomfort and panic.

Ischemic Heart Disease (IHD)

Epidemiology—Risk Factors and Diagnosis

Since not all coronary artery disease results in cardiac ischemia and since cardiac ischemia can result from noncoronary diseases, ischemic heart disease (IHD) is the preferable term to designate changes occurring in the myocardium from reduction of blood flow (ischemia) or reduction of oxygen supply (hypoxia). Beginning in 1968, the annual mortality from coronary heart disease has shown a progressive and modest decline for reasons that are not yet certain. However, in spite of this decline, IHD is the leading single cause of mortality in the western world and in the United States alone accounts for over 600,000 deaths annually. Obviously, it is a clinical and social problem of the highest magnitude. It primarily affects males in their forties or older. Unfortunately, the disease is usually "silent" in the sense that symptoms appear late, and early diagnosis is at present very difficult.

IHD's insidious nature is illustrated by the fact that approximately two-thirds of coronary deaths occur outside the hospital, usually without preceding symptoms and with little or no warning. The great majority of these acute deaths are precipitated by ventricular fibrillation, and at autopsy over three-fourths of the victims show advanced coronary disease. Curiously, only a minority of these patients appeared to have their ventricular fibrillation as a consequence of acute myocardial infarction, and most did not have antecedent chest pain. The instigation of disordered impulse conduction by aberrant autonomic reflexes has been suggested as a mechanism in these cases. The cardiac "sudden death" syndrome is currently the subject of intensive clinical investigation. The increasing therapeutic capabilities, which could now be applied if the existence of the disease were known, make it abundantly clear that one of the great deficiencies in modern preventive medicine is the lack of an adequate method for the early diagnosis of ischemic heart disease.

The primary factor contributing to IHD is coronary arteriosclerosis, a general term for thickening and hardening of the arterial wall. Atherosclerosis, the most prevalent type of arteriosclerosis, is the basic lesion, not only in coronary heart disease but also in cerebrovascular disease and most renal and peripheral vascular diseases. Atherosclerosis apparently begins with the deposition of cholesterol beneath the arterial intima. Why the process accelerates in IHD is not certain, but it appears to be related to hyperlipidemia, (i.e., increased triglyceride and low density lipoprotein, but most importantly, increased cholesterol levels of plasma). The tendency of hyperlipidemic subjects to coronary disease is illustrated in Figure 14.1.

Hypercholesteremia, increased low-density lipoprotein levels, hypertension, and cigarette smoking have been established as major risk factors in coronary artery disease. Increased plasma levels of high-density lipoproteins reportedly exert a protective effect on coronary artery disease. In addition to

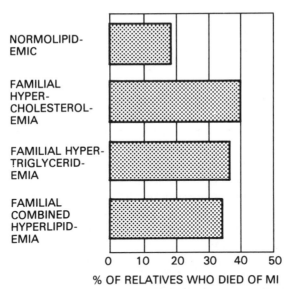

0   10   20   30   40   50

% OF RELATIVES WHO DIED OF MI

Figure 14.1. Predisposition of familial hyperlipidemic subjects to myocardial infarct (MI). MI death rates in adult, first degree relatives of hyperlipidemic MI patients were twice as high as relatives of normolipidemic patients. (Reprinted with permission from J.L. Goldstein, *The Myocardium: Failure and Infarction.* New York: HP Publishing Co., 1974.)

these major factors, diabetes mellitus, obesity, physical inactivity, and a positive family history of atherosclerosis are contributing risk factors for IHD.

Recently, emotional stress has been added to this select group, specifically a hyperactive behavior pattern termed "type A." Studies have shown that aggressive, competitive, impatient and sometimes hostile "time-fighters" may be statistically twice as apt to develop heart problems as are more passive individuals. It is believed that the common pathophysiological denominator in these individuals is catecholamine overdrive. Although catechol levels at rest or during sleep are not distinctive, type A individuals reportedly exhibit a much greater increase in arterial pressure and plasma catechols than do type B individuals in competitive or harassing situations. Present studies suggest that hostility and anger (rather than impatience and aggression) are the more significant coronary-prone characteristics.

Of the many recent developments in cardiovascular research, none is more important than the clear demonstration that different cultural patterns, lifestyles, and personal characteristics carry different degrees of risk of eventual heart attack or stroke.

Only when the arteriosclerotic process has progressed sufficiently to produce at least a 70% luminal narrowing of one or more of the three primary coronary arteries (or one of their larger branches) is the disease apt to manifest symptoms. Two of the most common clinical manifestations of ischemic heart disease are angina pectoris and myocardial infarction. Both are characterized by precordial chest pains, which may radiate to the left shoulder, arm and back. During periods of angina, the ECG may show S-T and T wave changes and in myocardial infarction, abnormal Q waves.

Recent studies in healthy elderly subjects have shown that the cardiovascular pathophysiology as well as circulatory responses to certain stresses are similar to those of coronary patients. Thus it is not always possible in ambulatory patients with mild to moderate symptoms to determine whether the cardiovascular changes are due to coronary artery disease or aging *per se*. Physiological changes due to age are further discussed in Chapter 12.

The diagnosis of IHD is generally made on the basis of a history of angina or myocardial infarction and is confirmed by noninvasive studies such as ECG, exercise stress tests, nuclear and ultrasonic imaging techniques and invasive procedures such as cardiac catheterization and angiography. Angiography involves the injection of radioopaque dye into the cardiac chambers (ventriculography) and the coronary arteries (arteriography) with the subsequent filming of the fluoroscopy for later review. From ventriculograms are determined end-diastolic volume (EDV), end-systolic volume (ESV), ejection fraction (EF), and, very importantly, any defects in ventricular wall motion such as akinesia (defective contraction) or asynergy (nonuniform contraction). These defects might indicate ischemia or a previous infarction. The arteriography allows visualization of the obstructive lesions. The diagnostic approach is tailored to the needs of the individual patient.

Angina Pectoris

Angina pectoris is a condition featured by attacks of sudden substernal discomfort or pain that may be described as "dull" or "burning" or as a "tightness." It may last several minutes and is the result of a transient, reversible, myocardial ischemia. The chest pain—sometimes severe—is associated with a temporary reduction of cardiac output, stroke volume, and ventricular contractility. It may be accompanied by dyspnea (shortness of breath) or other signs of early heart failure. Angina pectoris is the result of a temporary disparity between myocardial oxygen demand and supply and is classically associated with the clinical sequence of "exertion-pain" and "rest-relief." Prompt cessation of the pain usually follows administration of nitrites.

Angina may be induced by exertion, emotional stress, cold, isometric exercise, or by a meal. However, in some patients the attack may develop without any evident prior physical or emotional strain or other apparent inciting cause. Patients with angina may remain "stable" for many years with only an occasional attack; on the other hand the condition may become progressive, so that the attacks will become increasingly severe. While most angina patients have evidence of narrowing of the coronary arteries, a small percentage have, on angiography, anatomically normal coronary arteries.

In such cases, two possibilities exist. The first is that coronary arterial spasm is responsible for the myocardial ischemia. One form of this condition is "Prinzmetal's angina" in which arterial vasospasm may (but not necessarily) be superimposed on atherosclerotic coronary disease. In this variant, the patients develop chest pains at rest rather than during exertion and S-T segment elevation is more common than S-T depression. A second possible explanation of the occurrence of angina without apparent narrowing of coronary arteries is that the patient may have disease of the smaller vessels which are difficult to visualize. In any event, angina pectoris patients are more prone than normal subjects to an eventual myocardial infarct.

Myocardial Infarction

Pathogenesis

MI is a sudden, irreversible, ischemic injury due to coronary arterial narrowing or occlusion with sustained damage to a segment of the myocardium. Like angina, MI is primarily the result of an imbalance between a myocardial O_2 demand too great for the coronary artery to supply.

MI is associated with electrocardiographic, metabolic, and hemodynamic changes that depend on the size and location of the ischemic area. If the SA or AV nodes or a vital part of the conduction apparatus is affected, bradycardia, arrhythmia, or conduction defects such as AV block may result. If as much as 20 or 25% of the left ventricular mass ceases to contract, there is usually hemodynamic evidence of left ventricular failure. Involvement of 40% or more results in severe pump failure with cardiogenic shock or death.

It is thought that complete obstruction is initiated at the damaged inner surface of an already partially occluded vessel, probably by rupture of the subendothelial plaque, subsequent fibrin deposition, and finally thrombus formation. The exact sequence of events however is not certain, and some investigators believe that the thrombosis actually occurs after the infarct rather than preceding it.

Metabolic Changes in MI

Myocardium is dependent on aerobic metabolism for sufficient energy in the form of ATP to provide for the continuous contraction of the heart. As previously mentioned (Chapters 1 and 5), the myocardium contains very little reserve high-energy phosphate (HEP). ATP, together with creatine phosphate and adenosine diphosphate, supplies only enough to support about a minute of left ventricular contractile activity. This extraordinary dependence of myocardium on aerobic or mitochondrial metabolism is reflected in the fact that about 30% of the volume of a normal left ventricular myocyte is occupied by mitochondria. Glucose and amino and fatty acids can be oxidized to CO_2 and water with equal facility and yield large quantities of HEP. However, when substrates are equally available to the heart, fatty acids are preferentially oxidized and are the dominant mitochondrial substrate. The entry of glucose—the next most common substance—into the cell is facilitated by insulin. Amino acids are only a minor energy source.

Experimental studies have shown that if oxygen is cut off or perfusion is stopped in an isolated ventricle or working heart, depression of myocardial contractility begins within 15 seconds. Tissue Po_2 decreases, and when it falls below 5 mm Hg, HEP concentration (mainly creatine phosphate) decreases and myocardial energy metabolism promptly shifts to anaerobic glycolysis. The metabolic and functional consequences of this transition occur within seconds of the onset of the oxygen deficiency. Anaerobic glycolysis generates lactate at a high rate of speed during the first minute of ischemia, but the rate then quickly slows. The slowed rate is unable to provide enough HEP. If the ischemia is prolonged, the tissue ATP in the affected zones is reduced to a low level, and when anaerobic glycolysis ceases, the process becomes irreversible and myocyte death occurs. At this time, electron microscopy reveals intracellular edema and swelling of sarcoplasmic reticulum and mitochondria. While these metabolic and ultrastructural changes occur quite rapidly during the first few minutes, they progress relatively little during the next 10 to 24 hours. After the death of the myocytes there is phagocytosis, gradual removal of the dead fragments, and replacement with connective tissue, a process that takes about 30 to 40 days for completion.

Ischemia and hypoxia produce very different biochemical and pathological effects. During ischemia, the acid products of glycolysis are not washed out, lactic acid concentration rises, intracellular pH falls quickly, and the necrobiotic process is more rapid. Both oxidative metabolic and anaerobic production of ATP are diminished, and eventually glycolysis is inhibited and lactate production falls off. This lower glycolytic flux probably results from the acidotic inhibition of phosphofructokinase (PFK), a key enzyme in the glycolytic chain. Upon sudden experimental occlusion of a major coronary artery in the dog, a transmural gradient of ischemia results. Residual collateral flows are very low in the inner myocardium but are considerably greater in the outer layer. As might be expected, there are also lateral zones of tissue damage. Although the entire ischemic tissue is acontractile and may exhibit electrical abnormalities, cell death occurs quickly in inner zones of severe ischemia, more slowly in zones of moderate ischemia, and often does not develop at all in zones of mild ischemia. The result depends primarily on the collateral circulation.

The critical objective in clinical treatment is to limit the severely ischemic zone and salvage as much as possible of the border zones. Studies in experimental animals have suggested that the transition from reversible to irreversible ischemic injury occurs within 20 to 40 minutes after coronary occlusion. While this time limit is not certain, at least in the human heart, and obviously depends on the degree of cellular hypoxia, it appears very likely that significant salvage can only be achieved within the first few hours. Such studies have provided the basis for the occasional application of certain invasive treatment methods such as coronary artery bypass surgery, intracoronary infusion of fibrinolytic enzyme preparations, or PCTA (described later), shortly after acute myocardial infarction.

Myocardial Enzymes

Normally lactate is taken up by the heart and oxidized so that the coronary arterial concentration exceeds the coronary venous concentration. With the acceleration of glycolysis in hypoxia and ischemia, this lactate gradient is reversed. Furthermore, when MI occurs, the damaged cells become permeable to macromolecules, so that large molecular weight proteins and enzymes escape from their normal intracellular location and enter the circulation through either venous drainage or cardiac lymphatics. Consequently, there is an increased output of lactate as well as a release of certain enzymes such as glutamic oxaloacetic transaminase (SGOT), lactic dehydrogenase (LDH), and creatine kinase (CK) from the infarcted myocardium. Elevated serum levels and the time-concentration course of these enzymes (or their isoenzymes) are diagnostically useful in MI. The tests are sensitive but not specific and the false positive rate may be as high as 15%.

Effect on Ventricular Contractility

As mentioned in Chapter 11, the greater net perfusion pressure to epicardial coronary vessels is generally offset by the greater metabolic vasodilation (autoregulation) in the subendocardial vessels. In the presence of restricted coronary blood flow and hypotension, coronary autoregulation declines, and the subendocardium is further underperfused so that necrosis of subendocardium is much more common than that of the subepicardium. Thus, after coronary occlusion, contractility of the epicardium is better preserved than the endocardium, apparently as a manifestation of this preferential perfusion of the outer wall.

After severe hypoxia or ischemia, the deterioration of myocardial function is abrupt and profound. In the early ischemic state, this functional decline occurs while high-energy phosphate is still present in adequate amounts, so the latter does not appear to be the critical initiating factor. The metabolic, electrical and contractile activities cease as necrosis develops, and the myocardial changes are generally permanent with eventual scar formation. The

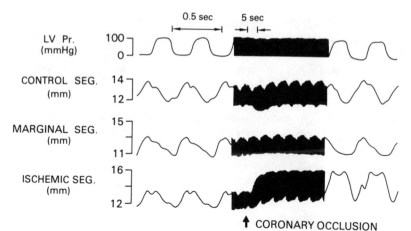

Figure 14.2. Regional responses of canine myocardium to experimental coronary occlusion. Occlusion was produced at the arrow; the degree of shortening (or lengthening) of muscle is indicated in the bottom three tracings. Within 15 seconds after occlusion, the ischemic segment bulged and remained expanded both in systole and diastole. The marginal segment showed some increase in end-diastolic length and decrease in systolic shortening. The control non-ischemic segment shows an initial increased shortening with a later increase in end-diastolic length and degree of shortening, a compensatory response of the uninvolved muscle. The left ventricular pressure (*top*) remained unchanged. (Reprinted with permission from P. Theroux, D. Franklin, J. Ross, Jr., and W.S. Kemper , *Circ Res* 35:896, 1974.)

critical factors in the prognosis are the size of the infarct, the ability to limit its spread, the general condition of the heart, and the assistance that can be rendered to the uninvolved myocardium.

Experimental ischemia of cardiac muscle usually results in a decrease or loss of contractile power with reduced contraction in the adjacent or marginal zones. In the uninvolved areas there are increased systolic, diastolic, and stroke volume excursions as these segments assume a greater share of the contractile burden (Fig. 14.2).

If more than about 25% of myocardial mass is involved, there is usually a decrease in left ventricular stroke volume, stroke work, and V_{max}. There is also an increase in ventricular EDV and EDP and a decrease in ventricular EF. With the loss of contractile power, the center of the ischemic zone may become immobile and, at first, bulges passively during ventricular systole, thus exhibiting "paradoxical" motion or dyskinesis.

However, shortly after the coronary occlusion, cellular swelling, edema, and fibrocellular infiltration take place so that now the infarcted, noncontracting myocardial segment becomes stiff and contributes to the rise in EDP.

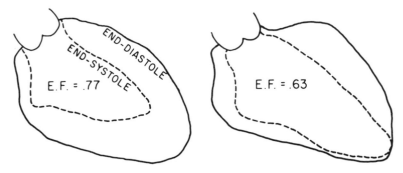

Figure 14.3. Left ventricular angiograms showing normal contraction pattern (*left*) and impaired contraction (*right*) because of hypokinesis of apical inferior area, with a fall in ejection fraction (EF). (Reprinted with permission from E.A. Amsterdam, R.R. Miller, D.H. Foley, and D.T. Mason, *Peripheral Circulation*, edited by R. Zelis. New York: Grune & Stratton, 1975.)

These changes may produce abnormalities in cardiac sounds and ventricular wall motion; accentuated presystolic sounds and large "a" waves become evident on the phonocardiogram and on the apex cardiogram. Because a part of the myocardium is not functioning, asynergy of the ventricular muscle may appear on the ventriculogram (Fig. 14.3).

At a later time in the postinfarct period, the systolic tension generated by the contracting myocardium may possibly stretch and eventually disrupt and weaken the tissue of the noncontracting segment with accentuated bulging during systole and aneurysm formation. In accord with Laplace's law (Chapter 1), the wall stress at these bulging sites will increase progressively and may further enlarge the ishemic zone.

Hemodynamic Response to MI: Autonomic Effects

The result of a myocardial infarct on systemic hemodynamics is not always predictable; sometimes a systemic pressor and sometimes a depressor response results. Randall and others have pointed out that this variability may be due to cardiopulmonary baroceptors and specifically to the cardiocardiac reflexes that are important in self-regulation of the heart. The role of the autonomic nervous system in determining the result of MI is indicated by the fact that experimental coronary occlusion in dogs after cardiac denervation resulted in a near zero incidence of ventricular ectopic activity and fibrillation and a reduced infarct size compared to normally innervated animals.

Upon coronary occlusion in experimental animals, there follows within 30 to 60 seconds bradycardia and frequently arrhythmia, efferent sympathetic inhibition with hypotension, and a prolonged renal vasodilation with inhibition of secretion of renin and ADH. This response is due to ischemia and bulging of the infarcted myocardial wall with a resultant chemical and mechanical stimulation of the ventricular sensory receptors whose fibers travel in the vagus nerve. Vagotomy will abolish the response (Chapter 10, Ventricular Receptors). Ischemia of the inferoposterior myocardium will produce a more pronounced cardioinhibitory and vasodepressor response than a comparable anterior myocardial ischemia, perhaps because of a denser population of these receptor endings in the inferoposterior cardiac region. Clinical studies have shown that bradyarrhythmias are seen more often in posterior than in anterior infarcts, suggesting that a comparable reflex mechanism exists in the human. This inhibitory reflex overrides that of the arterial baroceptors, which would be expected to induce a strong sympathetic stimulation in response to the reduced cardiac output and decreased arterial pressure that occur after coronary occlusion.

As mentioned in Chapter 10, there are chemosensitive endings not only in the ventricles but also in the atria and lungs which can be activated by veratrine, nicotine, and other chemicals. Such activation will induce brady-cardic and cardioinhibitory responses similar to those induced by ventricular mechanoceptors.

Afferent *sympathetic* fibers in the ventricles will also be stimulated fol-lowing coronary occlusion, but their precise role is less clear. They may be important in the generation of some cardiac arrhythmias, in the induction of cardiac pain, and perhaps in some cases in causing the tachycardic and hy-pertensive response sometimes seen in MI.

Patients who have recovered from MI or who have chronic angina pectoris have shown altered circulatory responses to certain autonomic stresses. Recent reports have indicated that in such patients there was a lesser heart rate slowing during phase IV of the Valsalva maneuver and a lesser vasoconstrictor re-sponse to upright tilt with a greater decline in systolic pressure. It is suspected that such changes in sympathetic and parasympathetic responses may be due to a decrease in the sensitivity of arterial or cardiopulmonary baroceptors; however, the underlying cause is not known. Investigations are currently underway to explore the possibility that these altered autonomic reflexes may be useful as adjunctive tests for the diagnosis and characterization of IHD.

Treatment of IHD

The general term, IHD, includes a wide spectrum of disease entities such as stable angina, MI, sudden death, and congestive heart failure. Obviously, the therapy will be tailored to the needs of the individual patient. The following is intended to be only an outline of some physiological principles in the treatment of IHD and not a treatise on clinical management. The immediate treatment objectives are (*a*) to relieve symptoms, (*b*) to detect and promptly treat any life-threatening complications such as arrhythmia or shock, and (*c*) to limit infarct size by reducing myocardial O_2 demand and increasing the supply. It has become standard practice to admit patients with acute MI into a coronary care unit (CCU) for close ECG and hemodynamic monitoring. The general objective in treating all coronary patients is to reduce the myocardial O_2 demand (MVO_2) and increase coronary blood flow.

As previously described (Chapter 5), the main work of the heart is expended in pressure energy, which is used to eject the stroke volume against the aortic afterload. Since aortic pressure is a key component of aortic impedance or afterload, an effective way to reduce cardiac work, and therefore myocardial oxygen demand, is through a reduction in mean arterial pressure consistent with maintenance of an adequate coronary perfusion pressure. An increase in myocardial oxygen supply must be achieved mainly by increasing coronary flow since myocardial oxygen extraction is normally at a high level. Since the pressure-rate (double) product is a close correlate of myocardial $\dot{V}o_2$ demand (Chapter 5), it is a useful clinical measure of cardiac work requirements.

Nitrates and Nitrites

Nitrates and nitrites (*e.g.*, nitroglycerin) are widely used to relieve anginal attacks by reducing venous tone and peripheral resistance and thereby lowering preload and afterload as indicated by aortic pressure. This, in turn, reduces myocardial O_2 requirements. The resulting decrease in left ventricular end-diastolic volume and myocardial tension override the disadvantages of the slight tachycardia and increased cardiac contractility, which result from the baroceptor response to the mild induced hypotension. The direct coronary dilator action of these agents is a secondary and less important one compared to the above effects.

β-Adrenergic Blockade

β-adrenergic blockade as induced, for example, by propranolol or timolol, improves survival from infarctions and exerts a beneficial effect by minimizing the increase in heart rate and myocardial contractility which may occur during stress. Its effectiveness in IHD is indicated by the fact that many patients receiving this drug will release less myocardial lactate during activity. This medication, however, is contraindicated in heart failure, since it would deprive the myocardium of the compensatory sympathetic stimulation that is a support of the weakened muscle in failure. Since it also decreases the atrial-ventricular conduction rate, it is also contraindicated in patients who have some conduction abnormalities (*e.g.*, heart block).

Calcium Channel Blocking Drugs

The slow-channel inhibitors (calcium antagonists) are important aids in the treatment of heart disease. Studies thus far indicate that agents such as verapamil, nifedipine, or diltiazem exert their effects by inhibiting transmembrane influx of extracellular calcium into cardiac and vascular smooth muscle. In isolated cardiac tissues, these drugs produce a depression of SA and AV node function and a negative inotropic effect. The peripheral effects consist mainly of an inhibition of excitation-contraction coupling in vascular smooth muscle and varying degrees of coronary and peripheral vasodilation. In patients, these drugs protect the myocardium (a) by a direct relaxant action on vascular smooth muscle, which increases blood flow through coronary and other beds, (b) through reduction of peripheral resistance, arterial pressure and, therefore, of left ventricular afterload, and (c) through prevention or reversal of coronary spasm. The inotropic action is countered by the afterload reduction so that the cardiac index is usually not decreased. The different agents have varying degrees of cardiac and peripheral vascular effects, and so the specific drug chosen depends on the individual hemodynamic problem.

Direct Myocardial Revascularization

The surgical construction of a bypass venous graft around the obstructed vessel will, in certain cases, reduce pain, alleviate anginal symptoms, preserve the myocardium, and improve survival. This procedure is frequently used for relief of symptoms or if medical therapy has not been successful. Coronary artery bypass surgery (CABS) seems well established in patients with left main coronary artery stenosis of 50% or more and in patients with 3-vessel disease and abnormal ventricular function. CABS usually relieves symptoms and increases exercise tolerance. The general mortality is low (1 to 3%) but is higher (5 to 10%) in patients with abnormal left ventricular function. However, within 10 years more than 50% of the transplanted vessel(s) will be restenosed. CABS and coronary angioplasty (described below) are at present the only treatment modalities that increase coronary artery blood flow. The other therapeutic maneuvers work by decreasing myocardial O_2 requirements. In any event, all methods have the common objective of improving the ratio of myocardial O_2 supply to needs.

Coronary Angioplasty

The most widely used procedure of this type, percutaneous transluminal coronary angioplasty (PTCA), consists of the percutaneous (through the skin) introduction of a dilating balloon catheter (via a brachial or femoral artery) into a stenosed coronary artery under fluoroscopic control. When the part of the slender catheter containing the balloon straddles the stenosis, the balloon is briefly inflated while balloon pressure and volume are carefully monitored. Successful dilation is indicated by enlargement of the coronary lumen and diminution of the pressure gradient across the stenosis. Patients with proximal, symmetrical, uncalcified coronary artery lesions are the best candidates for this procedure. In skilled hands, the technique has proven successful and complications have been minor.

Recent studies have shown the feasibility of more direct attacks on the coronary thrombus, which are sometimes termed coronary atherectomy. One technique consists of lysing of the thrombus by application (*via* catheter) of enzymes capable of dissolving the thrombus, for example, tissue plasminogen activator (TPA). Other methods involve cutting away the clot with a tiny, rotating, cutting blade at the end of a catheter or the use of a laser to dissolve the plaque. A recent long-term controlled study of 17,000 heart attack patients indicated that early administration of aspirin and IV streptokinase (a clot dissolver) resulted in a significant decrease in mortality. Further study is necessary to determine which of these procedures (or combination thereof) will be most effective in the treatment of acute coronary thrombosis.

Cardiac Rehabilitation

For the recuperating IHD patient, the most important part of therapy is this long-term, carefully planned program of cardiac rehabilitation. This includes: (*a*) early ambulation; (*b*) periodic exercise stress-testing; (*c*) a subsequent prescriptive exercise program; and (*d*) the coordinated, interdisciplinary efforts of psychosocial, educational, and vocational counseling aimed at returning the patient to a normal or near-normal life-style.

Early ambulation is intended to prevent the detrimental effects of prolonged immobilization (deconditioning) such as the decrease in physical work capacity, hypovolemia, the decrease in pulmonary ventilation, and a negative nitrogen and protein balance. In order to achieve the "training effect," there must be a minimum of two to three exercise periods per week lasting 30 to 40 minutes each, including warmup and cool down. The goal is to reach 70 to 85% of the exercise intensity level (as indicated by heart rate) that was safely achieved during the previous exercise testing. A successful exercise training program will result in a decrease in the resting heart rate and increases in $\dot{V}O_{2max}$ and maximal cardiac output. As a result, there is a lesser increase in heart rate and systolic pressure (*i.e.* a lower double product), less angina, fewer ischemic ECG changes and a more rapid slowing of the heart rate at any given level of submaximal work.

However, recent studies have shown that exercise programs of lesser intensity will also be of significant physical and psychosocial value to those patients. The exact mechanism of this improved circulatory performance is not certain but appears to involve peripheral adaptation since there is increased peripheral oxygen extraction. Whether or not there is improved myocardial contractility is uncertain. There is evidence, however, that a certain number of coronary patients are able, with high intensity training, to achieve endurance capacities almost equal to those of trained normal subjects.

There is currently little evidence that exercise training alters the natural history of atherosclerotic coronary artery disease or increases myocardial perfusion, but further study is required on these important issues. However, there is little question but that the great majority of patients who follow a planned rehabilitation regimen after MI are greatly benefited by improved working capacity, greater emotional stability, and a distinctly more productive and satisfying life. Exercise stress testing, physical training, deconditioning, arm *vs.* leg exercise, and isometric exercise are discussed in Chapter 12.

Congestive Heart Failure

Etiology

Congestive failure is a condition in which the heart is unable to pump blood at a rate commensurate with systemic metabolic requirements. It is not a single disease but rather a symptom complex (*i.e.*, a syndrome) with many causes. Although there is still a considerable knowledge gap, our understanding of the pathophysiology of this disorder has been greatly advanced in recent years. Some of these developments will be discussed in outline form in this section.

The basic cause of the cardiac output deficiency in congestive failure may be *cardiac* or *extracardiac*. The *cardiac* disturbance may be (*a*) a myocardial contractile failure due to ischemic heart disease, myocarditis, or cardiomyopathy (degeneration of the myocardium) or (*b*) a disorder that prevents proper filling or emptying of the heart such as a valvular stenosis, valvular regurgitation, or pericardial disease. *Extracardiac* disorders that may cause congestive failure are high-pressure overloads such as hypertension, or high-output overloads such as renal failure, anemia, AV fistula, or thyrotoxicosis. The apparent paradox of a heart failing because of increased output is the result of myocardial work demands in excess of coronary flow capabilities.

From a therapeutic standpoint it would be important to know whether the failure is due to an extracardiac, valvular, or pericardial disorder, which may be remediable, in contrast to a basic myocardial, contractile weakness, which is not.

As Cohn has pointed out, the heart failure syndrome has three important characteristics, reduced exercise tolerance, a high incidence of ventricular arrhythmias, and a shortened life expectancy.

Hemodynamic Mechanisms in Congestive Failure

Theory of the Failure

Controversy has long centered on the question of whether this disorder is primarily a *backward cardiac failure* in which the decreased ventricular output and the rising ventricular EDP produced, through retrograde action, increased venous and capillary pressures. The resulting fluid transudation into the tissue spaces contracts the plasma volume, which presumably "signals" an increase in tubular reabsorption of sodium and water. It was theorized that this combination of heightened capillary pressure and renal "hyperfunction" resulted in pulmonary and peripheral congestion and edema.

In contrast, the *forward-failure theory* held that the symptoms and signs stem from an inadequate left ventricular output with a reduction of renal perfusion pressure and glomerular filtration, and as a consequence, increased sodium and water reabsorption through the renin-angiotensin-aldosterone mechanism. Because it is now known that both mechanisms operate to varying degrees, this classification is not currently useful and has been generally abandoned.

While high cardiac filling and low cardiac output are hemodynamic hallmarks of this condition, the clinical manifestations of the syndrome are largely due to the compensatory responses rather than to the physiological changes of the disorder itself.

The signs and symptoms of the failure are ascribable to three main hemodynamic changes: *decreased cardiac output* with hypoperfusion of the peripheral bed, *increased left atrial pressure* with resulting pulmonary congestion, and *increased right atrial pressure* with resultant systemic and splanchnic congestion.

Decrease in Cardiac Output

Decreased cardiac output is primarily responsible for the limitation of physical activity, the renal hypoperfusion, the sodium and water retention, and the chronic fatigue that is characteristic of this condition. Fatigue may precede the other symptoms by many months. The *increased left atrial pressure*, the aftermath of the increased LVEDV and LVEDP, results in increased size of the atrium, increased pulmonary venous and capillary pressure, pulmonary congestion and edema and, if continued, decreased pulmonary air space and pulmonary compliance with resultant dyspnea and orthopnea. In addition to decreasing the available air space, congestion stiffens the lung and increases the work of breathing, leading to a feeling of breathlessness. In the upright position, some of the thoracic blood volume is displaced footward and central venous pressure is decreased. Thus, the patient may be able to breathe comfortably only when upright or propped up with several pillows (orthopnea). This is particularly true at night when, in the supine position, the dependent edema that has developed because of the gravity effect on the circulation (Chapter 6, Venous Pressure) tends to be reabsorbed into the circulation. This increases the central venous volume and congestion of the thoracic veins and leads to nocturnal dyspnea.

As described in Chapter 13, heart failure patients, unlike normal individuals, may show an increased stroke volume and cardiac output in the erect position (Fig. 13.4). If pulmonary capillary pressure becomes sufficiently high, fluid may transude from the plasma into the alveoli (pulmonary edema). The patient then becomes extremely breathless and may produce frothy sputum tinged with blood that has escaped from the capillaries.

Increase in Right Atrial Pressure

This will produce comparable changes in the systemic circulation, *i.e.*, increased volume and pressure in the vena cavae, peripheral veins, and capillaries with peripheral edema, particularly of the feet and ankles. There is also increased hepatic venous pressure with hepatic congestion and, if continued, liver dysfunction and intraperitoneal accummulation of fluid (ascites). Hepatic congestion, because of stretch of the liver capsule, may cause aching and tenderness in the region of the liver. Persistent hepatic congestion may also cause hepatic lobular necrosis. Increased right atrial pressure may develop from pulmonic valve stenosis or regurgitation, but more commonly it is a backward extension of left ventricular failure and pulmonary venous congestion.

In some cases, only one or two of these hemodynamic changes may occur, but all three frequently develop in the same patient. Signs and symptoms may vary considerably depending on the severity and rate of development of the underlying disorder. As mentioned earlier, a myocardial infarct involving over 40% of the myocardium will probably cause a hemodynamic collapse and cardiogenic shock. On the other hand, a patient may, from a lesser lesion, be in "compensated failure" for many years without severe disability.

Pathophysiological and Compensatory Changes

The most important manifestations of congestive failure are those involving (*a*) the myocardium, (*b*) fluid balance, (*c*) bioenergetics, and (*d*) the peripheral circulation. These will be discussed in the following sections.

Myocardial Failure and Compensatory Responses

In congestive failure, both clinical and experimental, there is usually a deficit in ventricular contractility as evidenced by depressed length-tension and ventricular function curves (Fig. 14.4, *curve c*).

In addition the myocardium usually shows a decreased force-velocity curve, thus clearly indicating inotropic inadequacy of the myocardium. This contractile defect may arise from a primary myocardial lesion such as MI or from a secondary ischemia resulting from a ventricular pressure or output overload.

The *ejection fraction* (EF) is an important measure of cardiac function in heart failure. The EF generally shows a positive correlation with the cardiac

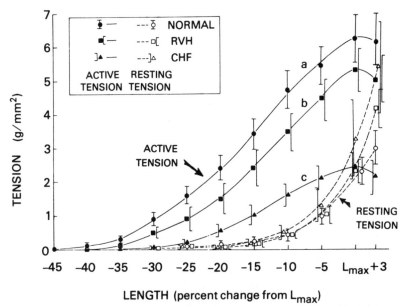

Figure 14.4.   Length-tension curves for normal (○), hypertrophied (□), and failing (△) ventricular muscle in the cat. *Bottom curves* show resting, passive tension and *top curves* show peak contractile tension. Tension is corrected for cross-sectional area. In heart failure, maximum tension is clearly depressed, but in hypertrophied muscle, depression is borderline. (Reprinted with permission from J.F. Spann, R.A. Buccino, E.H. Sonnenblick, and E. Braunwald, *Circ Res* 21:341, 1967).

index, although this relationship may not hold in certain conditions such as mitral regurgitation or congestive heart failure. With the decline in left ventricular performance, the EF decreases from its normal value of about 50 to 70% and in severe failure may be as low as 10 to 20%. A lesser ejection fraction is an important predictor of mortality.

The two compensatory mechanisms available to improve myocardial performance, the Starling effect and the sympathetic inotropic effect (Chapter 5), are both activated in congestive failure. As pointed out by McCall and O'Rourke, in the early stages these compensatory responses tend to improve cardiac output by increasing heart rate, contractility, and ventricular diastolic filling, but their continued presence often contributes to the progressive cardiac dysfunction seen in congestive heart failure. In addition to these two compensatory responses, ventricular volume and hypertrophy changes also occur. These adaptations are discussed in the following.

Starling Effect.   The decrease in cardiac output, aided by the increased sodium and water retention (discussed below), leads to progressive elevation of EDV and EDP. This increased diastolic stretch results in increased ventricular performance so long as the ventricle functions on the rising portion of the length-tension curve (Fig. 14.4, *curve c*). However this improved ventricular performance is achieved at the price of pulmonary congestion in the case of the left ventricle and systemic venous congestion in the case of the right. As the failure progresses, the heart is operating on a depressed ventricular function curve that is shifted down and to the right (Fig. 14.4).

Increased emphasis has been given recently to another effect of the increased EDV, namely the adverse influence of heightened EDV on ventricular diastolic compliance and the effect of the latter on the hemodynamics of congestive failure.

It will be noted in Figure 14.4 that as the ventricle fills and EDV and resting tension increase, the tension/length ratio, or stiffness, which under normal circumstances is considerably greater than that of skeletal muscle, increases disproportionately. This means that the diastolic or resting compliance (*i.e.*, the reciprocal of stiffness or the length/tension ratio) decreases sharply as the EDV rises. This decreased compliance, coupled in the case of MI with the decreased compliance incident to stiffening of the ischemic segment of the myocardium (mentioned earlier), tends to perpetuate the congestive state. Some investigators have suggested that in some cases the reduced diastolic compliance (*i.e.*, diastolic dysfunction) may be as important a factor in producing congestion as the impaired ventricular systolic contractility (*i.e.*, systolic dysfunction).

Ventricular Volume and Hypertrophy. If a cardiac chamber is subjected to continued distension from an increased preload or afterload stress, its internal capacity will increase. If it is required to consistently produce increased muscular work, either by a volume or pressure overload, it will hypertrophy (*i.e.*, the number of sarcomeres will increase, the wall will become thicker, and the muscle will increase in mass.) Pressure overload (*e.g.*, in hypertension or aortic stenosis) produces an increase in muscle mass and relatively little change in ventricular volume in the absence of heart failure. Volume overloads (*e.g.*, those resulting from abnormal shunts, such as atrial septal defects or incompetent valves as in aortic regurgitation) result mainly in ventricular dilation. Ordinarily, they would cause thinning of the wall but because some hypertension almost always develops, the wall thickness is maintained. In most cases, such as occurs physiologically in the endurance athlete and pathologically in congestive failure, there is an increase in both ventricular volume and mass. But changes in myocardial volume and mass are different phenomena and exert independent effects.

As the left ventricular chamber enlarges during early failure, it assumes a more spherical shape and the increased EDV, as described above, has a compensatory, supportive action. However, a continued EDV increase eventually becomes self-defeating because in an expanding, more spherical ventricle, the total force required for an equivalent systolic ejection against a comparable afterload will also increase as the radius increases (Laplace's law). Since myocardial $\dot{V}O_2$ is closely correlated with the ventricular wall stress that generates the cardiac force (Chapter 11), the oxygen demand becomes disproportionately greater than the stroke work produced, and the process becomes inefficient. This effect on wall stress is only partially offset by the fact that at a larger ventricular size a unit length of circumferential shortening will result in a larger stroke volume of the "spherical" ventricle.

Hypertrophy (*i.e.*, increased mass) is a compensatory mechanism that increases the force-generating capacity of the ventricle. But does hypertrophy lead to improved muscle function? The answer is not clear at present and seems to depend on the individual circumstances. The contractility of the hypertrophied muscle is reportedly only slightly less than that of a normal muscle (Fig. 14.4, *curve b*). Hypertrophy causes the increased pressure load to be distributed over a greater number of sarcomeres, and wall tension (T) becomes more normalized since the increase in pressure (P) is balanced by the increase in wall thickness (μ) (Laplace's theorem, Chapter 2). Therefore in conjunction with the Starling and other compensatory effects, hypertrophy helps to maintain overall circulatory compensation.

However, there is also a limit to this adaptive process, imposed mainly by an already borderline coronary perfusion pressure supplying a growing tissue mass. The net benefit will depend on the ability of a limited hypertrophy to establish compensation. Unfortunately, increased wall thickness will also decrease wall compliance, and in the case of failing heart, increased wall stiffness is an added disadvantage.

Gradually developing ventricular hypertrophy produced by intermittent volume overload (*e.g.*, the hypertrophy of endurance athletes engaged in sports that involve largely isotonic activity such as running or swimming) results in improved cardiac functioning. Abrupt pressure overload usually (but not inevitably) leads to depressed ventricular performance. Clinical and experimental studies have shown that myocardial hypertrophy is at least to some extent reversible. For example, in experimental animals a 50% increase in left ventricular mass was induced by 10 weeks of gradually developing experimental hypertension; reversal of this pressure overload resulted (in 10 more weeks) in the regression of all the mechanical and biochemical abnormalities. Recent animal studies have shown that aside from arterial pressure reduction, decline of myocardial mass also depends on sympathetic stimulation. A decrease in myocardial catecholamine levels favors regression of myocardial hypertrophy.

Autonomic Response to Congestive Failure

A key response to heart failure is the heightened sympathetic outflow to the heart and peripheral circulation. The mechanism of this effect is not certain.

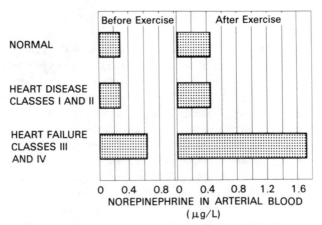

Figure 14.5. Norephinephrine levels in arterial blood are higher in severe heart failure patients (class III and IV) at rest and after exercise than in normal subjects or in patients with milder heart failure (I and II). (Reprinted with permission from E. Braunwald, *The Myocardium: Failure and Infarction.* New York: HP Publishing Co., 1974.)

Abboud *et al.* have suggested that the cardiac vagal afferent fibers, which at first are more active in response to cardiac distension, later adapt and have a lesser discharge frequency. This would theoretically result in an increased neurohormonal and sympathetic drive (Chapter 10). However, the sympathetic overdrive could also theoretically be due to a lessened arterial baroceptor stimulation secondary to a decreased arterial pressure. Heart failure is also associated with a marked deficiency of parasympathetic function as shown, for example, by a marked reduction in the bradycardic reflex response to both arterial hypertension and to the pressure overshoot phase of the Valsalva test. But whatever the cause, the result is associated with increased sympathetic outflow and elevated plasma norephinephrine, renin, aldosterone, and ADH. This increased sympathetic outflow is responsible for an increased inotropic effect on the myocardium and an increased peripheral vasoconstriction described below.

Sympathetic Inotropic Effect: Myocardial Response. During congestive failure, there is augmented sympathetic activity and increased concentration of plasma norepinephrine at rest and during exercise (Fig. 14.5). The resultant increase in the force and velocity of myocardial contraction exerts a considerable functional support for the heart. However, with continued sympathetic overactivity, the myocardial catecholamine stores become depleted, due mainly to a reduction in myocardial tyrosine hydroxylase activity, which is the rate-limiting step for the conversion of tyrosine to norepinephrine. This depletion is apparently not involved, however, in the pathogenesis of failure. It may

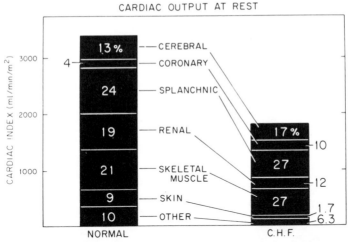

CARDIAC OUTPUT AT REST

Figure 14.6. Decrease in cardiac index (CI) and alteration in fractional distribution of CI in congestive failure patients (CHF). (Reprinted with permission from A.C. Hseih, *The Peripheral Circulation*, edited by R. Zelis. New York: Grune & Stratton, 1975.)

be that the residual catecholamines from the adrenal medulla and other sources remain effective because of the *de facto* denervation of the myocardium and the consequent hypersensitivity response to catechols (Chapter 9). The deleterious effect of the sympathetic overdrive is indicated by a positive correlation between the plasma catecholamine concentration and ultimate mortality.

Sympathetic Vasoconstriction Effect. The vasoconstriction results in a significant redistribution of left ventricular output, which, like hypervolemia and the inotropic effect, is an important compensatory mechanism (Fig. 14.6).

This redistribution diverts the renal and cutaneous portions of an already reduced cardiac output to the more critical cerebral and coronary beds. This occurs even at rest but is intensified in the presence of exercise, fever, or other stresses. There is a general increased tone of peripheral arteries and veins and, with only modest physical activity, a marked vasoconstriction of mesenteric and renal vascular beds as well. The heightened tone of the peripheral vessels is partially due to an increased infiltration of sodium and water into the arterial walls. The net result is a reduced ability of the vessels to dilate with increased activity so that oxygen extraction is limited (Fig. 14.7). Exercise or increased metabolic states will, therefore, produce lactic acidemia and an inability to dissipate heat. Consequently, the heart failure patient frequently has a heat intolerance.

Associated with the sympathetic hyperactivity is a blunting of both arterial and cardiopulmonary reflexes. This results in a diminished response by the heart failure patients to all circulatory stresses, including the ability to increase

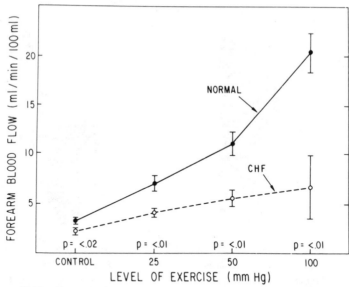

Figure 14.7. Forearm blood flow in congestive heart failure patients (CHF) increased less during handgrip exercise then that of normal subjects at all exercise levels, showing inability of peripheral vessels to dilate properly to metabolic stimulus. (Reprinted with permission from A.C. Hseih, *The Peripheral Circulation*, edited by R. Zelis. New York: Grune & Stratton, 1975).

the heart rate with postural change, cold, and exercise. Since these patients already have severe limitations in their ability to adjust stroke volume, the added rate limitation is an appreciable further handicap in meeting cardiac output needs.

Bioenergetics of Congestive Failure

The biochemical changes accompanying muscle contraction may be divided into three sequential processes: (*a*) energy production or the conversion of substrates to high-energy phosphates; (*b*) energy utilization or the translation of high-energy phosphates to contractile activity; and (*c*) excitation-contraction coupling, the mechanism by which the myocardial action potential results in calcium movement, which in turn mediates the contraction and relaxation (Chapter 5).

Studies have shown that even in severe failure, mitochondrial function is not disturbed, so that energy production appears adequate. ATP is converted to ADP primarily during the interaction of myosin and actin to produce shortening. The rate of this reaction correlates well with contractility. It has been shown that there is a deficiency in the myofibrillar-ATPase system in severe failure and some reduction of function in myocardial hypertrophy without failure, but the full implications of these defects are not yet known.

In some types of congestive failure, the ATP-dependent calcium pump of the isolated sarcoplasmic reticulum is defective. Both the amount and the rate at which calcium is pumped into the sarcoplasmic reticulum are deficient, and with the development of hypertrophy, the content of sarcoplasmic reticulum per muscle unit is reduced. Thus there may be a dilution of sarcoplasmic reticulum incident to the hypertrophy process itself. It is, therefore, evident that biochemical defects do exist in the failing muscle, but which are the critical ones is not yet known.

Fluid Balance in Congestive Failure

As cardiac output decreases in congestive failure, the reduced renal arterial hydrostatic pressure and the reflex renal vasoconstriction (described below) combine to reduce renal blood flow, particularly in the outer renal cortex. A reduction in glomerular filtration rate results, which leads to salt and water retention and eventually, if continued, to edema. The mechanism resembles the response to hemorrhage described in Chapter 13. The reduced renal blood flow leads to the liberation of renin, the elaboration of angiotensin II, and ultimately to the production of aldosterone by the zona glomerulosa of the adrenal cortex.

The hepatic dysfunction that accompanies severe congestive failure is responsible for a reduced catabolism of aldosterone so that aldosterone plasma levels are higher and more sustained, thus accentuating the fluid retention. Renal venous congestion plays a variable, but generally limited, role in the fluid balance disturbance.

Thus patients with congestive failure usually have increased blood volume, interstitial fluid volume, and total body sodium levels; although this may be associated with normal or even decreased serum Na^+ concentrations. Increased physical activity, because it causes increased sympathetic stimulation and heightened plasma norepinephrine, will result in further lowering of renal blood flow and the glomerular filtration rate and will increase the salt and water retention. Thus, during the decompensated phase of congestive failure, rest and restricted activity are an important part of therapy.

Treatment of Congestive Failure

Therapy will depend on the severity and rate of development of the disease and will be directed first toward the specific cause of the failure. The treatment of the congestive failure itself usually has three objectives: (a) reduction of cardiac work load, (b) enhancement of cardiac contractility, and (c) control of excessive fluid retention.

Reduction of Cardiac Work. This is done mainly by reducing afterload through rest, lessening of physical and emotional stress, and administration of vasodilators. The latter agents reduce peripheral vessel resistance and preload, thereby reducing ventricular EDV, EDP, and myocardial O_2 demands while increasing stroke volume and cardiac index. The reduction in EDV is highly beneficial since it is mechanically more advantageous to increase SV by increasing ejection fraction than by increasing EDV.

The objective is to reduce the cardiac work with a minimal reduction in aortic pressure. In attempting to manipulate aortic pressure, a balance must be struck between a relatively low value to reduce afterload and cardiac work and maintaining a sufficiently high level to insure reasonable perfusion of the coronary bed and peripheral tissues. As previously mentioned, the autoregulatory capacity of the coronary bed is often compromised in heart failure, so that flow is more directly dependent on perfusion pressure.

In some cases, the above forms of treatment will also relieve fluid retention. If not, more specific therapy is used in the form of (a) *thiazide diuretics* which reduce tubular reabsorption of sodium and thus increase its excretion, or (b) agents such as furosemide or aldactone (the latter because of its aldosterone-antagonist activity), which also exert powerful diuretic action.

Because of impaired capacity for renal excretion of Na^+, the restriction of Na^+ intake is important. Furosemide inhibits active Na^+ reabsorption and enhances renal K^+ excretion. Thus hyponatremia and hypokalemia are potential side effects of the more potent diuretics. Hypokalemia—because it may predispose to digitalis toxicity—must be guarded against.

Therapy must be carefully controlled. Although it is a pathological condition, hypervolemia is a compensatory change with a purpose. Rapid loss of fluid without improved cardiac performance might trade the edema for the increased fatigue of inadequate cardiac output. Overzealous use of diuretics with resultant hypovolemia must be particularly avoided.

Vasodilators. These unloading agents exert their effect through their ability to dilate arteries and veins. Some agents (*e.g.* hydralazine) are primarily arteriolar vasodilators and help to reduce afterload, while other agents (*e.g.*, nitrates) act mainly to dilate veins and help to reduce preload stress. Nitroprusside, prazosin, and isosorbide have both arterial-dilating and venous pooling effects. Hydralazine and isosorbide also improve survival. An afterload-reducing agent, captopril, an inhibitor of the enzyme that converts angiotensin I to angiotensin II, has also been reported as effective in congestive failure.

Glycosides. Digitalis and other glycosides have the fortuitous property of producing a more effective positive inotropic action in the failing rather than the normal heart. This is probably due to a combination of the direct myocardial effect with an arteriolar and venular dilation action. Positive inotropic agents shift the ventricular function curve upward, permitting reestablishment of some cardiac reserve and improvement of ejection fraction.

Suggested Readings

Ischemic Heart Disease

Abboud FM, Fozzard HA, Gilmore JP, and Reis DJ. *Disturbances in Neurogenic Control of the Circulation.* Bethesda, Md.: American Physiological Society, 1981.

Braunwald EA, Ross J, and Sonnenblick EH. *Mechanisms of Contraction of the Normal and Failing Heart,* 2nd ed. Boston: Little, Brown, 1976.

Brooks H, Holland R, and Al Sadir J. Right ventricular performance during ischemia: an anatomic and hemodynamic analysis. *Am J Physiol* 233:H500, 1978.

Cobb LA, Werner SA, and Trobaugh GB. Sudden cardiac death. *Mod Concepts Cardiovasc Dis* 42:31–42, 1980.

Coronary Artery Surgery Study (CASS). Randomized trial of coronary artery bypass surgery *Circulation* 68:939 and 951, 1983.

Ebert TJ, Hughes CV, Tristani FE, Barney JA, and Smith JJ. Effects of age and coronary heart disease on the circulatory responses to lower body negative pressure. *Cardiovasc Res* 16:663–669, 1982.

Elliot RS. *Stress and the Major Cardiovascular Disorders.* Mt. Kisco, N.Y.: Futura Publishing Co., 1979.

Ellrodt G, Chew CYC, and Singh BN. Therapeutic implications of slow channel blockade in cardiocirculatory disorders. *Circulation* 62:669–679, 1980.

Gross GJ. Antianginal drugs. In: *Modern Pharmacology,* edited by CR Craig and RW Stitzel. Boston: Little, Brown, 1982.

Gruntzig AR. Percutaneous transluminal dilation of chronic coronary stenosis. In: *Advances in Heart Disease,* edited by DT Mason. New York: Grune & Strattoon, 1980, Vol. III.

Heart Facts. Dallas: American Heart Assn. 1989.

Herman MV and Gorlin R. Pathophysiology of ischemic heart disease. In: *Clinical Cardiovascular Physiology,* edited by HJ Levine. New York: Grune & Stratton, 1976.

Hillis LD and Braunwald E. Coronary artery spasm. *N Engl J Med* 299:695–702, 1978.

Hurst J.W. (ed) *The Heart,* 7th ed. New York: McGraw-Hill, 1990.

Karliner JS, Gregoratos G, and Ross J. Myocardial infarction. In: *Internal Medicine,* edited by JR Stein, pp 439–451. Boston: Little, Brown, 1987.

Kirk ES and Jennings RB. Pathophysiology of myocardial ischemia. In: *The Heart, Arteries and Veins,* 5th ed., edited by JW Hurst, New York: McGraw-Hill, 1982, pp 976–1008.

McCall D, *et al.* Calcium entry blocking drugs: mechanisms of action, experimental studies and clinical uses. *Curr Problems Cardiol* 10:1, 1985.

Ogawa I, Wyden JK, Rose HB, Kanazana M, Seino V, and Swan HJC. Peripheral circulatory changes after physical conditioning in coronary artery disease patients. *J Cardiac Rehabil* 1:269–272, 1981.

Pantridge JF, Webb SW, Adgey AAJ, and Geddes JS. The first hour after the onset of acute myocardial infarction. In: *Progress in Cardiology,* edited by PN Yu and JF Goodwin. Philadelphia: Lea & Febiger, 1974, Chap. 5, Vol. 3, pp 173–188.

Pollack ML and Schmidt DH. *Heart Disease and Rehabilitation.* Boston: Houghton Mifflin, 1979.

Randall WC. *Nervous Control of Cardiovascular Function.* New York: Oxford University Press, 1984.

Shand DG. Beta adrenergic blocking drugs after acute myocardial infarction. *Mod Concepts Cardiovasc Dis* 51:103–106, 1982.

Thames MD, Klopfenstein HS, Abboud FW, Mark AL, and Walter JL. Preferential distribution of inhibitory cardiac receptors with vagal afferents to the inferoposterial wall of the left ventricle activated during coronary occlusion in the dog. *Circ Res* 43:512–519, 1978.

Tristani FE, Kamper DG, McDermott DJ, Peters BS, and Smith JJ. Alteration of postural and Valsalva responses in coronary heart disease. *Am J Physiol* 233:H694–H699, 1977.

Wenger NK and Hellertein HK. *Rehabilitation of the Coronary Patient*. New York: John Wiley & Sons, 1978.

Congestive Heart Failure

Abboud FM, Thames M, and Mark AL. Role of cardiac afferent nerves in regulation of circulation during coronary occlusion and heart failure. In: *Disturbances in Neurogenic control of the Circulation*, edited by FM Abboud, HA Fozzard, JP Gilmore, and DJ Reis. Bethesda, Md.: American Physiological Society, 1981, pp 65–68.

Braunwald E, Ross J, and Sonnenblick EH. *Mechanisms of Contraction of the Normal and Failing Heart*, 2nd ed. Boston: Little, Brown, 1976.

Brenner BM and Rector FC. *The Kidney*. Philadelphia: WB Saunders, 1976.

Capasso JM, Strobeck JE, Malhotra A, Scheuer J, and Sonnenblick EH. Contractile behavior of rat myocardium after reversal of hypertensive hypertrophy. *Am J Physiol* 242:H882–889, 1982.

Cohn JN. Current therapy of the failing heart. *Circulation* 78:1099–1107, 1988.

Francis GS, Goldsmith SR, Ziesche S, *et al.* Relative attenuation of sympathetic drive during exercise in patients with congestive heart failure. *J Am Coll Cardiol* 5:832–839, 1985.

Langer GA. Myocardial force development in health and disease. In: *Pathophysiology of the Heart*, edited by G Ross. New York: Masson Publishing Co., 1982, pp 1–39.

Levine HJ and Gaasch WJ. Diastolic compliance of the left ventricle. *Mod Concepts Cardiovasc Dis* 47:95–102, 1978.

McCall D and O'Rourke RA. Congestive heart failure—biochemistry, pathophysiology and neurohumoral mechanisms. *Mod Concepts Cardiovas Dis* 54:55–65, 1985.

Mason DT, Zelis R, and Wikman-Cottett J. Symposium on congestive heart failure. *Am J Cardiol* 32:395, 1973.

Sen S and Tarazi RC. Regression of myocardial hypertrophy and influence of the adrenergic system. *Am J Physiol* 244:H97–101, 1983.

Tillisch JH. Pump failure and cardiogenic shock. In: *Pathophysiology of the Heart*, edited by G Ross. New York: Masson Publishing Co., 1982, pp 225–256.

Zelis R *et al.* Vasoconstrictive mechanisms in congestive heart failure. *Mod Concepts Cardiovasc Dis* 58:7–18, 1989.

Zucker IH and Gilmore JR. Aspects of cardiovascular reflexes in pathologic states. *Fed Proc* 44:2400–2407, 1985.

chapter 15

Pathophysiology: Hypertension and Circulatory Shock

Hypertension
Definitions and Classification

About 20% of the adult population are afflicted with hypertension, the most common single disorder seen in the office of an internist. It is a major risk factor for coronary artery disease and a common cause of heart failure, kidney failure, stroke, and blindness. As Pickering has pointed out, the designation of a single dividing line between normotension and hypertension is somewhat artificial. The diagnosis is usually based on repeated resting levels of $\geq 140/90$ mm Hg in adults 18 to 49 years of age and $\geq 160/95$ mm Hg in adults over 50 years of age.

It is more common among males than females, and severe hypertension is four times more common in black men than in white. It has been suggested that this may be due to a higher renal vascular resistance in blacks, perhaps related to premature senescence in these patients.

Systolic hypertension (*i.e.*, the condition in which the systolic rise is more prominent,) increase with age, and in men over 45 years is considered a greater risk factor for coronary heart disease (CHD) than diastolic hypertension. Obesity is a strong predisposing factor, and hypertension is 10 times more common in persons 20% or more overweight. About 5% of adult hypertension is due to a specific, identifiable cause and is termed *secondary hypertension*. The remaining 95%, in which the cause cannot be determined, is classified as primary or *essential hypertension* (EH). The latter develops more often between the ages of 20 to 50 years. Hypertension developing during infancy or childhood or after the age of 50 is often of the secondary variety.

There are multiple ways in which arterial blood pressure can be raised, and almost each pressor mechanism has a representative example of a clinical type of hypertension. Only EH and a few of the more common types of secondary hypertension will be considered in this chapter. The renal circulation, which is closely involved in the pathogenesis of hypertension, was reviewed in Chapter 11.

Secondary Hypertension

Renovascular Hypertension

Renal diseases are the most frequent cause of secondary hypertension and include two clinical entities, *renovascular hypertension*, a disease of the renal arteries, and *renal parenchymal hypertension*. While kidney disease and hypertension have long been clinically associated, the relation between the two was obscure until Goldblatt showed that persistent hypertension could be produced experimentally by constriction of the renal arteries.

Renovascular hypertension is the result of stenosis of one or both renal arteries, usually caused by atherosclerosis or fibromuscular hyperplasia. Although these patients frequently have evidence of increased adrenergic drive to the circulatory system (*e.g.*, increased heart rate, cardiac output, left ventricular ejection, venoconstriction, or autonomic repsonsiveness) the underlying cause of hypertension is the increased production and release of renin and angiotensin II (Fig. 11.13). Angiotensin II raises arterial pressure through (*a*) its very potent systemic vasoconstrictor effect and (*b*) stimulation of aldosterone secretion with a resultant sodium retention and increase in interstitial fluid volume and plasma volume. Because β-adrenergic blockade can reduce renin activity, it is sometimes used in the treatment of renovascular hypertension.

Renal Parenchymal Hypertension

This occurs in a variety of acute and chronic renal parenchymal diseases such as pyelonephritis (inflammation and scarring of the kidney tubules) or chronic glomerulonephritis (inflammation and scarring of the glomeruli). It is thought that the underlying cause is a decreased renal perfusion due to inflammatory and fibrotic changes. In contrast to renovascular hypertension, patients with volume-loading hypertension, such as renal parenchymal hypertension, aldosteronism, or Cushing's syndrome (described below), usually have a normal cardiac output associated with elevated peripheral resistance and increased heart rate.

Endocrine Hypertension

Clinically and experimentally, it is known that when about 70% of the kidney mass has been destroyed and fluid and sodium intake increased, a "volume-loading hypertension" will be produced. It is basically the sodium which is responsible, since a persistent hypertension will not result if only water is retained. Similar types of hypertension will occur in certain endocrine disorders such as *primary aldosteronism*, a condition due to an adrenal tumor or hypertrophy with excessive aldosterone secretion and increased sodium reabsorption. There is frequently an associated muscle weakness due to potassium depletion.

Hypertension will also occur in *Cushing's syndrome*, which is characterized by excessive secretion of glucocorticoids and sodium rentention. Another cause of hypertension is *pheochromocytoma*, an adrenal medullary tumor in which there is increased secretion of epinephrine and norepinephrine associated with chronic peripheral vasoconstriction and myocardial hyperkinesis. In this disorder, heightened sympathetic tone rather than volume expansion is the main characteristic. *Mineralocorticoid hypertension* is characterized by low plasma levels of renin and aldosterone but elevated secretion of deoxycorticosterone (DOCA) or DOCA analogues, leading to NA^+ retention and often associated with hypokalemia. In some of these patients, the administration of an aldosterone antagonist such as spironolactone will result in a loss of sodium and a lowering of the blood pressure.

Other Types of Hypertension

There are other varieties of hypertension in which the inciting cause is known but the mechanism is uncertain. These include hypertension due to drugs such as oral contraceptives or monoamine oxidase and those due to hypercalcemia and to toxemia of pregnancy. Hypertension, primarily systolic in nature, can also be caused by coarctation of the aorta, hyperthyroidism, and decreased distensibility of the aorta.

Essential Hypertension

Hemodynamic Changes

Arterial pressure can rise because of an increase in cardiac output or vascular resistance or both. The fundamental defect in essential hypertension (EH) is the failure of the pressure-regulating mechanisms, although exactly where the failure lies is not yet known. The hemodynamic changes as well as the ensuing clinical picture depend on the stage and type of disease.

Borderline, mild, or labile hypertension include almost three-quarters of hypertensives. Most of these patients have increased heart rate, stroke volume (SV), cardiac output (CO), and rate of ventricular ejection but normal or only slightly elevated total peripheral resistance (TPR). In some patients, there is evidence of increased venomotor tone and decreased systemic venous compliance, which are undoubtedly responsible for the migration of blood toward the thorax with a resultant increased central blood volume (CBV). Since the total blood volume (TBV) is usually normal, these patients have an increased ratio of central to total blood volume (CBV/TBV). The increased CBV in turn, *via* the Starling mechanism, is probably responsible for the increased stroke volume and cardiac output, as suggested by clinical reports that show a highly significant, positive correlation between the CBV/TBV ratio and the cardiac output. These patients usually have low plasma renin activity (PRA) levels.

These hemodynamic findings indicate a hyperkinetic circulation with increased adrenergic drive to the heart and peripheral vessels. During head-up tilt, mental arithmetic, and other stresses, borderline hypertensives frequently respond with a greater rise in blood pressure than normal subjects. These increased autonomic reflex reactions are undoubtedly further manifestations of the sympathetic hyperkinesis that exists during this stage of EH.

About one-fourth of hypertensives fall into the *moderate, severe, or accelerated hypertension* classification. In these patients the pathophysiology

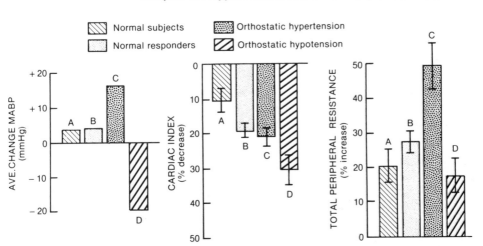

Figure 15.1. Responses of mean arterial blood pressure (MABP) (*left*), cardiac output (*middle*), and total peripheral resistance (*right*) to 50° head-up tilt and hypertensive patients. Normal subjects (*A*) and moderate hypertensives (*B*) showed similar arterial pressure changes. Patients with mild or early hypertension (*C*) showed increased arterial pressure (orthostatic hypertension) characterized by a moderate fall in cardiac output and a marked elevation n peripheral resistance— a hyperkinetic reaction. Severe hypertensives (*D*) had orthostatic hypotension which was the result of a marked fall in cardiac output and a lesser rise in vascular resistance. (Reprinted with permission from E.D. Frohlich et al.: Tilt test for investigating a neural component in hypertension. *Circulation* 36:387, 1967.)

depends on the level of the arterial pressure and the degree of TPR and cardiac enlargement. As the disease progresses, TPR rises. The left ventricular ejection rate and cardiac output decrease to normal or subnormal levels, and the left ventricle enlarges progressively in response to the increased afterload. Peripheral resistance rises in all vascular beds but most notably in the kidney. Plasma volume is reduced, and PRA values are often elevated.

In contrast to mild hypertension, there is in this stage little evidence of adrenergic stimulation. Autonomic responses to baroceptor stimulation, to the Valsalva test, and to head-up tilt (Fig. 15.1) are diminished in advanced hypertension.

There is a rapid resetting of baroceptors to the higher arterial pressure in hypertension, but the mechanism causing the resetting and chronic loss of baroceptor responsiveness is not well understood. While earlier investigators suggested that reduced compliance of the vasculature at the receptor site was responsible, it is now believed that defects in the receptor membrane, such as lag in the $NA^+ - K^+$ pump may be involved.

The atherosclerotic process is widespread and very closely linked to the pathology of EH. With continued pressure elevation, the atherosclerosis will be progressive regardless of the cause of the hypertension. Because of atherosclerosis, the hypertension, if unchecked, predisposes to ischemic heart disease, cerebrovascular accident, or renal disease with uremia (accumulation of urea and other protein metabolites in the blood). In some cases, for unknown reasons, the process becomes accelerated (malignant hypertension).

Pathogenesis

Only a brief outline will be given here of the immense investigative effort that continues to go into the etiology of EH. In this search, two features of the disease have loomed prominently, *viz.*, the strong genetic susceptibility and the self-perpetuating nature of the disease. The hereditary predisposition is polygenetically transferred as is evident not only from a study of clinical records but also from the emergence through inbreeding of spontaneously hypertensive rats (SHR) whose disease strongly resembles EH. In other genetic studies, rat strains have been developed that are supersensitive to salt feeding, (*i.e.*, strains in which hypertension will occur on salt diets that are innocuous to normal rats).

The concept of the almost inevitable progression of the disease is fostered by the evidence that hypertension begets arteriosclerosis, which in turn begets further pressure elevation. But what starts the process and why the arterial pressure-regulating system breaks down are not known. Among the many explanations for the initiation of EH are the *neurogenic theory*, proposed by Folkow and others, the *arterial pressure–urinary output theory* of Guyton, and the *regulatory imbalance* or mosaic theory of Page.

The *neurogenic theory* is supported in part by the considerable evidence that the nervous system is much involved in the regulation of arterial pressure. While emotional stress undoubtedly leads to an acute rise in arterial blood pressure, it has been difficult to document the role of stress in sustained clinical elevation of blood pressure. However, hypertension can be induced in experimental animals by transection of arterial baroceptor nerves, by lesions of the nucleus tractus solitarius (NTS) or lateral anterior hypothalamus, or by chronic stimulation of the posterior hypothalamus (Fig. 15.2). Normal animals can become chronically hypertensive when exposed to stressful learning situations, prolonged noise, or long-term psychogenic, emotional-frustration experiments. A recent interesting report indicates that carefully placed lesions in the preoptic region of the anterior hypothalamus will prevent a number of forms of experimental hypertension. Such a lesion will, for example, protect rats against subsequent development of renal hypertension, against deoxycorticosterone hypertension, and also against experimental hypertension produced by arterial baroceptor denervation or NTS lesions. Ob-

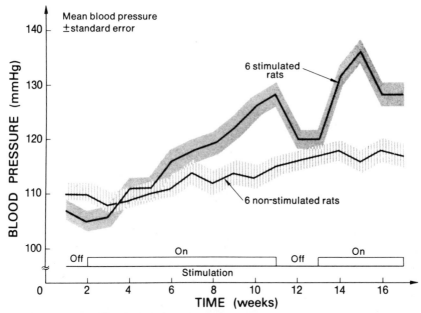

Figure 15.2. Enduring hypertension resulting from chronic stimulation of the hypothalamic defense area in the conscious rat. Stimulation was stopped during the 11th to 13th weeks. (Reprinted with permission from B. Folkow and E.H. Rubinstein, *Acta Physiol Scand* 68:48, 1966.)

viously considerable investigation is still required to unravel the basic role of the hypothalamus and other higher centers in the production of neurogenic hypertension.

The *arterial pressure–urinary output theory* suggests a relationship that has long been suspected between elevated levels of body sodium and hypertension. In countries where NA^+ intake is high, so is the frequency of hypertension and, as mentioned above, genetic strains have been developed in which ordinary innocuous high salt diets will cause hypertension. As previously described, certain types of renal pathology will induce persistent hypertension, but the mechanism is not known.

From an extensive application of computer techniques to renal and arterial pressure control systems, Guyton has developed a theory (previously described in Chapter 10) for the role of the kidney in blood pressure control. This theory proposes that the predominant long-term influence on the height of the arterial pressure is the urinary output of sodium and water, particularly the former. He suggests that even a minor disturbance in renal function can lead to a progressive increase in extracellular fluid and plasma volume, with a continued elevation in arterial pressure, because of the infinite gain of the system.

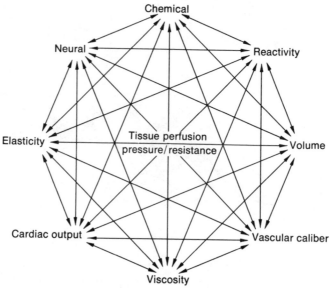

Figure 15.3.   Mosaic octagon illustrating multiple factors underlying the pressure/resistance control of tissue perfusion. (Reprinted with permission from I.H. Page, *Circ Res* 34:133, 1974.)

Guyton's theory holds, therefore, that EH begins as a renovascular deficiency and continues because of an obligatory arterial pressure–urinary output relation.

Cowley and his colleagues have extensively investigated the relationship between body fluid volumes and arterial pressure. They found that during the first 24 hours after acute expansion of blood volume in experimental animals, cardiac output increased, but arterial pressure changes were minimized by a decreased sympathetic tone and heightened urinary excretion. However, in the later stages of blood volume expansion (days and weeks) cardiac output and blood volume tended to remain near normal, but total peripheral resistance and arterial pressure rose substantially. The mechanism of the latter changes is not certain but probably involves local (not systemic) factors such as increased whole body autoregulation along with increased vasomotion and closure (rarefaction) of microcirculatory vasculature.

Page's *regulatory imbalance theory* assumes that a steady state exists among a number of factors that regulate blood pressure (Fig. 15.3). The different factors contribute, in varying degrees, to the maintenance of balance. One or more of these variables may be changed in an independent manner to produce hypertension. The theory assumes that EH is a "multifactorial disease of regulation" and that no single underlying cause is to be expected since no one mechanism dominates the regulatory process.

Page's theory has gained recent adherents among a number of investigators who have gradually abandoned the unitary theory. Folkow, for example, believes that aside from the undoubted hereditary influence, the two paramount environmental factors are: (*a*) psychoemotional (neurogenic) overstress and (*b*) high salt intake. He believes that either of these—or other factors—may initiate the hypertension but that the arteriosclerotic process perpetuates it. Folkow suggests that the early hypertrophy of the media layer of precapillary resistance vessels (induced by the beginning hypertension) increases internal wall thickness (w), which has been shown to decrease the internal vessel radius (r_i). According to Laplace's law, T (wall tension) = P (transmural pressure) $\times$ r_i/w. If P is increased, the quotient r_i/w tends to decrease in order to maintain equilibrium (Chapter 2). However, because of the 4th-power effect of radius change on vascular resistance, any r_i change instigated by the hypertension will induce an amplification effect on resistance. Thus further wall thickening and encroachment on r_i will lead to nonspecific hyperreactivity of the vessel to constrictor stimuli. This will, in turn, trigger a progressive structural adaptation (thickening) of the vascular muscle. It is theorized that in predisposed individuals, this positive feedback phenomenon may be the basis for enduring hypertension. Since arterial vasoconstriction is the undoubted primary final common pathway of the hypertension, other investigators have also studied vascular smooth muscle, particularly in spontaneously hypertensive rats. Winquist *et al.* found several primary changes in vascular smooth muscle (*e.g.*, deficiencies in excitation-contraction coupling). These were not related to the increase in wall stress but often preceded the development of high blood pressure. It is evident therefore that the pathogenesis of essential hypertension, one of our greatest public health problems, is still unknown.

Treatment of Hypertension

Among cardiovascular disorders, there are few that require greater skill in differential diagnosis or more diligent, constant attention to achieve successful treatment. Yet there are also very few in which the available treatment is as effective and the outlook as promising, provided the patient is cooperative. Because the symptoms are often minimal and the side effects of the drugs sometimes unpleasant, patients are frequently unwilling to follow their regimen.

The therapy for secondary types of hypertension is first of all directed at the specific cause. In the large exclusion group (i.e., *EH*), general measures would be instituted such as reduction of internal and external stress (so far as possible), moderate restriction of calories, alcohol, tobacco, cholesterol, saturated fat, and salt, and finally regular physical exercise within the limits of the patient's age and cardiovascular status. For specific therapy, it is sometimes possible to select antihypertensive medication with a mechanism of action that specifically fits the pressor mechanism involved. This usually means choosing between diuretics, sympathetic inhibitors, converting enzyme inhibitors, and Ca^{2+} channel blockers.

Thiazides, the most commonly used diuretics, lower arterial pressure by blocking sodium reabsorption at the distal nephron and thus cause salt and water depletion. Furosemide—a less commonly used diuretic—acts primarily to inhibit active chloride transport at the ascending loops of Henle. Diuretics are usually begun at moderate doses, the results followed, the dosage regulated and other agents substituted or added to achieve specific effects in individual patients. Careful attention is given to side effects, which include potassium loss, alkalosis, and elevated uric acid, glucose, and triglycerides. Because hypokalemia is a troublesome side effect, especially with longer-acting diuretics, K^+-sparing diuretics such as spironolactone (Aldactone) are also sometimes used in the treatment of essential hypertension, and K^+ supplements are often given.

Sympathetic inhibitors act at multiple sites through diverse mechanisms but affect particularly the heart, kidney, and vascular smooth muscle. Inhibition of arterial and venous vasoconstriction decreases both venous return and cardiac afterload thus lessening myocardial wall tension and arterial blood pressure and reducing myocardial O_2 demand.

Clonidine is a prototype of drugs that stimulate the α_2-receptors in the brain stem, thereby diminishing the sympathetic outflow to the vascular system. Prazosin and analogs produce relaxing effects on vascular smooth muscle through selective blockade of postsynaptic α_2-receptors in the peripheral vascular beds. Propranolol and other β-blockers act at multiple sites and also serve to reduce the renin secretion, thus inhibiting the renin-angiotensin-aldosterone (RAA) system.

A side effect of diuretic agents and sympathetic blockers is orthostatic hypotension induced partly by the decreased plasma volume and partly (in the case of the sympathetic inhibitors) because of the reduction in cardiac output and peripheral resistance. Elderly patients are often particularly vulnerable to orthostatic hypotension, so treatment should start at lower doses and the blood pressure should be reduced very gradually over a period of one to three months.

Vasodilating agents such as hydralazine and minoxidil, which relax vascular smooth muscle, cause fluid retention and reflex tachycardia. For this reason, they are not used alone but mainly as adjuncts. Angiotensin-converting enzyme (ACE) inhibitors such as captopril are commonly used in controlling hypertension. Calcium antagonists such as verapamil and nifedipine are also proving very useful in the treatment of hypertension.

The mortality in hypertension, which results mainly from myocardial failure, stroke, or renal failure, has in the last years been markedly reduced with the advent of effective antihypertensive drugs. While the lives of hypertensive patients are being prolonged, arteriosclerosis is still the cause of a high percentage of deaths. Thus antihypertensive therapy is blunting the disease but not preventing the eventual development of atherosclerosis.

The cornerstone of EH treatment is an individualized stepcare approach consisting of nonpharmacologic measures such as caloric, salt, and alcohol restriction and use of a diuretic, beta blocker, ACE inhibitor, or Ca^{2+} antagonist. This should be followed by addition or substitution of additional drugs and careful dosage regulations tailored to the individual patient's needs.

Circulatory Shock
General Characteristics and Classification

Circulatory shock is a failure of the circulation with decreased perfusion and/ or inadequate oxygenation of the vital organs and cells of the body. It is due to trauma, blood loss, myocardial failure, infection, or other serious bodily insult, and if untreated, has a tendency to progress toward general circulatory failure and death. The syndrome was named ('le choc') by a French physician, Le Dran, referring to patients who had undergone severe mechanical trauma. Samuel Gross in 1872 defined shock as a rude unhinging of the machinery of life—an introduction to death.

The cardinal feature of circulatory shock is inadequate tissue perfusion. Shock should not be equated with low blood pressure, although hypotension is usually present. Circulatory shock can occur without severe hypotension. In fact hypotension is usually a late sign in shock and indicates a failure of compensation. Although the causes of circulatory shock are multiple, there are three main clinical types: hypovolemic, cardiogenic, and septic shock.

In *hypovolemic shock*, a decrease in circulating blood volume is responsible for the fall in arterial pressure; in *cardiogenic shock* it is myocardial failure (*e.g.*, as a result of myocardial infarction) which causes the circulatory collapse. *Septic shock* often occurs incident to a massive infection, in which cardiac output and arterial pressure are usually normal or above normal, but the vital organs, because of a metabolic defect, are unable to extract adequate oxygen from the circulating blood.

While there are important clinical differences between the various types of shock, there are also many common features. A previously untreated patient after a severe trauma or blood loss will usually have a characteristic profound pallor of the skin and mucous membranes, a cold sweat, and a rapid, almost imperceptible, "thready" pulse (rate ≥ 140/min). The arterial pressure will be low (perhaps 85/60), the rectal temperature is often decreased to about 96 or 97°F, and respiration is feeble. The patient may be restless yet apathetic, and often semirational. Without early and proper treatment such a circulatory failure will frequently progress to irreversibility and death.

Among the earliest systematic investigations into the mechanism of circulatory shock were those of Dr. George W. Crile, a surgeon, who in 1899 reported his studies on shock in animals and the effect of different types of therapy. He described the low central venous pressure, the failure of venous return and cardiac output, and the response to infusion. He believed the ultimate failure of the circulation to be due to sympathoadrenal exhaustion.

In 1918 Cannon and his colleagues studied shock in wounded soldiers in France. Later in an extensive monograph they emphasized the correlation between low blood pressure and arterial acidosis as well as the beneficial effects of sodium bicarbonate infusion. These authors concluded that a histamine-like toxin, liberated from the traumatized cells, was the primary causative agent of the circulatory failure.

During the last 50 years, spurred initially by the need for improved treatment of military casualties, extensive studies have been made of the pathogenesis and treatment of shock. As a result, shock therapy has improved dramatically. Treatment is more ''aggressive'' with early and vigorous infusion of blood or blood substitutes, and more reliable autonomic and inotropic agents have become available. Particularly effective has been the segregation of these patients into a special intensive care unit (ICU) or coronary care unit (CCU) with trained personnel and facilities for continuous on-line recording of vital cardiopulmonary parameters. As a consequence, the recovery rate in severe shock has been greatly improved.

In studies of severely shocked patients, it has been noted that in order to achieve hemodynamic stability, it is frequently necessary to infuse much greater amounts of fluid or blood than would be anticipated (Fig. 15.4). This is because of excessive fluid loss through hemorrhage, sequestration into certain capillary beds, diffusion into interstitial tissues, or failure of venomotor tone (as described below).

Hypovolemic Shock

The pathophysiological changes and, therefore, the clinical picture, will vary somewhat in the different types of shock. In this section, hypovolemic shock, which is in a sense a prototype of clinical shock, will be described. Later in the chapter some of the specific features of cardiogenic and septic shock will be discussed. Hypovolemic shock may result from hemorrhage, trauma, burns, excess radiation, or any other injury that involves severe loss of body fluids, plasma, or blood. In many of these conditions (e.g., in burns or acute pancreatitis) the loss is not external but into the interstitial tissues; nonetheless it becomes unavailable to the cardiovascular system as circulating fluid.

Cardiovascular Changes

The circulatory alterations are due to the hypovolemia, and also, as will be noted later, to the compensatory changes resulting from the hypovolemia.

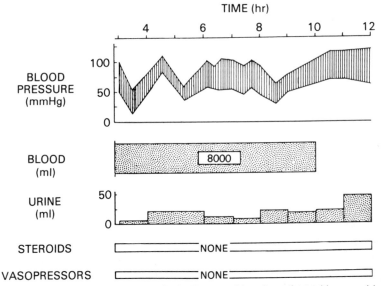

Figure 15.4. Posttraumatic shock. A 77-year-old male patient with a crushing injury of both legs and bilateral fractures of the femur, tibia, and fibula; the patient, who had very little external blood loss, required blood infusions totaling 8000 ml over 7 hours. (Reprinted with permission from L.D. MacLean, J.H. Duff, and A.P. McLean, *Can Med Assoc J* 105:78, 1971.)

The initial alterations are very similar to those seen early in hemorrhage, which were described in Chapter 13. In typical hypovolemic shock, the main circulatory effects are: (*a*) a decrease in central and peripheral venous pressure, in circulating blood volume, and in venous return; (*b*) a decrease in stroke volume and cardiac output, with particular reduction in flow to the skin, splanchnic area, and kidney; (*c*) a decrease in arterial blood pressure (mean, systolic, diastolic, and pulse pressure); (*d*) increased heart rate and myocardial contractility; (*e*) generalized vasoconstriction and venoconstriction with stagnant hypoxia; and (*f*) hemodilution, with increased $Paco_2$ and decreased pH. Within a few hours there follows a leukocytosis, a nonspecific stress response whose mechanism is not known.

The typical progression of the circulatory changes can be illustrated in an experimental animal, as shown in Figure 15.5. In this experiment, hypovolemic shock and hypotension were induced by hemorrhage; after a two-hour interval, the blood was reinfused and additional periodic transfusion given. In spite of this, the circulation failed progressively and the animal died. Whether the shock becomes irreversible depends mainly on the degree and duration of the hypotension and the adequacy of treatment. The possible causes of this irreversibility will be discussed later.

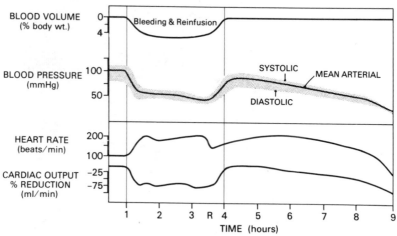

Figure 15.5. Experimental hemorrhagic shock. Two-hour hypovolemia and hypotension. Note the sharp fall in cardiac output (CO) and arterial pressure (AP), and rise in heart rate. With reinfusion of the withdrawn blood (at *R*), CO and AP recovered but later declined in spite of subsequent transfusion. (Reprinted with permission from C.J. Wiggers, *Physiology of Shock*. Cambridge: Harvard University Press, 1950.)

Compensatory Responses

The reactions to the stress—most of them reflex in nature—are an important part of the shock syndrome. The initial responses are directed particularly toward restoration of the two main deficiencies—the hypovolemia and the hypotension.

Almost immediately, the decreased central venous volume (and pressure) will initiate autonomic cardiopulmonary reflexes, and the falling arterial and pulse pressure will induce strong arterial baroceptor responses (Chapter 10). These reflexes will result in tachycardia, increased myocardial contractility, widespread vasoconstriction and venoconstriction, release of adrenal medullary catecholamines, and hyperventilation. When acidosis becomes evident, the arterial chemoceptors will also be activated and add an additional pressor effect. In deep shock the CNS ischemic reflex will provoke a still more intense sympathetic vasoconstriction (Chapter 10).

These reflex responses will tend to restore both cardiac output and arterial pressure, but they will not be maintained equally. As increasing fractions of blood volume are removed, the cardiac output will tend to fall, while arterial pressure may be temporarily maintained if the bleeding is not too rapid (Fig. 15.6).

Several important points should be noted in Figure 15.6. First, the maintenance of pressure at the expense of flow is the classic definition of resistance,

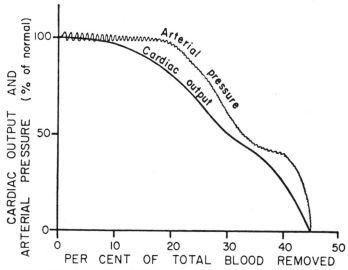

Figure 15.6.   Effect of graded hemorrhage on cardiac output and arterial pressure. Early in the bleeding, cardiac output (CO) falls but arterial pressure (AP) is maintained. After withdrawal of about 20% of the blood volume both AP and CO decline rapidly. (Reprinted with permission from A.C. Guyton, *Textbook of Medical Physiology*, 7th ed. Philadelphia: W.B. Saunders, 1986.)

and the ratio of the two is a measure of the extent to which total vascular resistance is being mobilized (as was discussed in Chapter 2). However, while the mean arterial pressure is being maintained, the pulse pressure steadily declines. If the heart rate is not changing greatly, this would suggest (if cardiac output determinations are not available) that stroke volume and cardiac output are declining. The graph also indicates that with about 15% of the blood volume removed, the bleeding still continuing, and the cardiac output declining, the mean arterial pressure may still be relatively normal. Thus in such a situation, with circulatory collapse imminent, the mean arterial pressure is not a good index of the state of the circulation. For this reason, pulse pressure, heart rate, central venous pressure, urine output, and other clinical signs must also be carefully monitored during shock.

Finally, the graph illustrates that when the arterial pressure reaches very low levels (*e.g.*, about 40 to 60 mm Hg), there is a temporary arrest in the decline of the arterial pressure and cardiac output resulting from a massive intensive sympathetic vasoconstriction—the CNS ischemic reflex (Chapter 10). This "last ditch" compensatory effort to maintain arterial pressure is thought to be initiated by ischemia of the brain stem.

Systemic vascular resistance is approximately doubled and pulmonary vascular resistance is increased about 5-fold in severe shock. As mentioned earlier, the sympathetic vasoconstriction is selective; constriction of the skin is responsible for the pallor and the renal vasoconstriction reduces glomerular filtration pressure, resulting in oliguria (decreased urine flow) or, if severe, anuria (cessation of urine output). The vasoconstriction in skeletal muscle and in the splanchnic area and the widespread venoconstriction will mobilize blood from these "reservoirs". This mobilization and the simultaneous shrinking of the general vascular capacity are very important aids to venous return and cardiac output.

Within minutes after hemorrhage or trauma, there is also a prompt tendency to restore *vascular volume*, mainly through: (*a*) influx of interstitial fluid into the capillaries through reduction of intracapillary hydrostatic pressure (Chapter 8); (*b*) renal vasoconstriction, which will not only reduce glomerular filtration pressure and urine output, but will also activate the renin-angiotensin-aldosterone mechanism (Chapter 11, Renal Circulation) and thus increase sodium and therefore also water reabsorption from the renal tubules; and (*c*) the release of vasopressin (ADH) from the posterior pituitary gland, which will increase the reabsorption of water from the renal tubules. ADH release will be instigated by (*a*) a decrease in atrial pressure and lesser stimulation of the cardiopulmonary receptors in the atria and (*b*) stimulation of osmoreceptors in the posterior pituitary gland by the increased osmolality of the blood (see Renal Blood Flow, Chapter 11). Some of the changes in circulatory shock are shown graphically in Figure 15.7.

The above responses are compensatory and protective. In severe and continued shock, decompensatory changes may supervene and lead to irreversibility and death. The relative importance of these various pathophysiological changes is discussed later in this chapter. There is evidence that venomotor tone, both in small and large vessels, fails in late shock; the resultant increased compliance in the large-capacity venous bed may be partly responsible for the excessive infusions of fluid often needed to restore central blood volume and pressure (Fig. 15.4).

Metabolic and Endocrine Changes

While the cardiovascular fluctuations in shock are dramatic and because of their urgency receive more attention, the metabolic and endocrine changes are in the long run, equally if not more significant since it is likely that irreversibility is due primarily to metabolic failure. The primary metabolic changes in moderate or severe hypovolemic shock are as follows.

1. Decreased metabolic rate and body temperature.
2. Alteration in carbohydrate metabolism: (*a*) an initial hyperglycemia, due to release of epinephrine (later in shock, hypoglycemia may occur because of depletion of hepatic glycogen and failure of gluconeogenesis); (*b*) an-

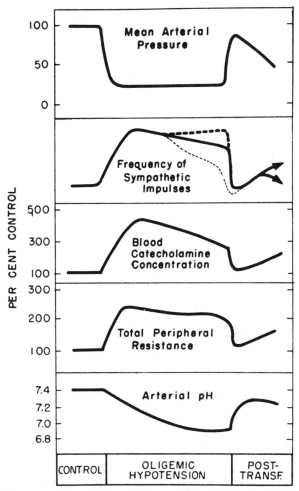

Figure 15.7.   Sympathoadrenal and blood pH responses to experimental hemorrhagic shock. The experimental procedure was similar to that shown in Figure 15.5 with reinfusion of the blood after the hypotensive period. In late shock, the frequency of sympathetic impulses may take different time courses as shown. Note the gradual decline in impulse frequency, catecholamine concentration, and vascular resistance and the progressive development of acidosis. (Reprinted with permission from S. Chien, *Physiol Rev* 47:252, 1967.)

aerobic glycolysis with increase in blood lactate and pyruvate. There is also depletion of high-energy phosphates, especially in the liver and kidney; however, those of brain and heart are well maintained.

3. Protein catabolism: (*a*) increase in blood amino acid nitrogen indicating

increased protein catabolism due to the stagnant hypoxia; (*b*) decrease in blood urea associated with a decline in the deamination function of the liver due to hepatic ischemia; (*c*) increase in liver and blood ammonia.
4. Blood: increase in $PaCO_2$ and decrease in pH, but the PaO_2 is usually well maintained; hemodilution, except in burns and in some cases of severe trauma, in which the hematocrit is high; increase in plasma catecholamines, 17-hydroxyketosteroids, and blood K^+.

The metabolic changes are mainly the result of (*a*) a generalized stagnant hypoxia, during which the intracellular PO_2 becomes very low with a resultant peripheral anaerobiosis, and (*b*) increased neuroendocrine activity, particularly of the sympathoadrenal and anterior pituitary-adrenal cortical systems.

Cardiogenic Shock

Cardiogenic shock usually denotes insufficient output of the heart despite an adequate ventricular filling pressure. While such a situation results primarily from myocardial infarction (MI), this type of shock can and does occur from a mechanical cardiac defect such as a large pericardial effusion (cardiac tamponade), a sudden valve failure, or as a later development in septic or hypovolemic shock.

In the classical case, however, it will result from an MI. Significant arterial hypotension and shock will develop if the myocardial damage is sufficient (about 30 to 40% of the myocardial mass) and if the systemic vascular resistance is not adequate to maintain the arterial pressure. The net result will depend mainly on (*a*) the effect of the MI on myocardial pump function and (*b*) the reflex response to the myocardial injury.

The reflex sympathetic vasoconstrictor response is of paramount importance for survival. As described in Chapter 10, the vascular impulses from cardiac receptors traveling *via* the vagus nerves may induce either pressure or depressor responses. Recent studies have also shown that experimental ventricular ischemia in the dog and monkey will result in afferent impulses carried *via* the dorsal sympathetic chain. These fibers can carry pain sensation but even more important, they can apparently inhibit sympathetic vasoconstrictors (Chapter 10, Ventricular Receptors).

Obviously the vasomotor and cardiac centers of the medulla are subjected to varied and sometimes conflicting influences. Aside from the afferent cardiac impulses, which are unpredictable (but generally depressor), the remaining cardiopulmonary afferents and the arterial baroceptors are strongly pressor. The net response is the result of the integration of these (and other) impulses by the medullary centers. An interesting recent finding is that efferent constrictor impulses to upper and lower limb skeletal muscle may elicit different responses, raising the possibility of more specific efferent control of vascular resistance than has been ordinarily visualized.

Septic Shock

Septic shock is usually the result of a severe infection and bacteremia, often with gram-negative organisms. The patient frequently has an increased central venous pressure (CVP) and cardiac output, hyperventiliation, and alkalosis along with hypotension, tachycardia, fever, and a low peripheral vascular resistance. The hyperventilation is an important, early and often unrecognized sign of impending septic shock.

In contrast to this hyperdynamic or "warm" phase, there is also a form of hypodynamic septic shock in which there is a decreased CVP and cardiac output, increased peripheral resistance, and cold, cyanotic extremities—the "cold" phase.

The syndrome of Gram-negative (GN) septic shock is the direct result of the endotoxin in the blood—or more precisely—the results of the action of lipopolysaccharides found in the cell walls of the GN organism. The "core" glycolipid of the endotoxin is linked to a lipoidal disaccharide termed lipid "A", which exhibits all the hemodynamic, pyrogenic, and inflammatory properties of the endoxtin. Soon after infection, endotoxin enters the reticuloendothelial system (RES), accumulating mainly in liver and spleen but also in the endothelium of the pulmonary alveoli and in neutrophils and platelets. The pathological consequences of endotoxin in man are myriad; the key reactions are (a) induction of fever due to release of endogenous pyrogen (b) generation of kinins and prostaglandins and release of β-endorphins, (c) activation of Hageman factor (XII) and complement, (d) injury of vascular endothelium through release of O_2 radicals by adherent leukocytes, and (e) indirect induction of the Schwartzman reaction through recruitment of white blood cells.

In the later or irreversible stage of septic shock, complement—apparently activated by endotoxin—recruits WBCs to endotoxin sites on pulmonary alveolar surfaces. The effort to phagocytize this material leads to liberation of toxic O_2 radicals onto the pulmonary endothelial surface with endothelial damage and fluid leakage into pulmonary parenchyma. The unfortunate result is the clinical picture of adult respiratory distress syndrome (ARDS) with high pulmonary arterial pressure, marked hypoxia, and pulmonary edema. Prostaglandins (PGs) and thromboxanes (TXs), which are potent vasoconstrictons and platelet aggregators, are believed to be important contributors to the pulmonary pathology. Cook and his coworkers have shown, for example, that TX inhibitors reduce shock mortality in rats.

Endotoxin may (aside from producting TX) also disturb the clotting mechanism through endothelial damage, activation of the Hageman factor, and depletion of fibrinogen, prothrombin, and factors, V, VII, and VIII to XII. The result is further thrombus formation and disseminated intravascular coagulation (DIC) with associated glomerular capillary thrombosis. DIC is an extensive disorder of the blood-clotting mechanism characterized by frequent occurrences of bleeding due to consumption of clotting factors and tissue hypoxia due to microemboli. While septic shock is frequently the direct result of infection, it may also occur as an aftermath of cardiogenic or hypovolemic shock, perhaps because of the temporary deleterious effect of the latter on the body's bacterial defense mechanisms or on the integrity of mucous membrane surfaces.

Mechanism of Irreversible Shock

The hemodynamic and metabolic changes in early hypovolemic and cardiogenic shock are the result of low cardiac output, hypotension, and generalized stagnant hypoxia. However, in many cases of septic shock the cardiac output is normal or even elevated, but the cellular damage leads to similar metabolic results. The changes are due to the initial tissue damage, so the pathogenesis of early shock is reasonably understandable.

However, the search for the mechanism of the later changes in shock, particularly the irreversibility, has been unsuccessful in spite of enormous research efforts. Two special difficulties complicate the shock problem. First, as Wiggers has pointed out, shock not only stops the machine, but also wrecks the machinery. So many processes are simultaneously affected that it is difficult to determine which is the primary disorder. There have been innumerable theories about the irreversibility, with the evidence frequently being only circumstantial. The second difficulty lies in finding a common denominator for a process that can be initiated in many different ways and in which the only endpoint is a fatality. However, while a single cause has not yet been found, our understanding of circulatory shock has been considerably advanced in recent years.

Site of the Failure in Shock

From the standpoint of etiology, many investigators have been concerned with the question of which organ or system initiates the irreversibility. Others have concentrated on which process might be responsible. In earlier studies, the excessive splanchnic vasoconstriction and hepatic ischemia, especially in dogs, drew attention to the liver as a possible critical site. However, this approach has limited application to clinical medicine since the pronounced hepatic congestion and intestinal necrosis, which characterize irreversible canine shock, are not usually found at autopsy in fatal human shock.

The role of other organs has also been studied. The main issue of the failure site has, however, revolved around the question of whether it is basically of cardiac or peripheral circulatory origin. Jones et al. have advocated the primary role of the heart. Zweifach and Froneck, in their extensive analysis of shock mechanisms, stated that in their opinion the issue was unsettled, but they favored the view that peripheral failure was responsible. Undoubtedly one of the reasons for the conflicting evidence on the role of the heart is the great difficulty—if not impossibility—of achieving with present methods the conditions necessary for making a valid assessment of cardiac contractility during severe circulatory shock.

There is considerable evidence to implicate peripheral vascular mechanisms as critical factors in shock survival. Stekiel and his colleagues have reported adrenergic neurotransmitter depletion in mesenteric arteries in hemorrhagic shock and believe that loss of such compensatory vasoconstriction may be a key defect. Haglund *et al.* have presented evidence that the ischemic intestine releases into the blood materials "toxic" to the circulatory system, probably from ulcerated villi. Rothe and Selkurt emphasized the role of skeletal muscle vascular failure in irreversible shock in dogs, and recently Bond *et al.* found that the terminal decompensatory skeletal muscle vasodilation was probably caused by the inhibitory action of locally released prostaglandins on the peripheral sympathetic endings. Kovach and his group have found marked reduction of blood flow and loss of responsiveness in the hypothalamus and reticular formation of dogs in hypovolemic shock and have indicated the potential importance of this central neurogenic influence on irreversibility.

It is evident that severe tissue damage occurs in many different organ systems in shock, and it may be that the irreversibility can be initiated at any one of multiple sites.

Cause of the Circulatory Failure in Shock

Many investigators have focused their efforts, not on a target organ, but on a basic metabolic process or toxic substance in an effort to discover the cause of death in shock. While a number of metabolic deficiencies have been identified, none of these have thus far been proved to be an instigating factor in the irreversibility. Studies by Filkins and coworkers and Hinshaw and others have emphasized the importance of certain aspects of carbohydrate metabolism, particularly in endotoxin shock.

Irreversibility is usually characterized by a marked hypoglycemia and a profound depression of gluconeogenesis. Shock mortality is also found to be increased in situations of enhanced insulin secretion, suggesting an important role for hyperinsulinemia as well as hypoglycemia in endotoxin and perhaps septic shock.

Toxic Factors in Shock

A number of circulating toxins have been proposed as causative agents for the irreversibility in shock. Fine and his colleagues were the first to suggest that bacterial endotoxins absorbed from the ischemic gut might play a role in the pathophysiology of shock. This view was given support by the finding that very small doses of endotoxin could produce in experimental animals a circulatory failure resembling hypovolemic and traumatic shock. While the overall role of endotoxins in shock is uncertain, they are undoubtedly concerned in the circulatory failure in septic shock, particularly of the Gram-negative type.

Lefer and coworkers have accumulated considerable evidence for a causal relationship between a myocardial depressant factor (MDF) and mortality in experimental shock. MDF is a low molecular weight, dialyzable polypeptide apparently produced in the pancreas and recoverable from the blood of animals suffering shock. Further studies indicate that this agent has a strong myocardial depressant effect. These investigators believe MDF to be a key factor in the circulatory failure of shock.

Reticuloendothelial System (RES) in Shock

In early studies, Zwiefach and others noted a correlation between RES function and the mortality from trauma, as well as increased shock mortality following RES blockade. Filkins *et al.* demonstrated that administration of zymosan, a yeast extract with potent RES-modulating properties, significantly lowered the mortality of rats to traumatic shock. Loegering and Saba have reported that in experimental shock, there was a depression of RES phagocytic function. The evidence indicates that both humoral and cellular factors may be involved in the decreased functional capacity of the RES in shock. It has been suggested that such a decline in the body defense mechanism may play a role in septic shock and particularly in its occurrence as a sequela to other types of circulatory failure. There is also recent evidence that the RES is concerned with the depression of gluconeogenesis and the hyperinsulinism characteristic of late endotoxin shock.

Lysosomes in Shock

Lysosomes are cytoplasmic granules present in almost all body cells. They contain a variety of potent hydrolytic enzymes enclosed within a relatively impermeable membrane. Following the pioneer work of De Duve on the role of lysosomes in cellular function, investigations have been made of their possible role in shock. Studies have indicated that hypoxia and mechanical trauma cause disruption of lysosomes *in vitro*. Furthermore after hemorrhage, endotoxin injection, or trauma, lysosomal proteases escape from ischemic cells and are found in high concentration in the plasma. Some investigators have ascribed the role of the RES in shock to the fact that RES tissue is rich in lysosomes. The interaction of proteases from disrupted lysosomes with certain plasma proteins is thought to be the source of several biologically active protein derivatives, (*e.g.*, the myocardial depressant factor (MDF) described above). These lines of evidence have led a number of investigators

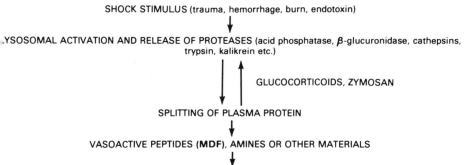

Figure 15.8. Schema illustrating a possible mechanism for the development of irreversible shock. Glucocorticoids and zymosan (an extract of brewers' yeast) have both been shown to lower mortality in experimental shock, presumably through their ability to stabilize lysosomal membranes.

to propose that lysosomes may play a key role in the etiology of lethal shock as outlined in Figure 15.8.

Monokines and the Pathogenesis of Septic Shock

Recent interesting investigations—which in a sense are outgrowths of the previous RES and lysosome studies described above—have focused on a "monokine theory" for septic shock, advanced by Filkins and his colleagues. Monokines are regulatory peptides produced by stimulated mononuclear phagocytes. The concept that they were key mediators of the septic process arose from early studies of the RES and its role in endotoxin shock. Although the RES is highly important in host defense against bacteremia and endotoxicosis, somewhat paradoxically, stimulation of the RES often led not to the expected decreases in endotoxin lethality but rather to an enhanced sensitivity to endotoxin. This paradox was resolved by the realization that macrophages are not solely endocytic but also are exocytic cells endowed with synthetic capabilities that become active during tissue injury, infection, or inflammation. These macrophage mediators were then given functional names such as pyrogens, lymphocyte activators, tumor necroses, glucoregulators, and insulinreleasers.

A further breakthrough was the isolation, purification, and synthesis *via* recombinant technology of two unique peptide mediator systems from appropriately stimulated monocytes and macrophages. These two macrophage regulatory peptides were named interleukin-1 (IL-1) and tumor necrosis factor (TNF). It was soon discovered that IL-1 and TNF possessed a remarkable spectrum of physiologic and pathologic effects. It is now recognized that working both individually and in concert, IL-1 and TNF are key initiators of tissue injury incident to infection and inflammation. The final development in the monokine hypothesis of septic shock pathogenesis was the finding that TNF and/or IL-1 injected into various animal models induced a septic shock-like state and septic-like signs and symptoms in humans. As mentioned above, it is believed that the end process of circulatory failure in many non–septic shock patients may be *via* sepsis and an increase in endotoxin titers. If so, it is possible that monokines may also play a significant role in the pathogenesis of other forms of irreversible shock.

Treatment of Shock

The treatment of circulatory disorders such as shock is highly complex and requires the maximum of diagnostic and clinical management skills. The following brief description is intended only to illustrate some of the general physiological principles used to treat these patients; it is in no sense intended as a guide to specific therapy.

Fluid Replacement and Central Venous Pressure

Because in the great majority of shock patients, there is a fluid deficit, treatment is first directed toward replacement therapy with crystalloids, colloids, plasma, blood substitutes, or whole blood depending on individual needs. If there is no known or apparent cardiopulmonary disease, such therapy can be monitored *via* central venous pressure (CVP). Clinical CVP monitoring usually refers to central vena caval or right atrial pressure determinations which provide a general index of *right* ventricular filling pressure and *right* ventricular end-diastolic pressure (RVEDP).

As discussed in Chapter 2, pressure in the central veins (as in any blood vessel) depends on the distensibility (or compliance) of the vessel and the volume contained. Heightened sympathetic tone will decrease the distensibility. However, at any given distensibility level, CVP will depend on the contained volume, which will in turn, reflect the balance of inflow and outflow. If there is no abnormality of right ventricular function or of intrathoracic pressure, CVP will be an index of venous return and serve as a rough guide to circulating blood volume and the need for fluid replacement therapy. CVP is normally about 5 to 10 cm saline and in shock usually is less than 3 to 4 cm saline. The goal is to achieve about 8 to 10 cm saline CVP with additional fluid, provided other signs do not contraindicate such treatment. The general objective is to improve ventricular function through greater diastolic filling (the Starling effect).

Monitoring of Ventricular Function in Cardiogenic Shock

In cardogenic shock, in contrast to the above, factors other than circulating blood volume will influence ventricular filling pressure and, therefore, must be taken into consideration. As mentioned in Chapter 14, after an MI with left ventricular involvement, there will be a gradual decrease in LV compliance, with a concomitant rise in LVEDP. The latter development is generally beneficial since it improves ventricular function, but it has two potential disadvantages. Since the ventricular diastolic curve rises steeply (Fig. 14.4), diastolic volume and, therefore, stroke volume will be limited. The second additional factor is that a rising LVEDP increases the possibility of pulmonary congestion.

In such a situation, left ventricular monitoring obviously becomes of prime importance in the treatment of cardiogenic shock. However, CVP is a poor reflection of LVEDP. Fortunately, Swan, Ganz, and their colleagues reported in 1970 the development of a double-lumen, flow-directed catheter that could be guided *via* a peripheral vein into the pulmonary artery without fluoroscopy. This permits the monitoring of pulmonary arterial pressure for the detection of any developing pulmonary congestion and, by gently "wedging" the catheter into a pulmonary arterial branch, also provides a reasonable estimate of left atrial pressure and thus of left ventricular filling pressure.

Using this technique, clinical studies have indicated that fluid replacement therapy can safely be continued up to left ventricular filling pressures of about 20 to 24 mm Hg. This will provide a reasonable level for improvement of ventricular function *via* the Starling effect without undue risk of inducing pulmonary congestion. Thus in cardiogenic, and sometimes in other forms of shock, a pulmonary artery catheter as well as a central venous catheter may be employed. In this way both right and left sides of the heart may be monitored.

Specific Therapy

The treatment of metabolic acidosis in shock is best accomplished by restoring tissue perfusion, rather than simply by loading with buffer. In severe acidosis (arterial blood pH under 7.2) sodium bicarbonate should be given intravenously. Shock patients usually are administered oxygen by mask to improve PaO_2.

Drug therapy will depend on the type of shock and the hemodynamic and metabolic condition of the patient. If there is evidence of diminished myocardial contractility (*e.g.*, in cardiogenic shock), inotropic agents such as dopamine or dobutamine may be given. The intent is to enhance arterial pressure by increasing left ventricular ejection rather than by increasing peripheral resistance. Dopamine is reasonably effective in this regard since at low doses its β-adrenergic effect is more prominent than its α-adrenergic action. Dobutamine is theoretically preferable since it is exclusively a β-agonist, but experience with this drug has been rather limited thus far. The renal vasodilation effect of these β-adrenergic agents may be useful in increasing urine flow.

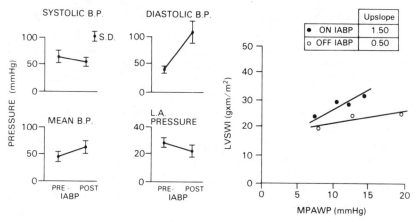

Figure 15.9. Effect of intraaortic balloon counterpulsation (IABC) on aortic and left atrial pressure and left ventricular stroke work index. *Left*, values immediately before and after IABC; *right*, the relationship of mean pulmonary artery wedge pressure (MPAWP) and left ventricular stroke work index (LVSWI) before and after IABC. In a critically ill patient, MPAWP is equivalent to left atrial filling pressure. Note the improved ventricular function during IABC. (Reprinted with permission from R.L. Berger, V.K. Saini, T. J. Ryan, D. M. Sokol, and J.F. Keefe, *J Thorac Cardiovasc Surg* 66:906, 1973; and R.D. Weisel, R.L. Berger, and H.B. Hechtman, *N Engl J Med* 292:682, 1975.)

α-Vasoconstrictors, such as methoxamine or norepinephrine, are sometimes given for short periods in hypovolemic shock if severe hypotension persists. Their disadvantages are that they further restrict peripheral tissue perfusion and increase cardiac afterload. Vasodilator agents—formerly believed to be contraindicated in shock—are now used selectively in some cases of cardiogenic shock. One of the factors limiting ventricular ejection is afterload (*i.e.*, aortic pressure). The success of a vasodilator, such as nitroprusside which has a direct relaxant effect on vascular smooth muscle, is based on the expectation that the reduced cardiac pressure work and the increased cardiac index that results will override the disadvantage of a somewhat lower aortic perfusion pressure. Obviously, such medication must be carefully monitored and controlled. Reports have indicated, however, that combinations of inotropic agents and vasodilators have proven effective in selected cases of circulatory shock. Because of its sometimes fulminating nature and high mortality, septic shock is challenging and often difficult to treat. Administration of high doses of appropriate intravenous antibiotics is the cornerstone of treatment.

The use of corticosteriods in pharmacological doses in septic shock remains controversial. Although recent large-scale studies revealed no therapeutic benefit from corticosteroids, some clinicians favor their use as adjunct therapy in certain instances. The basis of corticosteriod use is their ability to stabilize cellular and subcellular membranes, and thus prevent the escape of lysosomal hydrolases into the circulation.

Intraaortic Balloon Counterpulsation (IABC)

In very severe shock, in which arterial pressure cannot be maintained despite all available methods, additional circulatory support is sometimes given by introduction *via* catheter of an inflatable balloon into the upper thoracic aorta (Fig. 15.9). The balloon is inflated during diastole and rapidly deflated at the end of diastole. Thus central diastolic pressure is increased, which assists coronary flow, and systolic peak pressure is decreased, which reduces the afterload work of the left ventricle. With this procedure, cardiac output is increased with relatively little change in mean arterial pressure. Counterpulsation has proven helpful in certain circumstances in achieving hemodynamic stability, although it provides only temporary assistance.

Suggested Readings

Hypertension

Brest AN. Antihypertensive therapy in perspective *Mod Concepts Cardovasc Dis* 57:65–67 and 58:1–3, 1988–89.

Brod J, Fencl V, Hejl Z, and Jirka J. Circulatory changes underlying blood pressure elevation during acute emotional stress. *Clin Sci* 18:269, 1959.

Brody MJ, Haywood JR, and Touw KB. Neural mechanisms in hypertension. *Annu Rev Physiol* 42:441–453, 1980.

Brody MJ and Johnson AK. Role of forebrain structures in models of experimental hypertension. In: *Disturbances in Neurogenic Control of the Circulation*, edited by FM Abboud, HA Fozzard, JP Gilmore and DJ Reis. Bethesda, Md.: American Physiological Society, 1981, pp 105–117.

Chobanian AV. Pathophysiology of systemic hypertension. In: *Clinical Cardiovascular Physiology*, edited by HJ Levine. New York: Grune & Stratton, 1976, pp 563–596.

Chobanian AV (ed.). *Detection, Evaluation and Treatment of High Blood Pressure*, US Dept of Health and Human Services. NIH Pub. No 88–1088, May 1988.

Coleman TG, Cowley AW Jr., and Guyton AC. Experimental hypertension and long-term control of arterial pressure. In: *Cardiovascular Physiology, MTP International Review of Science*, edited by AC Guyton and CE Jones. Baltimore: University Park Press, 1974, Vol. I, pp 259–298.

Cowley AW, Barber WS, Lombard JH, Osborn JL, and Liard JF. Relationship between body fluid volumes and arterial pressure. *Fed Proc* 45:2862–2870, 1986.

Dustan HP. Pathophysiology of hypertension. In: *The Heart, Arteries and Veins*, 5th ed., edited by JW Hurst. New York: McGraw-Hill, 1982, pp 1171–1181.

Folkow B. Physiological aspects of primary hypertension *Physiol Rev* 62:347–504, 1982.

Folkow B and Karlstrom G. Age and pressure-dependent changes in vascular smooth muscle. *Data Physiology Scand* 122:17–33, 1984.

Hagberg JM and Seals DR. Exercise training and hypertension. *Data Med Scand Supp* 711:131–136, 1986.

Harder DR, Contney SJ, Willems WJ, and Stekiel WJ. Norepinephrine effect on in situ venous membrane potential in spontaneously hypertensive rats. *Am J Physiol* 240:H837–842, 1981.

Itskovitz HD, Kochar MS, Anderson AJ, and Rimm AA. Patterns of blood pressure in Milwaukee. *JAMA* 238:864–868, 1977.

Laragh JH, Letcher RL, and Pickering TG. Renin profiling for diagnosis and treatment of hypertension. *JAMA* 241:151–156, 1979.

Moorthy AV and Kochar S. Nephrology and hypertension. In: *Concise Textbook of Medicine*, 2nd ed, edited by MS Kochar. New York: Elsevier, 1990, pp 520–537.

Mancia G, Ludbrook J, Ferrari A, Gregorini L, and Zanchetti A: Baroceptor reflexes in human hypertension. *Circ Res* 43:170–177, 1978.

Page IH. Arterial hypertension in retrospect. *Circ Res* 34:133–142, 1974.

Safar ME, Weiss YA, Levenson JA, London GJ, and Milliez PL. Hemodynamic study of eighty-five patients with borderline hypertension. *Am J Cardiol* 31:315–319, 1973.

Whelton PK and Russell RP. Systemic hypertension. In: *Principles and Practice of Medicine*, edited by AM Harvey. Norwalk, Conn.: Appleton and Lange, 1988.

Winquist RS, Webb RC, and Bohr DF. Vascular smooth muscle in hypertension. *Fed Proc* 41:2387–2393, 1982.

Zucker IH and Gilmore JP. Aspects of cardiovascular responses in pathologic states. *Fed Proc* 44:2400–2407, 1985.

Circulatory Shock

Abboud FM. Pathophysiology of hypotension and shock. In: The *Heart, Arteries and Veins*, 5th ed., edited by JW Hurst. New York: McGraw-Hill, 1982, pp 452–463.

Altura BM. Reticuloendothelial cells and host defense. *Adv Microcirc* 9:252–294, 1980.

Beckman CB, Geha AS, Hammond GL, and Bave AE. Results and complications of intra-aortic ballon counter-pulsation. *Ann Thorac Surg* 24:550–559, 1977.

Bond RF, Bond CH, Peissner LC, and Manning ES. Prostaglandin modulation of adrenergic vascular control during hemorrhagic shock. *Am J Physiol* 241:H85–90, 1981.

Bond RF and Green HD. Peripheral circulation. In: *Handbook of Shock and Trauma, Vol. 1, Basic Science* edited by BM Altura *et al.* New York: Raven Press, 1983, pp 29–49.

Bone RC, Fisher CJ, Clemmer TP, *et al.* Controlled clinical trial of high dose methyl-prednisolone in the treatment of severe sepsis and septic shock. *NEJM* 317:653–658, 1987.

Cohn JN. Recognition and management of shock and acute pump failure. In: *The Heart, Arteries and Veins*, 5th ed., edited by JW Hurst. New York: McGraw-Hill, 1982, pp 463–476.

Cook JA *et al.* Elevated thromboxane levels in the rat during shock; protective effects of imidizole. *J Clin Invest* 65:227–230, 1980.

Dole WP and O'Rourke RA. Hypotension and cardiogenic shock. In: *Internal Medicine*, edited by SH Stein. Boston: Little, Brown, 1986, pp 407–417.

Fejes-Toth G, Brinck-Johnsen T, and Fejes-Toth AN. Cardiovascular and hormonal response to hemorrhage in conscious rats. *Am J Physiol* 254:H947–53, 1988.

Filkins JC. Monokines and the metabolic pathophysiology of septic shock. *Fed Proc* 44:300, 1985.

Filkins JP. Role of RES in the pathogenesis of endotoxic hypoglycemia. *Circ Shock* 9:269–280, 1982.

Filkins JP, Smith PM, and Smith JJ. Glucocorticoid treatment of septic shock. In: *Pharmacology and Physiology of Shock*, edited by M Hamamdic, AFB Kovach, *et al.* New York: Plenum Press (in press).

Goldfarb RD. Cardiac mechanical performance in circulatory shock: a critical review of methods and results. *Circ Shock* 9:633–653, 1982.

Guntheroth WG, Jacky JP, Kawabori I, Stevenson JG, and Moreno AH. Left ventricular performance in endotoxin shock in dogs. *Am J Physiol* 242:H172–176, 1982.

Guyton AC. Physiology and treatment of circulatory shock. In: *Textbook of Medical Physiology*, 7th ed., edited by AC Guyton. Phil., P.A. 1986, pp 326–335.

Haglund U, Jodal M, and Lundgren O. The small bowel in arterial hypotension and shock. In: *Physiology of the Intestinal Circulation*, edited by JP Shephard and DN Granger. New York: Raven Press, 1984.

Hinshaw LB. Concise review: the role of glucose in endotoxin shock. *Circ Shock* 3:6–10, 1976.

Hinshaw, LB, Beller-Todd BK, and Archer-LI. Current management of the septic shock patient: experimental basis for treatment. *Cir Shock* 9:543–553, 1982.

Jones CE, Smith EE, and Crowell JW. Cardiac output and physiological mechanisms in circulatory shock. In: *Cardiovascular Physiology, MTP International Review of Science*, edited by AC Guyton and CE Jones. Baltimore: University Park Press, 1974, pp 233–258.

Kostreva DR, Hess GL, Zuperku EJ, Neumark J, Coon RL, and Kampine JP. Cardiac responses to stimulation of thoracic afferents in the primate and canine. *Am J Physiol* 231:1279–1284, 1976.

Kovach AGB and Sandor P. Cerebral blood flow and brain function during hypotension and shock. *Physiol Rev* 38:571–596, 1976.

Lefer AM. Eicosanoids or mediators of ishcemia and shock. *Fed Proc* 44:275, 1985.

Loegering DJ and Saba TM. Hepatic Kupffer cell dysfunction during hemorrhagic shock. *Circ Res* 3:107–113, 1976.

Lombard JH, Loegering DJ, and Stekiel WJ. Effects of prolonged hemorrhagic hypotensive stress on catecholamine concentration of mesenteric blood vessels. *Blood Vessels* 14:212–228, 1977.

McLean LD. Shock: causes and management of circulatory collapse. In: *Textbook of Surgery*, 12th ed., edited by DC Sabiston. Philadelphia: W.B. Saunders, 1981, pp 58–90.

Old LJ. Tumor necrosis factor. *Sci Am* 258:59–73, 1988.

Rock P, Furman WR, and Sylvester JT. Circulatory and ventilatory management of the critically ill patient: general aspects. In: *Principles and Practice of Medicine*, 22nd ed., edited by AM Harvey. Norwalk, Conn.: Appleton and Lange, 1988.

Rothe CF and Selkurt EE. Cardiac and peripheral failure in hemorrhagic shock in the dog. *Am J Physiol* 207:203–214, 1964.

Smith JJ, Loegering DJ, McDermott DJ, and Bonin ML. The role of lysosomal hydrolases in the mechanism of shock. In: *Neurohumoral and Metabolic Aspects of Injury*, edited by AGB Kovach, HB Stoner and JJ Spitzer. New York: Plenum, 1973, pp 535–543.

Swan HJ, Ganz W, Forrester J, Marcus H, Diamond G, and Chonette D. Catheterization of the heart in man with the use of a flow directed balloon-tipped catheter. *N Engl J Med* 283:447–450, 1970.

Tillisch JH. Pump failure and cardiogenic shock. In: *Pathophysiology of the Heart*, edited by G Ross, New York: Masson Publishing Co., 1982, pp 225–256.

Wolski BM, Smith EM, Meyer WJ, Fuller GM, and Blalock JE. Corticotropin-releasing activity of monokines. *Science* 230:1035–1037, 1986.

Zweifach B and Froneck A. Interplay of central and peripheral factors in irreversible hemorrhagic shock. *Prog Cardiovasc Dis* 18:147–180, 1975.

Index

Acetyl choline
  and pulmonary circulation, 219
  effect on circulation, 54–55, 144–147
Acidosis in shock, 312, 314–318
Action potential, cardiac, **47–54**
  ionic conductance and AP, 49–55
  spread and velocity, 47–49
Adenosine
  and active hyperemia, 15
  and coronary flow, 197
ADH (*see* Antidiuretic hormone)
Adrenergic blockers (*see* Sympathetic
  nervous system, blockade)
Afterload of heart, 78–79 (*see also* Aortic
  pressure)
  effect on stroke volume, 117–118
Aging, **242–251**
  and arterial distensibility, 12–13
  and baroceptor sensitivity, 167
  and coronary heart disease, 234, 242
  and Na depletion, 247–248
  and orthostatic tolerance, 247–248, 257
  and stress response, 247–248
  and $\dot{V}_{O_{2max}}$, 234, 242–243
  aortic changes, 243–244
  aortic impedance in, 21–22
  autonomic responsiveness, 246–247
  circulatory effects, general, **242–249**
  relation to heart disease, 242
Aldactone in heart failure, 298
Aldosterone, **202–204** (*see also* Renin-
  angiotensin-aldosterone system)
Aldosteronism, primary, 303
Alpha receptors, 145–150
  alpha$_1$ and alpha$_2$ receptors, 147
Altitude, effect on blood O_2, 15
Anemia, **5–6**
  and blood viscosity, 22–24
  and heart failure, 288
Anesthesia
  and blood-brain barrier, 185

  and cerebral blood flow, 190
Aneurysm, aortic, 27–28
Angina pectoris, **278–279**
  and cold pressor test, 174
Angiography, 278
  and Bezold-Jarisch reflex, 171
Angiotensin, 155, **202–204** (*see also* Renin
  and Renin-angiotensin-aldosterone
  system)
Angular acceleration, 174
Anomalous viscosity, 23–24
Anouxia, 275
Anrep effect, 79
Antidiuretic hormone (ADH), 153, **202–204**
  ADH (vasopressin) mechanism, 202–204
  and cardiopulmonary reflex, 170–171
Anuria, in shock, 316
Aortic aneurysm, 27–28
Aortic diastolic pressure, 90–92, 94
Aortic distensibility, **10–13**, 94
Aortic flow, 89–90
  in Valsalva test, 252
Aortic incompetence, 43
Aortic pressure, 3–4, 8–9, **89–95**
  curve, 90–94
  determinants, 93–94
  effect on stroke volume, 117–118
  mean, 91–92
Aortic stenosis, 42, 44
  and cardiac work, 86
  and muscle blood flow, 228
  and ventricular hypertrophy, 292
Arrhythmias, cardiac, **63–69**
  and diving reflex, 266
  lidocaine in, **69**
  treatment of, 68–69
Arterial baroceptors (*see* Baroceptors,
  arterial)
Arterial chemoreceptors (*see*
  Chemoreceptors)
Arterial pressure, 4, 8–12, **95–96**

Page numbers in **boldface** indicate more definitive discussions of the topic.

Page numbers in **boldface** indicate more definitive discussions of the topic.

Page numbers in **boldface** indicate more definitive discussions of the topic.

Page numbers in **boldface** indicate more definitive discussions of the topic.

Page numbers in **boldface** indicate more definitive discussions of the topic.

Page numbers in **boldface** indicate more definitive discussions of the topic.

Page numbers in **boldface** indicate more definitive discussions of the topic.

Page numbers in **boldface** indicate more definitive discussions of the topic.

Page numbers in **boldface** indicate more definitive discussions of the topic.

Page numbers in **boldface** indicate more definitive discussions of the topic.

Page numbers in **boldface** indicate more definitive discussions of the topic.

Page numbers in **boldface** indicate more definitive discussions of the topic.

Page numbers in **boldface** indicate more definitive discussions of the topic.

344 Index

Page numbers in **boldface** indicate more definitive discussions of the topic.